An Introduction to
Cardiovascular Physiology

An Introduction to Cardiovascular Physiology

Second Edition

J R Levick, DSc, MA, BM, BCh (Oxon)
Professor of Physiology, St George's Hospital Medical School, London

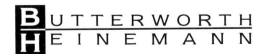

Butterworth-Heinemann
Linacre House, Jordan Hill, Oxford OX2 8DP
225 Wildwood Avenue, Woburn, MA 01801-2041
A division of Reed Educational and Professional Publishing Ltd

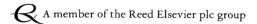 A member of the Reed Elsevier plc group

OXFORD   BOSTON   JOHANNESBURG
MELBOURNE   NEW DELHI   SINGAPORE

First published 1991
Reprinted 1992
Second edition 1995
Reprinted 1996, 1998

British Library Cataloguing in Publication Data
Levick, J. R.
    Introduction to cardiovascular
    Physiology. - 2Rev.ed
    I. Title
    612.1

ISBN 0 7506 2167 2

Library of Congress Cataloguing in Publication Data
Levick, J. R. (J. Rodney)
    An introduction to cardiovascular physiology/J. R. Levick. - 2nd ed.
    p. cm.
    Includes bibliograhical references and index.
    ISBN 0 7506 2167 2
    1. Cardiovascular system-Physiology. I. Title
    [DNLM: 1. Cardiovascular System-physiology. WG 102 L664i 1995]
    QP101.L47 1995
    612.1-dc20   94-45631
                                                                      CIP

Printed and bound in Great Britain by Bath Press

Preface to the second edition

Four years have passed since the manuscript for the first edition was written. In the intervening period cardiovascular research has continued apace, resulting in important new pathophysiological findings and the elucidation of mechanisms underlying some familiar physiological processes. These advances, coupled with a dwindling stock of the reprinted first edition (for which the publishers and I heartily thank the medical public), led to the production of this second edition.

The exercise has been more than cosmetic, I believe. The book has been revised and updated throughout, over 20 new or revised illustrations incorporated, and new references added. Important changes include the splitting of a single chapter on cardiac excitation into two updated chapters, one on the cardiac myocyte and one on the cardiac electrical system and its regulation. A brief account of important subtypes of ion channels in cardiac and vascular smooth muscle has been added (e.g. K-ATP channels) and new summary tables provided. There are new sections on intracellular mechanisms of vasodilatation, the role of adhesion molecules in white cell migration in inflammation, the role of endothelial cell Ca^{2+} in inflammation, vessel wall mechanics, shear-related viscosity changes, mechanisms of action of metabolic vasodilators (hypoxia, CO_2, adenosine, etc.), flow-induced and ascending vasodilatation, the role of inducible NO synthase in endotoxin shock, migraine, and hypoxic vasoconstriction in the lung. Sections on cardiac and coronary mechanoreceptor reflexes and on decompensated shock have been updated and completely new accounts added of integrated cardiovascular responses to feeding, ageing, systemic hypoxia and high altitude.

I should like to thank all those who wrote to me with comments about the first edition, and those who have helped with expert comments during preparation of the new edition. The latter include Paul Andrews, Mark Cannell, Dave Eisner, Peter Gaehtgens, William Large, Janice Marshall, Mike Mulvany, Clive Orchard, Jeremy Pearson, Garry Scroop, Jeremy Ward and Brian Whipp.

Despite some simplifications and deletions, the advance of science has had the usual, undesirable effect of increasing the size of the book, albeit modestly. In order to compensate for this and, hopefully, help the hard-pressed medical student revising for examinations, a set of learning objectives has been added at the end of the book, and a summary has been added after every chapter. I hope that the gains outweigh the disadvantage of increased length and that the book continues to serve its original purpose, namely to act as a readable *introduction* to the fascinating and complex world of cardiovascular physiology.

Rodney Levick
St. George's Hospital Medical School
December 1994

Preface to the first edition

This is an introductory text designed primarily for students of medicine and physiology. The teaching style is necessarily didactic in many places ('The way it works is like this, . . .') but also, where space permits, I have tried to show how our knowledge of the circulation is derived from experimental observations. The latter not only puts flesh on the didactic bones, but ultimately keeps the student (and the writer) in contact with reality. Human data are presented where possible, and their relevance to human disease is emphasized. The occasional anecdotes and doggerel betray a deplorable levity on my part, but will have earned their place if they interest the reader, and doubly so if they help to make a point memorable. The undergraduate will find a useful guide to learning objectives in the coloured box at the beginning of each chapter.

The traditional weighting of subject matter has been re-thought, resulting in a fuller account of microvascular physiology than is usual. This reflects the explosion of microvascular research over the past two decades. Even setting aside these advances, it seems self-evident that the culminating, fundamental function of the cardiovascular system – the transfer of nutrients from plasma to the tissue – merits more than the few lines usually accorded to it in introductory texts. Major advances continue apace in other fields too, for example the elucidation of the biochemical events underlying Starling's law of the heart, the discovery of new vasoactive substances produced by endothelium, the exploration of non-adrenergic, non-cholinergic neurotransmission, rapid advances in vascular smooth muscle physiology, and new concepts on how the central nervous control of the circulation is organized.

I would like to thank many friends and colleagues – Tom Bolton, John Gamble, Max Lab, William Large, Janice Marshall, Charles Michel, Mark Noble, Peter Simkin, Laurence Smaje, Mike Spyer and John Widdicombe – for helpful comments on sections of the text. Any mistakes or muddles that remain are, of course, entirely my own; please do not hesitate to point them out to me. Perhaps I should thank the cardiovascular system too, for proving to be even more fascinating than I had realized before writing this book!

Rodney Levick
St. George's Hospital Medical School
September 1990

Contents

Chapter 1
Overview of the cardiovascular system

The heart and blood vessels have evolved to provide rapid transport of oxygen, nutrients, waste products and heat around the body. Small primitive organisms lack a cardiovascular system, because their needs can be met by direct diffusion from the environment, and even in man diffusion remains the fundamental means of transport between blood and tissue. To appreciate properly the need for a cardiovascular system, the limitations of diffusion need to be considered.

1.1 Diffusion: its virtues and limitations

The 'drunkard's walk' theory Diffusion is a passive process: it is driven not by metabolic energy but by the random thermal motion of molecules in a solution of gas. Each movement of an individual molecule is random in direction (the 'drunkard's walk'), but this gives rise to a net movement of solute when a concentration gradient is

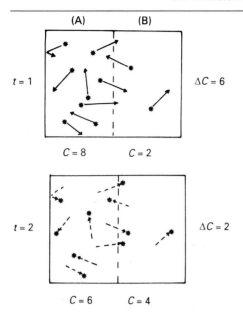

Figure 1.1 Sketch illustrating how random molecular steps result in a net movement of solute down a concentration gradient. At time 1 (upper sketch) there are 8 molecules per unit volume in (A) and 2 in (B). At time 2 (lower sketch) each molecule has moved a unit step in a random direction. Because there was a greater density of molecules in A, there was a greater probability of random movement from A to B, resulting in a net 'downhill' flux

present. The arrows in Figure 1.1 show how this happens. Notice that although the net transfer of solute is from compartment A into compartment B, there is also a smaller backflux into compartment A. This can be proved by adding a trace of radiolabelled solute to compartment B; some labelled molecules appear in compartment A despite net diffusion from A to B.

Importance of diffusion distance The *rate* of transport by diffusion is critically important because the delivery of nutrients to cells must keep up with demand. Unfortunately, as Albert Einstein showed, the time (t) that it takes a randomly jumping particle to move a distance x in one specific direction increases with the square of distance:

$$t \propto x^2 \tag{1.1}$$

(see footnote to Table 1.1). As a result, diffusional transport is extremely slow over large distances. Over a short distance such as the neuromuscular gap (0.1 μm) diffusion takes only 5 millionths of a second, whereas across the heart wall (about 1 cm) it is hopelessly slow, taking over half a day (Table 1.1). Sadly, Nature often proves the validity of Einstein's equation and Figure 1.2 is an example of this. It shows the heart of a patient who suffered a coronary thrombosis (obstruction of the blood supply to the heart wall). The pale area is muscle that died from lack of oxygen, despite the fact that the adjacent cavity was full of richly oxygenated blood. The patient died simply because a distance of a few millimetres reduced diffusional transport to an inadequate rate.

Table 1.1 Time taken for a glucose molecule to diffuse a specified distance in one direction

Distance (x)	Time (t)*	Comparable distance in vivo
0.1 μm	0.000005 s	Neuromuscular gap
1.0 μm	0.0005 s	Capillary wall
10.0 μm	0.05 s	Cell to capillary
1 mm	9.26 min	Skin, artery wall
1 cm	15.4 h	Ventricle wall

*Times are calculated by Einstein's equation $t = x^2/2D$. 'D' is the solute diffusion coefficient. For glucose in water at 37°C, D is 0.9×10^{-5} cm²/s (Einstein, A. (1905) *Theory of Brownian Movement* (trans. and ed. by R. Fürth and A. D. Cowper, 1956), Dover Publications, New York)

Convective transport for speed over long distances Clearly then, for distances greater than about 0.1 mm a faster transport system is needed. This is provided by the cardiovascular system (Figure 1.3). The cardiovascular system still relies on diffusion for the uptake of molecules at points of close proximity to the environment (e.g. oxygen uptake into lung capillaries), but it then transports material rapidly over large distances by sweeping it along in a stream of

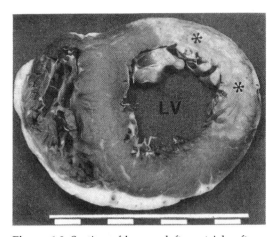

Figure 1.2 Section of human left ventricle after a coronary thrombosis, stained for a muscle enzyme. Pale area (asterisks) is an 'infarct' – an area of muscle badly damaged or killed by oxygen lack; the pallor is due to the intracellular enzyme having leaked out of the dying cells. The infarct was caused by a blockage of the coronary artery that halted blood flow to the wall and hence oxygen delivery. Oxygen diffusion from blood in the main chamber (LV) is unaffected, yet only a thin rim of adjacent tissue (about 1 mm) survived. (Courtesy of Professor M. Davies, St George's Hospital Medical School, London)

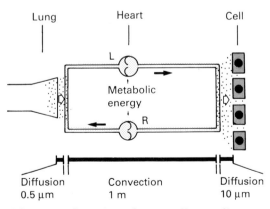

Figure 1.3 Overview of mammalian cardiovascular system, illustrating the roles of diffusion and convection in oxygen transport. L, left side of heart. R, right side of heart

pumped fluid. This mode of transport is called bulk flow or convective transport. Convective transport requires an energy input and this is provided by a pump, the heart. In man, convection takes only 30 s to carry oxygen over a metre or more, from the lungs to the smallest blood vessels of the limbs (capillaries), whereas diffusion would take over 5 years! Over the final 10–20 μm between capillary and cell, diffusion is again the main transport process.

1.2 Functions of the cardiovascular system

First and foremost is the *rapid convective transport* of oxygen, glucose, amino acids, fatty acids, vitamins, drugs and water to the tissues, and the rapid washout of metabolic waste products like carbon dioxide, urea and creatinine. In addition, however, the cardiovascular system is part of a *control system* in that it distributes hormones to the tissues, and even secretes some hormones itself (e.g. atrial natriuretic peptide). It also plays a vital role in *temperature regulation*, by delivering heat from the core of the body to the skin; and a vital role in *reproduction*, providing the hydraulic mechanism for penile erection.

1.3 Circulation of blood

The heart consists basically of two intermittent muscular pumps, the right and left ventricles (Figure 1.4). Each pump is filled from a reservoir, the right or left atrium. The right ventricle pumps blood through the lungs to the left side of the heart (the *pulmonary circulation*) and the left ventricle simultaneously pumps blood through the rest of the body and back to the right side (the *systemic circulation*). The blood is compelled to follow a circular pathway by one-way valves in the heart and veins, as first established by the London physician William Harvey, in a celebrated book

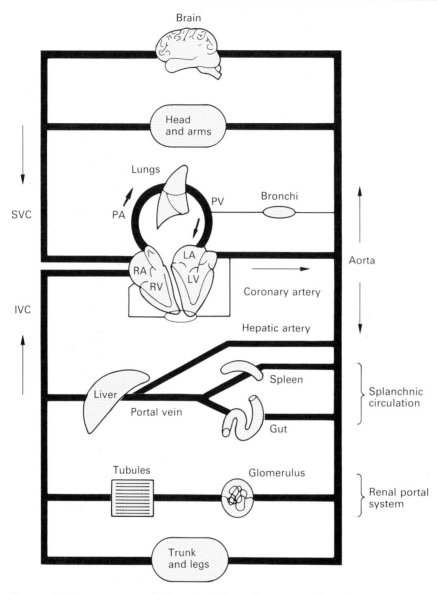

Figure 1.4 Arrangement of the circulation. Systemic and pulmonary circulations are 'in series'. Circulations to individual organs are mostly in parallel (e.g. cerebral and coronary circulations) but a few are in series (e.g. liver, renal tubules). Bronchial venous blood drains anomalously into the left rather than the right atrium. PA, PV, pulmonary artery and vein; RA, LA, right and left atrium (an 'atrium' was a Roman hall); RV, LV, right and left ventricle; SVC, IVC, superior and inferior vena cava

entitled *De Motu Cordis* (Concerning the Movement of the Heart, 1628).

Pulmonary circulation Venous blood enters the right atrium from the two major veins, the superior and inferior venae cavae, then flows through a valve into the right ventricle. The ventricle is composed mainly of cardiac muscle and it receives the blood while its muscle is relaxed. Cardiac relaxation is called diastole (pronounced dia-stol-i). Contraction then follows, called 'systole' (pronounced sis-tol-i). Systole expels some of the blood into the pulmonary artery at a fairly low pressure, whence it flows into the lungs. In the air sacs (alveoli) of the lungs, gaseous exchange occurs by diffusion, raising the blood's oxygen content from approximately 150 ml/l (venous blood) to 195 ml/l. The oxygenated blood returns through the pulmonary veins to the left atrium and left ventricle.

Systemic circulation   The left ventricle contracts virtually simultaneously with the right and ejects the same volume of blood, but does so at a much higher pressure. The blood flows through the aorta and a branching system of arteries to reach microscopic thin-walled tubes called capillaries. Here the ultimate function of the cardiovascular system is fulfilled; dissolved gases and metabolites pass between the capillary blood and tissue by diffusion. The circulation of the blood is then completed by the venous system, which conducts blood back to the venae cavae.

1.4 Cardiac output and its distribution

The cardiac output is the volume of blood ejected by one ventricle during one minute. This depends on the volume ejected per contraction (*stroke volume*) and the number of contractions per minute (*heart rate*). In a resting 70 kg adult, the stroke volume is 70–80 ml and the heart rate around 65–75 beats/min, so the resting cardiac output is approximately 75 ml × 70 per min, or roughly 5 litres per min. The output is not fixed, however, and adapts rapidly to changing internal or external circumstances. In strenuous exercise for example, when oxygen demand can increase tenfold or more, the heart responds with a fourfold increase in output, or even

more in athletes. These changes imply that control systems must exist for regulating the heart beat, and these are the subject of Chapters 3, 4 and 7.

Distribution of cardiac output   The output of the right ventricle passes exclusively to the lungs. The output of the left ventricle is distributed to the peripheral tissues in proportion to their metabolic rate, as a rather rough rule. Resting skeletal muscle, for example, accounts for some 20% of human oxygen consumption and receives roughly 20% of the cardiac output (Figure 1.5). This egalitarian principle is overridden, however, in organs whose particular function requires a high blood flow, notably the kidneys. The kidneys account for only 6% of total oxygen consumption, yet they receive 20% of the cardiac output, because this is necessary for their excretory function. As a result, some other tissues are relatively ill supplied and, rather surprisingly, cardiac muscle is one of these. To make up for this, cardiac muscle extracts an unusually high proportion of the oxygen in the blood, namely 65–75%.

The distribution of the cardiac output is not fixed, however; it is actively adjusted to match demand. Heavy exercise provides a good example of this; the proportion of the cardiac output going to skeletal muscle increases to 80% or more in heavy exercise due to a widening of the arterial vessels supplying blood to the muscle (vasodilatation).

1.5 Introducing hydraulics: pressure and flow

Blood pressure   What drives blood along the blood vessels after it has left the heart? The main factor is a gradient of blood pressure. Ventricular ejection raises aortic blood pressure to approximately 120 mmHg above atmospheric pressure, whereas the pressure in the great veins is close to atmospheric pressure. This pressure difference drives blood from artery to vein.

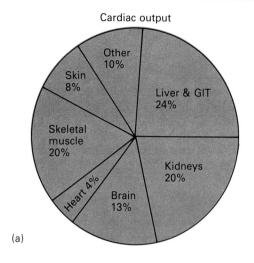

Cardiac output

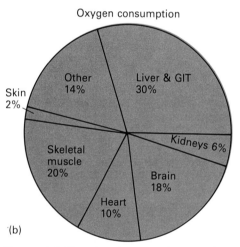

Oxygen consumption

(b)

Figure 1.5 The distribution of left ventricular output in a resting man (top) compared with oxygen consumption (bottom). GIT = gastro-intestinal tract. (From Wade, O. L. and Bishop, J. M. (1962) *Cardiac Output and Regional Blood Flow*, Blackwell, Oxford, by permission)

Arterial pressure is pulsatile, because the heart ejects blood intermittently. Between successive ejections, systemic arterial pressure decays from 120 mmHg to approximately 80 mmHg, while pulmonary pressure decays from 25 to 10 mmHg (Figure 1.6). The conventional way of writing this is 120/80 mmHg and 25/10 mmHg. The con-

ventional units are mmHg above atmospheric pressure, because human blood pressure is measured clinically with a mercury column, taking atmospheric pressure as the reference or zero level (see Appendix II, 'Pressure').

A simple 'law of flow' Blood flow is pulsatile (Chapter 8) but it is useful at this stage to consider a much simpler situation, namely water flowing steadily along a rigid tube, driven by a steady pressure gradient. Under these conditions flow ($\dot{Q}$) is directly proportional to the pressure difference between the inlet (pressure P_1) and outlet (P_2):

$$\dot{Q} \propto P_1 - P_2 \tag{1.2}$$

Flow is often represented by $\dot{Q}$ because Q stands for quantity of fluid and the dot denotes rate of passage. (This was Newton's original calculus notation.) It should be noted that flow is by definition a rate (the passage of a volume or mass per unit time) and the common expression 'rate of flow' is therefore rather nonsensical and best avoided. By inserting a proportionality factor (K) into the above expression we can change it into an equation describing flow:

$$\dot{Q} = K(P_1 - P_2) \tag{1.3}$$

where K is called the *hydraulic conductance* of the tube. Conductance is the reciprocal of *resistance* (R), so we can also write:

$$\dot{Q} = \frac{(P_1 - P_2)}{R} \tag{1.4}$$

This is a form of Darcy's law of flow, analogous to Ohm's law for an electrical current ($I = \Delta V / R$). It states that flow is proportional to driving pressure ($P_1 - P_2$) and inversely proportional to hydraulic resistance. The total resistance of the systemic circulation in man is around 0.02 mmHg per ml/min, while that of the pulmonary circulation is only 0.003 mmHg per ml/min. The low resistance of the pulmonary circulation explains why a very low pressure suffices to drive the cardiac output through the lungs.

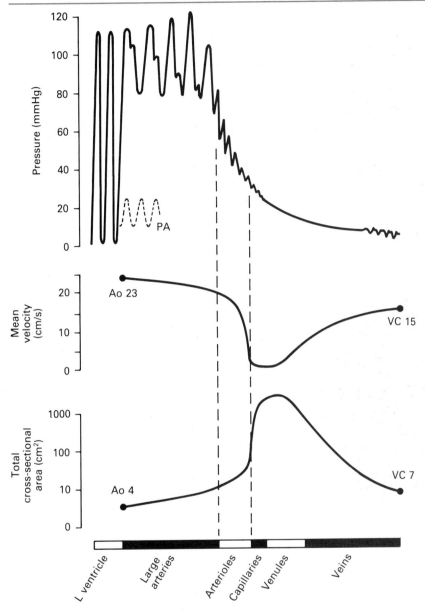

Figure 1.6 The profile of blood pressure and velocity in the systemic circulation of a resting man. The abscissa is distance along the vessels. The greatest fall in pressure occurs across arterioles and the tiniest arteries. Velocity is the cardiac output divided by total cross-sectional area of the vascular bed at that point. Pressure in the pulmonary artery is shown as a dotted line. Ao, human aorta; VC, human vena cava.

The law of flow helps us to understand how the blood flow to an organ is regulated. Equation 1.4 shows that there are in principle two ways to alter flow: either the driving pressure or the vascular resistance can be changed. In normal subjects, blood pressure is in fact kept roughly constant and it is changes in *vascular resistance* that regulate local blood flow. During salivation, for example, blood flow to the salivary gland can increase tenfold due to a fall in vascular resistance to one-tenth its former value, while the driving pressure (arterial pressure) does not change. Changes in vascular resistance are brought about by contraction or relaxation of the vessel walls, and the structure of these is described next.

1.6 Classification of blood vessels

The aorta and pulmonary artery divide into smaller arteries, which branch progressively to form narrow high-resistance vessels called arterioles (see Figure 1.8). Arterioles branch into innumerable capillaries which then converge to form venules and veins. Because of the increase in vessel number with branching, the *total cross-sectional area* of the vascular system increases despite the progressive fall in vessel size (Table 1.2). This slows the *velocity* of the blood (cm/s), because velocity is flow (cm^3/s) divided by cross-sectional area (cm^2). Similarly, a river slows down where the river bed broadens. Thus, in the capillaries the blood velocity is <1/200th of that in the aorta

(see Figure 1.6). The total *flow* (cm^3/s) through the capillaries is velocity × cross-sectional area and this is of course the same as through the aorta. The greatest *volume* of blood is found in the venous system at any one instant (Table 1.2).

Structure of the blood vessel wall

Except for capillaries, all blood vessels have a three-layered plan as shown in Figure 1.7. The wall consists of a tunica intima (innermost layer), tunica media (middle layer) and tunica adventitia (outer layer). The *intima* is a sheet of flat endothelial cells resting on a thin layer of connective tissue. The endothelial layer is the main barrier to plasma proteins and also secretes many vasoactive products, but it is mechanically weak. The *media* supplies mechanical strength and contractile power. It consists of spindle-shaped smooth muscle cells arranged circularly and embedded in a matrix of elastin and collagen fibres. Sheets of elastin (the internal and external elastic laminae) mark each boundary of the media. In places, the endothelial cells of small arteries project through gaps in the internal elastic lamina to make contact with smooth muscle cells. This may allow some transfer of information, but the exact significance of this remains unclear. The

Table 1.2 Average dimensions of blood vessels in dog mesentery*

Vessel	Number	Length (mm)	Diameter (mm)	Total cross-sectional area (mm^2)	Volume (% of total)
Main artery	1	60	3	7	2.5
Arterioles and smallest arteries	1 380 000	1.5–2	0.024–0.031	739	8.1
Capillaries	47 300 000	0.4	0.008	2378	5.7
Venules	2 100 000	1.0	0.026	1151	6.9
Small veins	180 000	1–14	0.075–0.28	1019	21.3
Large veins	61	39–60	1.5–6	174	46.7

*The vessels are easily seen here for counting, unlike most circulations. (After Scleier, J. (1918) *Archiv Gesamte Physiologie*, **173**, 172.) Largest area and therefore slowest flow is in the capillaries. Largest volume is in the veins

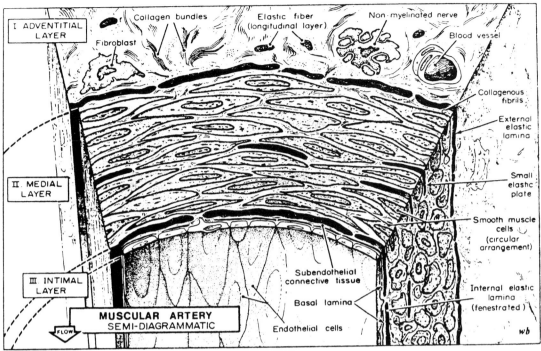

I ADVENTITIAL LAYER — Collagen bundles — Elastic fiber (longitudinal layer) — Non-myelinated nerve — Blood vessel — Fibroblast — Collagenous fibrils — External elastic lamina — Small elastic plate — II. MEDIAL LAYER — Smooth muscle cells (circular arrangement) — III. INTIMAL LAYER — Subendothelial connective tissue — Basal lamina — Endothelial cells — Internal elastic lamina (fenestrated) — MUSCULAR ARTERY SEMI-DIAGRAMMATIC — FLOW — w b

Figure 1.7 Sketch of the structure of a muscular artery. (From Rhodin, J. A. G. (1980), see Further Reading, by permission)

adventitia is a connective tissue sheath with no distinct outer border. It serves to tether the vessel loosely in place. The adventitia of the larger arteries contains small blood vessels, the vasa vasorum (literally 'vessels of vessels'), and in the largest arteries these penetrate into the outer media too. Their task is to nourish the thick media of large vessels. Some large vessels (e.g. limb veins) contain small-diameter nociceptive sensory fibres: these probably mediate pain in such conditions as thrombophlebitis.

Functional classification

The circulation is constructed on the sound economical principle that each vessel must fulfil at least one extra function besides conducting blood. Vessel structure is specially adapted for this extra function, as follows.

Elastic arteries (diameter 1–2 cm in man) The pulmonary artery, aorta and major branches, like the iliac arteries, have very distensible walls because their tunica media is particularly rich in elastin (Table 1.3), a protein six times more extensible than rubber. This allows large arteries to expand and receive the stroke volume during ventricular ejection, and to recoil during diastole. This converts the intermittent ejection of blood by the heart into a continuous flow through the more distal vessels. Another protein, collagen, forms a meshwork of strong fibrils in the media. Collagen is 100 times stiffer than elastin and its role is to prevent overdistension.

Conduit (muscular) arteries (diameter 0.1–1 cm in man) In medium to small arteries such as the popliteal, radial, cerebral and coronary arteries, the tunica media is thicker relative to the lumen diameter (Figure 1.8), and it contains more smooth muscle (Table

Table 1.3 The changing composition of the blood vessel wall (%)

	Endothelium	*Smooth muscle*	*Elastic tissue*	*Connective tissue*
Elastic artery	5	25	40	27
Arteriole	10	60	10	20
Capillary	95	–	–	5 (basal lamina)
Venule	20	20	–	60

(After Caro, C. G., Pedley, T. J., Schroter, R. C. and Seed, W. A. (1978) *The Mechanics of the Circulation*, Oxford University Press, Oxford, and Burton, A. C. (1972) *Physiology and Biophysics of the Circulation*, Year Book Medical Publishers, Chicago)

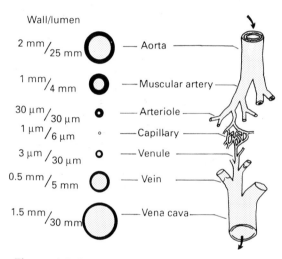

Figure 1.8 Approximate thickness of the wall relative to the diameter of the lumen in the various types of blood vessel. The ratio varies, however, with blood pressure and vascular tone. The large-vessel dimensions are for man. (Sources as for Table 1.3)

1.3). The muscular arteries act as low-resistance conduits and their thick walls help prevent collapse at sharp bends like the knee joint. They have a rich autonomic nerve supply and can contract or relax. Their ability to contract can be life-saving on occasion, as demonstrated by a motor-cycle crash victim brought into Casualty with one leg almost completely severed at the knee. The popliteal artery was torn in half, yet the proximal stump was scarcely bleeding: intense contraction of the media had prevented the patient from bleeding to death. Contrac-tion of muscular arteries can also occur physiologically in cerebral arteries (Chapter 13) and in the limbs of diving animals (Chapter 15), and dilatation occurs in arteries feeding exercising muscle (Chapter 12).

Resistance vessels The main resistance to blood flow resides in the smallest, terminal arteries (diameter 100–500 μm) and arterioles (<100 μm). This is proved by the large drop in pressure as blood traverses these vessels (see Figure 1.6). Definitions are a little unsatisfactory here; some workers reserve the term arteriole for vessels with only a single layer of muscle in the media, while others define it by size, e.g. <100 μm diameter. The latter meaning is used here. The proximal resistance vessels have thick walls relative to their lumen (Figure 1.8) and are richly innervated by vasoconstrictor nerve fibres. The terminal arterioles or metarterioles (diameter 10–40 μm) are poorly innervated and possess only 1–3 layers of smooth muscle cells. The high resistance is due to the narrow lumen and limited number of these vessels (see Table 1.2). Because arterioles dominate resistance to flow they are able to act as the 'taps' of the circulation, turning local blood flow up or down to match local needs. When they dilate (*vasodilatation*) the resistance to flow falls, so blood flow increases. *Vasoconstriction* has the reverse effect. The terminal arteriole also has a further role: by contracting hard it can temporarily prevent blood from flowing through the group of capillaries that it feeds, and can thus influence capillary exchange. (This task used to be attributed to 'precapillary sphincters', but it now seems that discrete sphincters exist only in a few tissues, such as mesentery.)

Exchange vessels The capillaries are so tiny (diameter 4–7 μm) and numerous that few cells are further than 10–20 μm from a capillary. The wall is reduced to a single layer of endothelial cells and its thinness (0.5 μm) facilitates the rapid transfer of metabolites between blood and tissue. Some exchange also takes place across slightly larger, downstream vessels called postcapillary or pericytic venules (diameter 15–50 μm); these are microscopic venules that lack a complete smooth muscle coat. Some gas exchange also occurs across the walls of small arterioles before blood even reaches capillaries, so the functional category of 'exchange vessel' actually embraces both sides of the true capillary network.

Although capillaries are extremely narrow, the capillary bed as a whole offers a surprisingly modest resistance to flow. This is partly because of a special pattern of blood flow in capillaries (bolus flow, Chapter 8) and partly because the total cross-sectional area of the capillary bed is very large (see Table 1.2). The large area also reduces blood velocity to 0.5–1 mm/s (under 1/200th of mean blood velocity in the aorta), as noted earlier. The slowing allows the red cell about 1–2 s in the capillary (the transit time), which is more than sufficient to unload O_2 and take up CO_2.

The arteriovenous anastomosis In a few tissues, notably the skin and nasal mucosa, there are wide shunt vessels (diameter 20–135 μm) that connect arterioles to venules directly, bypassing the capillaries. Their thick muscular walls are richly innervated by sympathetic nerves and, in skin, they are involved in temperature regulation (Chapter 13). They are not present in all tissues.

Capacitance vessels Venules (diameter 50–200 μm) and veins differ principally in size and number rather than wall structure. The

wall is thin and comprises an intima, a thin media composed of smooth muscle and collagen, and an adventitia. In limb veins, the intima possesses pairs of semilunar valves (discovered by the gloriously named Hieronymous Fabricius ab Aquapendente in 1603) and these prevent backflow of venous blood. The large central veins and veins of the head and neck lack functional valves. Venules and small veins are more numerous than arterioles and arteries (see Table 1.2), so they offer a low resistance to flow; indeed, a pressure of just 10–15 mmHg suffices to drive the cardiac output from venule to vena cava.

Because of their large number and size, veins contains about two-thirds of the circulating blood at any one instant (Figure 1.9). They are therefore called 'capacitance vessels'. Being thin-walled, they are easily distended or collapsed, so they act as a variable reservoir of blood. Moreover, many veins are innervated by vasoconstrictor nerve fibres, so the volume of blood in the reservoir can be actively controlled. At times of physiological stress the veins are

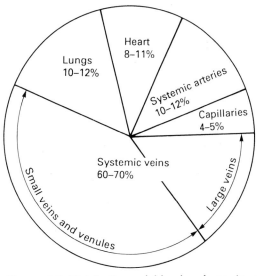

Figure 1.9 Distribution of blood volume in a resting man (5.5 litres). (From Folkow, B. and Neil, E. (1971) *Circulation*, Oxford University Press, London, by permission)

constricted, which displaces blood into the heart and arterial system.

1.7 Plumbing of the vascular circuits

The systemic circulation is made up of numerous specialized individual circuits supplying the brain, kidneys, gut, etc. Usually the blood supply to an organ arises directly from the aorta so that each organ is supplied at full pressure, without any interference by other organs (see Figure 1.4). This form of plumbing is called 'in parallel'. A few organs, however, are connected 'in series' with another organ; that is to say, they obtain their blood secondhand from the venous outflow of another organ. This is called a *portal system.*

The largest portal system in the body is that of the liver. Around 72% of the liver's blood supply is venous blood from the intestine and spleen, carried in the portal vein (Figure 1.4). The portal vein enters the liver at the 'porta hepatis', or gateway of the liver, which is how the term 'portal system' arose. The liver also receives arterial blood directly via the hepatic artery, so its circuitry is partly in series and partly in parallel. Portal systems have the advantage of transporting a valuable commodity directly from ·one site to another – for example, products of digestion from intestine to the liver. Portal systems also exist in the kidney, where effluent blood from the glomerulus supplies the tubules, and in the brain, where a portal system carries hormones from the hypothalamus to the anterior pituitary gland. A portal system has one serious weakness, however; the downstream tissue receives partially deoxygenated blood under a reduced pressure head, and as a result the downstream tissue is very vulnerable to damage during episodes of hypotension (low arterial pressure). Renal tubular damage, in particular, is a not uncommon medical complication of severe hypotension.

1.8 Central control

The behaviour of the heart and blood vessels has to be constantly adjusted in order to deal with varying environmental and internal demands. This is achieved by nervous and neuroendocrine reflexes, which are coordinated by the brain. One of the most important cardiovascular reflexes is the arterial baroreceptor reflex, which safeguards blood flow to the brain by maintaining a stable blood pressure. The reflex is initiated by 'baroreceptors' in the walls of major arteries, which sense changes in blood pressure. Nerve impulses are sent to the brainstem and reflexly alter the activity of autonomic nerves that control the heart and blood vessels. This results in changes in cardiac output, peripheral resistance and venous capacitance that restore blood pressure to normal.

What's next? In a system as complex as the cardiovascular system there is a real danger of 'not seeing the wood for the trees'. The above outline should help avoid this. In Chapters 2-12 (cardiac electricity, haemodynamics, etc.) we bump into the trees and even peep under the bark. In Chapters 13–16, we again stand back to gain the broader view of how the system reponds as a whole to physiological and medical challenges.

1.9 Summary

Because the time taken for transport by diffusion increases with the square of distance, animals larger than 1 mm or so require a cardiovascular system. Metabolic energy (the heart beat) is used to produce rapid *convective transport* of oxygen, nutrients, waste products, hormones and heat; and the branching vascular tree ensures delivery to within 10 µm or so of most cells. Over the final 10 µm or so, *diffusion* takes over. In the absence of convective transport, cell death occurs, as in a myocardial infarct or ischaemic leg.

The right ventricle, primed via the right atrium, pumps deoxygenated blood at low pressure (~ 15 mmHg) through the lungs for oxygenation (*pulmonary circulation*). The left ventricle, primed via the left atrium, pumps the oxygenated blood at high pressure (~ 90 mmHg) to the rest of the body (*systemic circulation*). The *cardiac output* (heart rate × stroke volume) is about 5 litres/min in a resting man, resting rate being 60–70 beats/min and stroke volume 70–80 ml. The *distribution* of the cardiac output to tissues is actively controlled, so that in general tissues receive blood in proportion to their activity; skeletal muscle is a good example. The kidneys, however, receive an unusually high proportion of the cardiac output (20%), to satisfy their excretory role.

Flow through a given tissue ($\dot{Q}$) is driven by the pressure difference between artery and vein, $P_a - P_v$. This is stated by the basic *law of flow*, $\dot{Q} = (P_a - P_v)/R$, where R is resistance to flow. The main resistance lies in the arterioles and tiny terminal arteries, as proved by the large pressure loss in these vessels. It is these '*resistance vessels*' that, by constricting or dilating, actively regulate local blood flow to match local demand. Other functional categories of vessel are as follows: *elastic arteries* (e.g. aorta) receive the intermittently ejected stroke volume and convert it into a continuous albeit pulsatile peripheral flow; *exchange vessels* (capillaries, postcapillary venules) allow solute and water exchange with the tissue; *capacitance vessels* (venules, veins) have an actively-controlled, variable blood capacity and normally contain about two-thirds of the circulating blood volume.

Except for capillaries (comprising a single layer of endothelial cells), all blood vessels comprise three main layers, the *intima* (primarily the endothelial lining), the *media* (vascular smooth muscle, collagen and elastin) and the *adventitia* (connective tissue). The smooth muscle regulates the diameter of resistance and capacitance vessels, and thereby regulates local blood flow, arterial pressure and blood volume distribution.

Vascular smooth muscle is, in general, *controlled* by autonomic nerves, circulating hormones and local factors. The rate and force of the heart beat too are controlled by autonomic nerves and circulating hormones. The cardiovascular system is thus under the control of the *central nervous system and neural reflexes* (e.g. the baroreflex).

Most special circulations (coronary, cerebral, etc.) are 'plumbed' in parallel so that each receives fully oxygenated arterial blood. A few circulations, however, lie in series with an upstream tissue and receive venous blood. These are called *portal circulations*; the portal vein supplying the liver with blood drained from the intestine is a good example.

Further reading

Cliff, W. J. (1976) *Blood Vessels*, Cambridge University Press, Cambridge

Harvey, W. (1628) *The Movement of the Heart and Blood* (trans. by G. Whitteridge) (1976), Blackwell Scientific Publications, Oxford

Henderson, J. R. and Daniel, P. M. (1984) Capillary beds and portal circulations. In *Handbook of Physiology, The Cardiovascular System*, Vol. IV, Part 2 (eds E. M. Renkin and C. C. Michel), The American Physiological Society, Maryland, pp. 1035–1046

Neil, E. (1983) Peripheral circulation: historical aspects. In *Handbook of Physiology*, Vol. III, Part 1 (eds J. T. Shepherd and F. M. Abboud), American Physiological Society, Maryland, pp. 120

Rhodin, J. A. G. (1980) Architecture of the vessel wall. In *Handbook of Physiology, Cardiovascular System*, Vol. II (eds D. F. Bohr, A. P. Somlyo and H. V. Sparks), American Physiological Society, Bethesda, p. 132

Chapter 2
Cardiac cycle

The adult human heart weighs only 300–350 g, yet most of us can reasonably expect it to pump out around 200 million litres of blood over our allotted 'three score years and ten'. In this chapter the mechanical events underlying this remarkable performance are described.

2.1 Gross structure of the heart

The mature heart is built upon a collagenous 'skeleton' in the shape of a fibrotendinous ring (the *annulus fibrosus*) which is located at the atrioventricular junction (Figure 2.1). The muscular atria and ventricles are attached to either side of this ring, and the ring is perforated by four apertures, each containing a valve. As well as functioning as the mechanical base of the heart, the fibrotendinous ring insulates the ventricles electrically from the atria.

Right atrium and tricuspid valve The right atrium is a thin-walled muscular chamber which receives the venous return from the venae cavae and the coronary sinus (the main vein draining heart muscle; Figure 2.2a). The wall near the entrance of the superior vena cava also contains the cardiac pacemaker, the 'sparking plug' that initiates each heart beat. The right atrium communicates with the right ventricle through the tricuspid valve which, as its name implies, has three cusps, although it is sometimes difficult to distinguish all three. The large anterior cusp is mainly responsible for valve closure. Each cusp is a flexible flap of connective tissue, roughly 0.1 mm thick, covered by endothelium. The free margin of the cusp is tethered by tendinous strings (*chordae tendineae*) to an inward projection of the ventricle wall, the papillary muscle. The *papillary muscle* contracts and tenses the chordae tendineae during systole and this

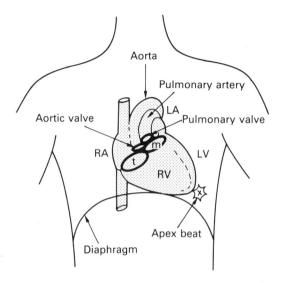

Figure 2.1 The heart lies obliquely across the chest. The fibrotendinous ring (black) acts as a base for the heart. It contains the tricuspid (t), mitral (m), aortic and pulmonary valves grouped in an oblique plane beneath the sternum. The apex of the heart is formed by the left ventricle (LV), and the anterior surface is formed by the right ventricle (RV) and right atrium (RA). The inferior surface of the heart and the pericardium (not shown) rest on the central tendon of the diaphragm

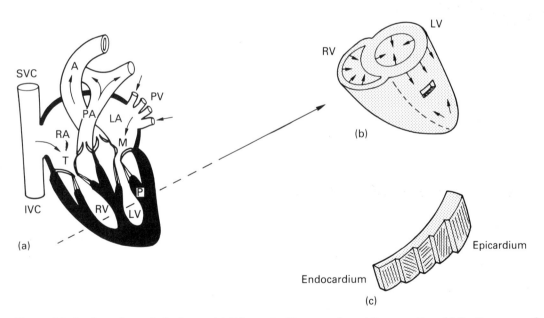

Figure 2.2 Sections through the heart. (a) Schematic diagram of an oblique section. (b) Section across the ventricles to illustrate mode of emptying. (c) Arrangement of muscle fibres in the ventricle wall. RA, LA, right and left atrium. The opening just below the label RA is the coronary sinus. RV, LV, right and left ventricle; T, M, tricuspid and mitral valves; P, papillary muscle with chordae tendineae; A, aorta; PA, PV, pulmonary artery and veins; SVC, IVC, superior and inferior venae cavae

helps to prevent the valve from inverting into the atrium during ventricular systole.

Right ventricle and pulmonary valve The anterior wall of the right ventricle is about 0.5 cm thick in man, and resembles a pocket tacked around the septum (Figure 2.2b). Expulsion of blood is produced chiefly by the free anterior wall approaching the septum, rather like an old-fashioned bellows. The outlet from the ventricle into the pulmonary artery is guarded by the pulmonary valve which, like the aortic valve, consists of three equal-sized, baggy cusps.

Left atrium and mitral valve The left atrium receives blood from the pulmonary veins and transmits it into the left ventricle through a bicuspid valve. The large anterior and small posterior cusps are thought to look like a bishop's mitre, hence the name 'mitral valve'. The cusp margins are tethered by chordae tendineae to two papillary muscles in the left ventricle.

Left ventricle and aortic valve The chamber of the left ventricle is conical and ejection of blood is produced by a reduction in both diameter and length. The wall is around three times thicker than that of the right ventricle, because it has to generate higher pressures. The innermost (endocardial) muscle fibres are orientated longitudinally, running from the base of the heart (the fibrotendinous ring) to the apex (tip of left ventricle); the central fibres run circumferentially; the outermost or epicardial fibres again run longitudinally; and intermediate fibres run obliquely (Figure 2.2c). In other words the muscle orientation changes progressively across the wall. When the chamber contracts, it twists forwards and the apex taps against the chest wall, producing the *apex beat*. This can be felt in the fifth, left intercostal space, about 10 cm from the midline (mid-clavicular line). The root of the aorta contains a three-cusp valve similar to the pulmonary valve.

The heart is enclosed in a fibrous sac or pericardium, which is lined by a layer of mesothelium and is lubricated by pericardial fluid. The lower surface of the pericardium is fused to the diaphragm, and as the diaphragm descends during inspiration it pulls the heart into a more vertical orientation.

2.2 Mechanical events of the cardiac cycle

The atria and ventricles contract in sequence, resulting in a cycle of pressure and volume changes, and a thorough knowledge of the cycle is needed for the diagnosis of valvular defects. The cardiac cycle has four phases and we will begin, arbitrarily, at a moment when both the atria and ventricles are in diastole (relaxed). The timings below refer to a human cycle of 0.9 s duration (67 beats/min) and the data have been acquired by a combination of echocardiography (Section 2.5), cardiac catheterization (Section 2.5), electrocardiography (see Chapter 5) and cardiometry (Section 7.3).

Ventricular filling

Duration: 0.5 s
Inlet valves (tricuspid and mitral): open
Outlet valves (pulmonary and aortic): closed

Ventricular diastole lasts for nearly two-thirds of the cycle at rest, providing ample time for refilling the chamber. Initially the atria too are in diastole and blood flows passively from the great veins through the open atrioventricular valves into the ventricles. There is an initial phase of rapid filling, lasting about 0.15 s, as shown by the cardiometer volume trace in Figure 2.3. This phase has a curious feature; even though ventricular volume is increasing, ventricular pressure is falling (see region Y of the ventricle pressure trace in Figure 2.4). The reason is that the ventricle wall is recoiling

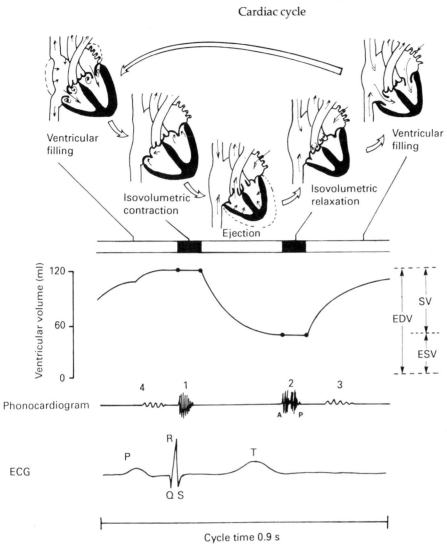

Figure 2.3 The changes in valve setting and ventricular volume during one cardiac cycle lasting 0.9 s. EDV, end-diastolic volume; ESV, end-systolic volume; SV, stroke volume. The ejection fraction is SV/ EDV. The heart sounds on the phonocardiogram are numbered 1 to 4 and the second sound is split here into an aortic component (A) and pulmonary component (P). The electrocardiogram (ECG) waves are described in the text

elastically from the deformation of systole, and is in effect sucking blood into the chamber. As the ventricle reaches its natural volume, the rate of filling slows down and further filling requires distension of the ventricle by the pressure of the venous blood; ventricular pressure now begins to rise. In the final third of the filling phase, the atria contract and force some additional blood into the ventricle. In resting subjects, this atrial boost is quite small and enhances ventricular filling by only 15–20%: indeed,

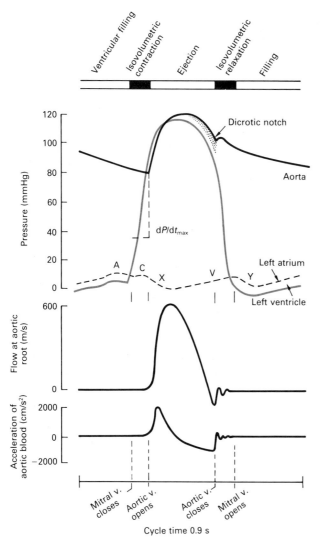

Figure 2.4 Diagram of pressure and outflow on the left side of the human heart, based on data from intracardiac catheters and velocity measurements at the aortic root. $(dP/dt)_{max}$ is the maximum rate of rise of ventricular pressure, a measure of myocardial contractility. The stippled region highlights the pressure gradient that decelerates outflow during the late ejection phase. Note the slight reversal of aortic flow at aortic valve closure. For explanation of the atrial waveform see Section 2.3. The waveforms in the right heart are of similar shape but the pressures are lower. (After Noble, M. I. M. (1968) *Circulation Research*, **23**, 663–670)

the absence of an atrial boost in patients suffering from atrial fibrillation (ineffective atrial contractions; Section 5.8) makes little difference to resting cardiac output. During exercise, however, heart rate is high, the time available for passive ventricular filling is curtailed (as explained later) and the atrial boost then becomes important.

The volume of blood in a ventricle at the end of the filling phase is called the *end-diastolic volume*, or EDV, and is typically around 120 ml in an adult human. The corresponding *end-diastolic pressure*, or EDP, is a few mmHg. As Table 2.1 shows, the EDP is a little higher in the left ventricle than in the right, because the left ventricle wall is thicker and therefore needs a higher pressure to distend it.

Table 2.1 Mean pressures during the human cardiac cycle in mmHg*

	Right	Left
Atrium	3	8
Ventricle –		
end of diastole	4	9
peak of systole	25	120

*Adult, resting supine.

Isovolumetric contraction

Duration: 0.05 s
Inlet valves: closed
Outlet valves: closed

As atrial systole begins to wane, ventricular systole commences. It lasts 0.35 s and is divided into a brief isovolumetric phase and a longer ejection phase. As soon as ventricular pressure rises fractionally above atrial pressure, the atrioventricular valves are forced shut by the reversed pressure gradient. Backflow during closure is minimal because the cusps are already approximated by vortices behind them in the late filling phase. The ventricle is now a closed chamber, and the growing wall tension causes a steep rise in the pressure of the trapped blood; indeed the maximum rate of rise of pressure, $(dP/dt)_{max}$, is frequently used as an index of cardiac contractility.

Ejection

Duration: 0.3 s
Inlet valves: closed
Outlet valves: open

When ventricular pressure exceeds arterial pressure, the outflow valves are forced open and ejection begins. Three-quarters of the stroke volume is ejected in the first half of the ejection phase (phase of rapid ejection, approximately 0.15 s), and at first blood is ejected faster than it can escape out of the arterial tree. As a result, much of it has to be accommodated by distension of the large elastic arteries, and this drives arterial pressure up to its maximum or 'systolic' level. Vortices behind the cusps of the open aortic valve prevent the cusps from blocking the adjacent entrances into the coronary arteries.

As systole weakens and the rate of ejection slows down, the rate at which blood flows away through the arterial system begins to exceed the ejection rate, so pressure begins to fall. Active ventricular contraction actually ceases about two-thirds of the way through the ejection phase, but a slow outflow continues for a while owing to the momentum of the blood. As the ventricle begins to relax, ventricular pressure falls below arterial pressure by 2–3 mmHg (see stippled zone in Figure 2.4) but the outward momentum of the blood prevents immediate valve closure. The reversed pressure gradient, however, progressively decelerates the outflow, as shown in the bottom trace of Figure 2.4, until finally a brief backflow closes the outflow valve. Backflow is less than 5% of stroke volume. Valve closure creates a brief pressure rise in the arterial pressure trace called the *dicrotic wave*. For the rest of cycle, arterial pressure gradually declines as blood runs away into the periphery.

It must be emphasized that the ventricle does not empty completely but only by about two-thirds. The average *ejection fraction* in man is 0.67, corresponding to a *stroke volume* of 70–80 ml in adults. The residual *end-systolic volume* of about 50 ml acts as a reserve which can be utilized to increase stroke volume in exercise.

Isovolumetric relaxation

Duration: 0.08 s
Inlet valves: closed
Outlet valves: closed

With closure of the aortic and pulmonary valves, each ventricle once again becomes a closed chamber. Ventricular pressure falls very rapidly owing to the mechanical recoil of collagen fibres within the myocardium, which were tensed and deformed by the contracting myocytes. When ventricular pressure has fallen just below atrial pressure, the atrioventricular valves open and blood floods in from the atria which have been refilling during ventricular systole.

The ventricular pressure–volume loop

A plot of pressure in the ventricle versus its volume forms a closed loop, as shown in Figure 2.5. This is a particularly useful way of representing the cardiac cycle, combining features of Figures 2.3 and 2.4 in a single figure, and it will be used to explain the control of stroke volume in Chapter 7. Starting at a point where the mitral valve has just opened (bottom left corner), the bottom curve shows ventricular filling. In the initial phase of rapid filling the pressure is actually falling, because the walls of the relaxing ventricle recoil elastically and exert a suction effect. In the later slow-filling phase, a rise in pressure drives the increase in volume, and the line now coincides with the passive pressure–volume curve of the relaxed ventricle. With onset of systole, the mitral valve closes (bottom right) and isovolumetric contraction raises ventricular pressure. When ventricular pressure reaches diastolic blood pressure, the aortic valve

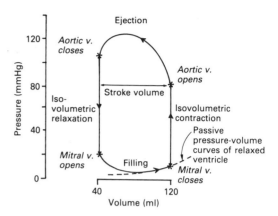

Figure 2.5 Pressure–volume cycle of human left ventricle

opens (top right) and volume decreases as ejection occurs. As the systole weakens, the aortic valve closes (top left) and isovolumetric relaxation leads to mitral opening and refilling of the ventricle.

The atria refill with blood during ventricular systole, which leads us to consider next the atrial cycle.

2.3 Atrial cycle and central venous pressure cycle

The cycle of events in the atria produces a cycle of pressure changes in the veins of the thorax and neck (jugular veins) because these veins are in open communication with the atria. A direct recording of pressure in the atrium or jugular vein reveals that there are two main pressure waves per cycle, called the A and V waves, and a third smaller wave, the C wave (see dashed line in Figure 2.4).

The *A wave* is an increase in pressure caused by atrial systole, and the 'A' stands for atrial. Atrial systole produces a slight reflux of blood through the valveless venous entrances: this briefly reverses the flow in the venae cavae and raises central venous pressure to its maximum point (3–5 mmHg).

The next event, the *C wave*, occurs earlier in the right atrium than in the neck. In the atrium, it is caused by the tricuspid valve bulging back into the atrium as it closes. In the internal jugular vein, the C wave is caused partly by expansion of the carotid artery, which lies alongside the vein and presses on it during systole; 'C' stands for 'carotid'. After the C wave there comes a sharp fall in pressure, called the *X descent*, which is caused by atrial relaxation. Venous inflow reaches its peak velocity during this phase (see Figure 8.20, Chapter 8). As the atria fill, atrial pressure begins to rise again, producing the *V wave*; the 'V' refers to ventricular systole, which is going on at this time. Finally, the atrioventricular valves open and the atria empty passively into the ventricles, producing the sharp *Y descent*.

The cycle of right atrial pressure is mirrored in the internal and external jugular veins of the neck, because the latter are in open communication with the superior vena cava. The pulsating jugular veins are readily visible in a recumbent lean subject and this enables the physician to assess the central venous pressure cycle by simple inspection. What the eye particularly notices in the neck are two sudden collapses of the vein, corresponding to the X and Y descents. Examination of the jugular pulse is a regular clinical procedure because certain cardiac diseases produce characteristic abnormalities in the pulse. Tricuspid incompetence, for example, can produce exaggerated V waves, because blood leaks back through the incompetent valve during ventricular systole.

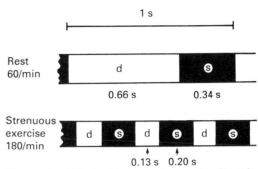

Figure 2.6 Effect of heart rate on the diastolic period available for filling. d, diastole; s, systole. Diastole is curtailed more than systole as heart rate increases

phases do not, however, all shorten to an equal degree (Figure 2.6). Ventricular systole does shorten, but only to about 0.2 s, and this leaves a mere 0.13 s for refilling during diastole. Passive filling remains important, but atrial systole contributes relatively more than at rest. Even with the help of atrial systole, 0.12 s is about the minimum interval that allows an adequate refilling of the human ventricle. Further increase in heart rate, such as the pathological tachycardia which occurs in the Wolff–Parkinson–White syndrome (>250 beats/min), actually causes cardiac output to decline rather than increase, because refilling during diastole becomes inadequate. Diastolic interval is thus the chief factor limiting the maximum useful heart rate.

2.4 Effect of heart rate on phase duration

The timings given earlier for the cardiac cycle refer to a resting subject, but when the heart is beating 180 times per min (which is close to the normal maximum), the duration of the entire cycle is only 0.33 s, and all phases of the cycle have to be shortened. The various

2.5 Clinical aspects of the human cardiac cycle

The cardiac cycle is assessed in routine clinical practice by examining various physical signs, such as the *arterial pulse*, the *jugular venous pulse* and the *apex beat*. Another important sign, not yet described, is the *sound* generated by closing valves.

The heart sounds

When a heart valve closes, the cusps balloon back as they suddenly check the momentum of refluxing blood. The sudden tension in the cusps sets up a brief vibration, rather as a sail slaps audibly when suddenly filled by a gust of wind. The vibration is transmitted to the chest wall, where it can be heard through a stethoscope. Provided that the valve is normal, it is only closure that is audible: opening is silent, as with a well-oiled door.

Two heart sounds are normally clearly audible per beat, the first and second heart sounds. They are usually represented as lubb-dupp followed by a pause, roughly in waltz time; the first heart sound (lubb) is the one immediately after the pause. (Lubb-dupp should not be taken too seriously, for it appears that only English-speaking hearts go lubb-dupp, while German ones go doop-teup and Turkish ones rrupp-ta). The heart sounds can be recorded by a microphone placed on the precordium, and a tracing of the sound is called a phonocardiogram (see Figure 2.3). The *first heart sound*, a vibration of roughly 100 cycles/s (100 Hertz), is caused by closure of the tricuspid and mitral valves. They close virtually simultaneously. The *second sound*, of similar frequency, is caused by closure of the aortic and pulmonary valves.

The second sound is sometimes audibly *'split'*, with an initial aortic component and a fractionally delayed pulmonary component; the sounds might then be represented as lubb-terrupp. Splitting of the second sound is common in healthy young people during inspiration, because inspiration has two effects on stroke volume. (1) It increases the filling of the right ventricle. This raises its stroke volume, which in turn prolongs the right ventricular ejection time and slightly delays pulmonary valve closure. (2) At the same time, inspiration expands the lung's blood vessels, temporarily reducing the rate of return of blood to the left side of the heart. This reduces left ventricular stroke volume, shortens the left ventricle ejection time and so hastens closure of the aortic valve. The second sound thus 'splits' because of an equal and opposite movement of its two components.

Two additional sounds besides the first and second sounds can be detected by phonocardiography, but they are of low frequency and difficult for untrained ears to detect. The third heart sound is common in young people and is caused by the rush of blood into the relaxing ventricles during early diastole. The fourth sound occurs just before the first sound and is caused by atrial systole.

Anatomically, the four heart valves lie very close together under the sternum (see Figure 2.1) but fortunately each valve is best heard over a distinct *'auscultation area'* some distance away, because the vibration from each valve propagates through the chamber fed by the valve. The mitral valve is best heard in the mid-clavicular line of the 4th–5th left intercostal space, the tricuspid valve in the 5th interspace at the left sternal edge, the aortic valve in the 2nd interspace at the right sternal edge, and the pulmonary valve in the 2nd interspace at the left sternal edge.

Valvular abnormalities

There are two fundamental classes of valvular abnormality, stenosis and incompetence. *Stenosis* is a narrowing of the valve. A high pressure-gradient is needed to force blood through a stenosed valve. *Incompetence* is failure of the valve to close tightly, thus allowing a regurgitation of blood.

With either abnormality, blood passes through the valve in a turbulent jet, setting up a high-frequency vibration which is heard as a *'murmur'* through the stethoscope. Given four valves and two pathologies, there are eight basic murmurs, but just one example must suffice here. In mitral valve incompetence there is regurgitation into the left atrium during ventricular systole, producing a murmur that occurs throughout systole (a pansystolic murmur) and sounds loudest over the mitral area. The heart sounds may then be represented, roughly, by a lu-shshshsh-tupp. Hypochondriacs should note, however, that a *benign murmur* is not uncommon during the ejection phase in the young. It is not caused by a valve lesion but by turbulence in the ventricular outflow tract. This 'benign systolic murmur' is especially marked during pregnancy, strenuous exercise and anaemia (Section 8.2).

Electrocardiography

The electrocardiogram (ECG) is a record of cardiac electrical events obtained from the body surface. The ECG is described fully in Chapter 5, so here we will simply note the relation between the electrical blips of the ECG and the mechanical events (see Figure 2.3). The P wave of the ECG is produced by electrical activation of the atria, and its peak coincides with the onset of atrial contraction. The QRS complex is produced by electrical activation of the ventricles, so the QRS complex is followed almost immediately by the onset of ventricular contraction and the first heart sound. The T wave is produced by electrical recharging of the ventricles, and since this marks the onset of diastole it is closely followed by the second heart sound.

Echocardiography

Echocardiography is an invaluable tool for the non-invasive assessment of the human cardiac cycle. A beam of ultrasound is directed across the heart from a precordial ultrasonic emitter (a piezoelectric crystal), and reflections of the sound from the walls and valves are collected and used to build up a record of their motion. An example is shown in Figure 7.20.

Cardiac catheterization

This is a direct and powerful investigative procedure. Under local anaesthesia, a fine catheter is threaded through the antecubital vein in the crook of the elbow and advanced under X-ray guidance through the right atrium into the right ventricle, or even into the pulmonary artery. The aorta and left ventricle can be reached by a catheter introduced through the femoral artery. The intracardiac catheter can then be put to one of the following uses.

Cine-angiography A radio-opaque contrast medium is injected through the catheter and the progress of the medium through the cardiac chambers is followed by X-ray cinematography (cardiac angiography). This displays the movement of the heart wall and reveals any valvular regurgitation.

Radionuclide angiography A recent extension of the angiographic method is to inject a gamma-ray emitting isotope into a central vein and record the gamma emission with a scintillation camera placed over the precordium. Not only can images of the heart in diastole and systole be computed but also, from the fall in counts produced by each ejection, the ventricular ejection fraction can be measured.

Intracardiac pressure measurement Chamber pressures can be recorded by connecting the catheter to an external pressure transducer, or by mounting a miniature transducer in the tip of the catheter. The pressure drop across a closed valve serves as an excellent test of its competence. A pulmonary artery catheter can also be wedged in the pulmonary arterioles, and the recorded 'wedge pressure' is often used as an estimate of pulmonary capillary pressure.

Intracardiac pacing This is a therapeutic application of the cardiac catheter, in which a wire catheter is wedged in the ventricle and used to stimulate each heart beat from an external electrical device, thereby replacing the heart's own pacemaker.

2.6 Summary

The four muscular chambers of the mammalian heart are built upon a fibrotendinous ring that contains four apertures with valves. The ring also isolates the atria electrically from the ventricles, except at the bundle of His. Each chamber ejects blood through a valved outflow aperture. The cardiac cycle comprises four phases of unequal duration, with events on the right and left sides almost synchronous. In the *filling phase* the heart is in diastole; the arterial outlet valves are closed (aortic and pulmonary valves) and the atrioventricular inlet valves are open (tricuspid and mitral valves), allowing rapid, passive filling of the ventricles. This is boosted by atrial systole towards the end of the phase. In the *isovolumetric contraction phase* the onset of ventricular systole raises ventricular pressure, which closes the atrioventricular valves (first heart sound); pressure then rises very rapidly. This is quickly terminated by opening of the arterial outlet valves and onset of the *ejection phase*. Two-thirds of the ventricular blood is now ejected (resting subject). As ejection rate wanes, pressure falls until the outlet valves are closed by a slight back-flow (second heart sound, sometimes split). In the *isovolumetric relaxation phase* ventricular pressure now falls rapidly, until less than atrial pressure, at which point the atrioventricular valves open and rapid filling begins. The ventricular *pressure–volume loop* diagram is a particularly useful way, physiologically, of representing this cycle.

The cycle of pressure changes in the right atrium is reflected in the jugular veins and can be seen on inspection of the neck. There is an *A wave* (atrial systole) and *C wave* (closure of tricuspid valve) followed by the *X descent* (atrial diastole). Pressure then rises again due to continuing venous return (*V wave*) and falls when the tricuspid valve opens (*Y descent*), emptying the atrial contents into the ventricle.

Ventricular diastole occupies two-thirds of the cycle at rest, but is reduced to only one-third of the cycle at high heart rates. This restricts the time available for refilling the ventricle and limits the maximum useful heart rate in man to 180–200 beats/min.

Abnormalities of the cardiac cycle can be detected clinically by inspection of the venous pulse in the neck, measurement of arterial blood pressure, auscultation for heart sounds (valvular stenosis or incompetence create characteristic 'murmurs'), electrocardiography, echocardiography, radionuclide angiography and diagnostic cardiac catheterization.

Further reading

Braunwald, E. and Ross, J. (1979) Control of cardiac performance. In *Handbook of Physiology, The Cardiovascular System*, Vol. I *The Heart* (ed. R. M. Berne), American Physiological Society, Bethesda, pp. 533–579

Caro, C. G., Pedley, T. J., Schroter, R. C. and Seed, W. A. (1978) *The Mechanics of the Circulation*, Oxford University Press, Oxford

Parmley, W. W. and Talbot, L. L. (1979) Heart as a pump. In *Handbook of Physiology, The Cardiovascular System*, Vol. I *The Heart* (ed. R. M. Berne), American Physiological Society, Bethesda, pp. 429–460

Robinson, T. F., Factor, S. M. and Sonnenblick, E. H. (1986) The heart as a suction pump. *Scientific American* (June), 62–69

Chapter 3

Excitation and contraction of a cardiac myocyte

Overview The heart beat is initiated by a special electrical system, the pacemaker–conduction system, situated within the wall of the heart. This system is composed of specially modified muscle cells, not nervous tissue. When the electrical signal generated by the pacemaker–conduction system reaches the muscle cells that form the bulk of the heart, the latter are excited and fire off an action potential. This leads to a rise in intracellular calcium concentration, which in turn activates the contractile machinery of the cell.

Cardiac muscle cells can thus be divided into two categories. The vast majority are specialized to perform mechanical work, i.e. to contract, and these are usually referred to simply as 'myocytes'. These cells do not contract, however, unless stimulated electrically. A minority of the muscle cells are specialized for the task of initiating and conducting an electrical impulse in order to excite the myocytes. Such cells form a specialized *cardiac electrical system*, consisting of a stimulus initiator (the pacemaker or sino-atrial node), a delaying device (atrioventricular node), conduction bundles and a fast distributing network of Purkinje fibres in the ventricles. The task of the electrical system is to initiate and coordinate the heart beat. This chapter describes the structure and function of the contractile myocytes, while Chapter 4 describes the pacemaker and conduction system.

3.1 Ultrastructure of myocyte

Branching cells and their junctions

The human myocyte (the contractile, working cell) is typically 10–20 μm in diameter and 50–100 μm long, with a single central nucleus. The cell is branched and is attached to adjacent cells in an end-to-end fashion (Figure 3.1). The end-to-end junction, or intercalated disc, has a characteristic stepped profile in cross-section, and it contains two kinds of smaller, specialized junctions, namely desmosomes and gap junctions. *Desmosomes* hold the adjacent cells together,

probably by means of a proteoglycan glue located in the 25 nm wide space between the cell membranes. The *gap junction*, or nexus, is a region of very close apposition of the adjacent cell membranes and is thought to be an electrically-conductive region through which ionic currents can pass from one cell to another. The gap (2–4 nm) is spanned by protein particles called connexons which have a central channel running through them, i.e. they form molecular tubes. Ions can pass through these tiny channels, allowing transmission of impulses from cell to cell. As a result of these electrical connections the myocardium acts as an electrically

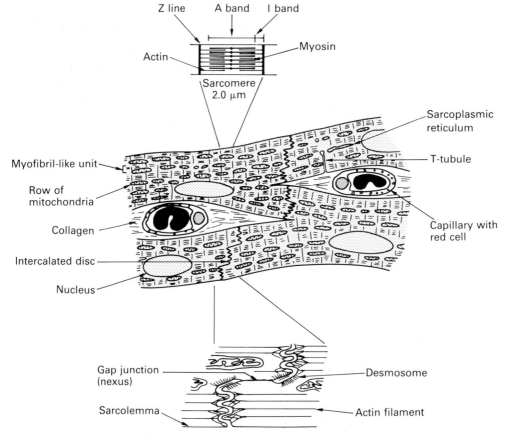

Figure 3.1 Section of myocardium parallel to fibre axis, based on electron microscopic studies. The width of the sarcomere (2 μm) and red cell (7 μm) indicate the scale. The enlargement of part of the intercalated disc at the bottom shows a gap junction or nexus along the horizontal step (interplicate segment) and two desmosomes

continuous sheet, and this enables excitation to reach every cell. Gap junctions are progressively uncoupled in ischaemic disease (inadequate oxygen delivery by blood), and this is thought to contribute to poor conduction in ischaemic myocardium.

The myofibril and the sarcomere

The myocyte is packed with long contractile bundles whose diameter is around 1 μm. They are called myofibril-like units (because of their resemblance to the myofibrils of skeletal muscle) or myofibrils for brevity. Each myofibril is composed of smaller units called sarcomeres, joined end to end. Sarcomeres are aligned across the cell, giving the myocyte its characteristic striated appearance under the microscope. The sarcomere is the basic contractile unit and is defined as the material between two Z lines: a Z line is a thin dark-staining partition composed of a protein, α-actinin. The sarcomere is 1.8–2.0 μm long in resting myocytes and contains two kinds of interdigitating filament: a thick filament made of the protein myosin and a thin filament composed chiefly of actin, another protein. The thick filaments, of diameter 11 nm and length 1.6 μm, lie in parallel in a central region of the sarcomere called the A band. (The 'A' stands for 'anisotropic', a reference to its appearance through a polarizing microscope.) The thin filaments, of diameter 6 nm and length 1.05 μm, are rooted in the Z line and form the pale I band (isotropic band); the latter is only approximately 0.25 μm wide because most of the length of the thin filament protrudes into the A band inbetween the myosin rods. In other words, the actin and myosin filaments overlap. As well as actin, the thin filaments contain the proteins troponin and tropomyosin. The cell also contains non-contractile cytoskeletal filaments (connectin or titin), which contribute to its stiffness.

Transverse tubular system

The surface membrane, or sarcolemma, is invaginated opposite the Z line into a series of fine transverse tubules (T tubules) which run into the cell interior (Figure 3.2). The T-tubules transmit the electrical stimulus rapidly into the interior of the cell and thus help to activate the numerous myofibrils almost simultaneously. This system is well developed in ventricular myocytes but is scanty in atrial and Purkinje cells. The T-tubules are lined by membrane throughout, so the extracellular fluid is never in direct contact with intracellular fluid.

Sarcoplasmic reticulum

Within the cell there is a second, quite separate system of tubular structures called

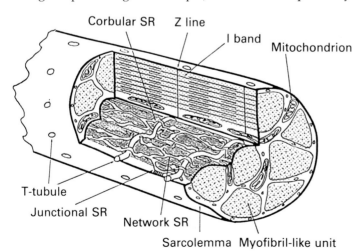

Figure 3.2 Three-dimensional reconstruction of the transverse tubular system (T tubules) and sarcoplasmic reticulum (SR). The latter forms about 5% of the cell volume. For subdivisions of SR, see text

the sarcoplasmic reticulum (SR). This is developed from endoplasmic reticulum and is of major importance because it contains a store of Ca^{2+} ions. This store is released into the cytoplasm (sarcoplasm) following electrical excitation, and activates the contractile machinery there. The SR consists of a closed set of anastomosing tubules coursing over the myofibrils. Electron micrographs show that it can be subdivided into several distinctive regions, each possessing, probably, separate functions. *Network SR* courses over the myofibrils and is 20–60 nm in diameter. *Junctional SR* lies very close to the sarcolemma (cell surface) or a T tubule; it appears to be connected to these by dense strands ('feet') and is very electron dense. *Corbular SR* comprises sac-like expansions of diameter 50–100 nm along the network SR in the I band. These sacs are very electron dense, but are not apposed to the sarcolemma or T tubule. Both junctional and corbular SR have a high content of Ca^{2+} and calcium-storage protein (calsequestrin), so they are thought to be potential sites of Ca^{2+} release. Network SR, by contrast, possesses abundant Ca^{2+}-ATPase pumps, plus their regulator protein, phospholamban (which junctional SR lacks). Network SR is therefore thought to be responsible for Ca^{2+} re-uptake after release.

As indicated above, when the myocyte is excited electrically, calcium ions are released from the SR and activate the contractile machinery. This brings us to the question of how contraction is produced.

3.2 Mechanism of contraction

Contraction of the myocyte is caused by shortening of its sarcomeres. Direct inspection shows that the I bands shorten, but the A band does not. This is one of the key observations indicating that contraction is caused by the thin filaments of the I band sliding into the spaces between the thick filaments of the A band – the *sliding filament mechanism*. The filaments are propelled past

each other by the repeated making and breaking of crossbridges between the thin and thick filaments. These crossbridges are actually the heads of myosin molecules, which protrude from the side of the thick filament as illustrated in Figure 3.3. At rest the actin sites, with which the myosin heads would react, are blocked by tropomyosin. Contraction is initiated by a sudden rise in the concentration of free intracellular calcium ions. Some of these ions bind to troponin C, a component of the troponin complex. This alters the position of the adjacent tropomyosin molecule and thereby exposes a specific myosin-binding site on the actin chain, allowing the myosin head to bind to the actin. Force and movement is produced by a subsequent change in the angle of this crossbridge (i.e. the attached myosin head), after which the head disengages and the process repeats itself at a new actin site. This process occurs at numerous similar sites along the filament, and in this way the thick filament 'rows' itself into the space between the thin filaments. The most important point about the whole process from the physiological point of view is that the number of crossbridges formed, and therefore the force of the contraction, depends directly on the concentration of free calcium ions within the myocyte.

Energy supply and oxygen

The energy for crossbridge cycling is provided by adenosine triphosphate (ATP), which is broken down during the process into inorganic phosphate and adenosine diphosphate (ADP) by an ATPase site on the myosin head. In order to maintain an adequate supply of ATP, the myocyte possesses an exceptionally high density of mitochondria, which lie in rows between the myofibrils and form 30–35% of the cell volume. ATP is manufactured in mitochondria by oxidative phosphorylation, for which oxygen is obligatory, and this is why cardiac performance is directly dependent on coronary blood flow. Myocyte Po_2 is in the range 5–20 mmHg, so there is a large oxygen

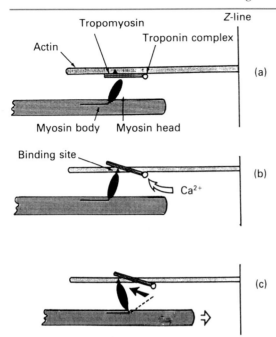

Figure 3.3 Diagram of the contractile proteins at three stages during the crossbridge cycle. (a) Resting state. The actin binding site is blocked by tropomyosin and the myosin heads are disengaged. (b) Calcium ions bind to troponin C of the troponin complex, displacing the tropomyosin. The myosin head cross-links to the exposed actin binding site. (c) The angle of the myosin head changes, 'rowing' the thick filament towards the Z line. The head then disengages and the cycle repeats at a new actin site. Only one myosin molecule is shown here but the thick filament contains approximately 400. Similarly, there are many binding site along the actin filament

gradient from blood to cell to drive transport. The sarcoplasm itself contains the protein myoglobin, which functions as a small store of oxygen; it is about 50% saturated at a P_{O_2} of 5 mmHg. Myoglobin also facilitates the diffusional transport of O_2 throughout the sarcoplasm. It is present at a concentration of about 3.4 g/l.

The release of calcium from the SR store, which activates the contractile machinery, is triggered by the cell's action potential, so we must consider next the nature of the electrical potential in a myocyte.

3.3 Resting membrane potential

The potential difference between the interior and exterior of a myocyte can be measured by driving a fine microelectrode into the cell (a microelectrode is simply a piece of glass tubing which has been heated, drawn out and filled with a conducting solution). The intracellular electrode is connected to an amplifier and a voltmeter, and the other lead of the voltmeter is connected to an electrode outside the cells. The intracellular potential of the resting myocyte is then found to be −60 mV to −90 mV (i.e. 60–90 mV lower than the extracellular potential). In atrial and ventricular cells this 'resting membrane potential' is stable, until external excitation is applied (Figure 3.4a), but in sino-atrial (SA) node cells and many conduction fibres it is unstable, drifting towards zero with time; this more complex situation is considered in Chapter 4.

Electrical potentials arise from differences in ion concentration across the cell membrane, coupled with the presence of selective, ion-conducting channels spanning the membrane. An increasing variety of ion channels has been recognized in recent years following the introduction of a method called '*patch clamping*', in which a segment of cell membrane (the patch) is 'glued' across the end of a micropipette, allowing the activity of just the few channels in the attached patch to be investigated. By using ion substitution, channel blockers and voltage–current–time plots, a large number of specific channels have now been identified. The following description concentrates on the three main classes of channel, K^+-, Na^+- and Ca^{2+}-conducting channels, and touches only briefly on subtypes when necessary.

Potassium: generator of the resting membrane potential

The resting potential is due primarily to two factors: the high concentration of potassium ions in the intracellular fluid and the high

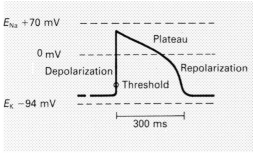

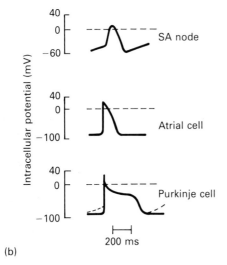

(b)

Table 3.1 Concentration of ions in myocardial cells

	Intracellular (mM)	Extracellular (mM)	Nernst equilibrium potential (mV)
K$^+$	140	4	−94
Na$^+$	10	140	+70
Ca^{2+}	0.0001*	1.2†	+124
Cl$^-$	30	120	−37
pH	7.0–7.1	7.4	–

*Value at rest
†The total Ca^{2+} concentration in plasma is about double this, but only 1.2 mM is in the ionic form

Figure 3.4 Intracellular potential of a ventricular work cell (a) measured by a glass microelectrode. The stable baseline potential of −80 mV is the resting membrane potential. The depolarization stage of the action potential is so rapid (500 V/s) that it appears vertical. The theoretical potassium equilibrium potential E_K and sodium equilibrium potential E_{Na} are marked. (b) Three records to illustrate the different shapes of action potential at other sites. Note the unstable resting potential in the pacemaker cell (SA node). Some Purkinje fibres also have unstable resting potentials (dotted line). In *man*, the atrial action potential has a distinct spike and plateau (cf. triangular in other species) and resembles the action potential labelled 'Purkinje' here

permeability of the cell membrane to potassium ions compared with other ions. The latter property is due to the fact that, at resting membrane potential, many K$^+$ chan-

nels are open, whereas Na$^+$ and Ca^{2+} channels are mostly closed. The intracellular K$^+$ concentration is about 35 times higher than the extracellular K$^+$ concentration (Table 3.1), so there is a continuous tendency for K$^+$ to diffuse out of the cell down its concentration gradient, via open K$^+$ channels. However, the negative intracellular ions, mainly organic phosphates and charged proteins, cannot accompany the K$^+$ ions because the cell membrane is impermeable to them (Figure 3.5). The outward diffusion of a small number of potassium ions therefore creates a very slight separation of charge and leaves the cell interior negative with respect to the exterior. Because the electrical charge on a single ion is very large indeed (see Faraday's constant, Appendix II), just one excess negative ion per 10^{15} ion pairs is sufficient to produce the resting potential. A numerical imbalance of this size is of course far too tiny to be detected by chemical methods.

Potassium equilibrium potential

If the negative intracellular potential were big enough, the electrical attraction of the cell interior for the positive potassium ions could fully offset the outward diffusion tendency of the ions, creating a dynamic equilibrium in which there would be no further net movement of K$^+$ out of the cell. The

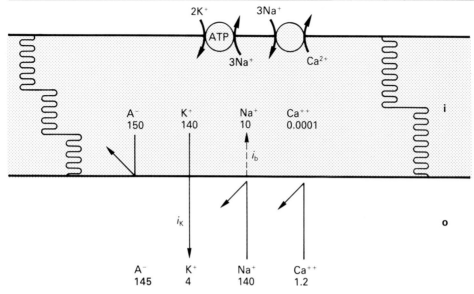

Figure 3.5 Chemical gradients and currents across the resting membrane (i, inside. o, outside). A⁻ inside cell refers to impermeant intracellular anions. Straight arrows show concentration gradients for ions permeating the sarcolemma. Reflected arrows indicate ions unable to penetrate the resting membrane. i_b is the inward background current and i_K the outward background current. Cell membrane pumps are shown at the top.

electrical potential at which this would happen is called the potassium equilibrium potential. This *electrical potential* is, by definition, equal in magnitude to the outward-driving effect of the concentration gradient, or *chemical potential* as it is called. The chemical potential depends on the ion concentration outside the cell (C_o) relative to that inside (C_i). The exact relation between equilibrium potential of ionic species X (E_x) and the ionic concentration ratio is given by the *Nernst equation*, namely:

$$E_x = \frac{RT}{zF} . \log_e(C_o/C_i) \qquad (3.1)$$

where z is the ionic valency, R is the gas constant (Appendix II), T is absolute temperature and F is Faraday's constant. For a monovalent ion at body temperature (310 K), and switching to 'ordinary' logarithms, this works out in millivolts as $61 \times \log(C_o/C_i)$. Since the potassium ratio is 1:35, the potassium equilibrium potential works out to be −94 mV. Experimentally, it is found that the myocyte's resting potential is indeed close to

the potassium equilibrium potential (but never quite equal to it) – see Figure 3.6. It is also found that when the extracellular potassium concentration is increased, as can happen in certain medical conditions, the myocyte resting potential declines (grows less negative) in proportion to the logarithm of the extracellular potassium concentration, as predicted by the Nernst equation (Figure 3.6).

Non-equilibrium due to background currents

Figure 3.6 shows that the resting membrane potential always falls a little short of the potassium equilibrium potential. This is due to a small inward current of positively charged ions, mainly sodium ions, which is known as the 'inward background current' (i_b). Although the permeability of the resting membrane to sodium is only 1/10th to 1/100th of its permeability to potassium, both the electrical gradient and the chemical gradient for Na⁺ are directed into the cell (see Table 3.1), and their sum, the 'electrochemical gradient', drives

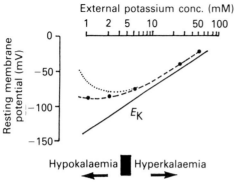

Figure 3.6 Dependence of resting membrane potential on extracellular K^+ concentration in cat papillary muscle (data points joined by dashed line) and Purkinje fibres (dotted line). Solid line is Nernst equilibrium potential for K^+, E_K. Membrane potential is smaller than E_K due to inward background current (i_b). [In hypokalaemia, the deviation from E_K increases, especially in Purkinje fibres. This is because potassium conductance declines, reducing outward current i_{K1} (see Table 4.2, Chapter 4) and making i_b relatively more important. Also, the outward current contributed by the $3Na^+-2K^+$ pump is reduced at very low K^+.] After Page, E. (1962) *Circulation* **26**, 582–595, and Noble, D. (1979), see Further Reading.

a small inward current of Na^+ into the cell (see Figure 3.5). As a result, the resting membrane potential is 10–20 mV more positive than the potassium equilibrium potential. Moreover, because the resting potential is not quite negative enough to fully counteract the outward diffusion of K^+ ions, there is a continuous trickle of K^+ out of the cell, producing an 'outward background current' of potassium ions (i_K). The net outward current (i_K) plus a smaller outward current due to the Na^+-K^+ pump (see later) is equal to the inward current I_b, so the resting membrane potential is stable despite the continuous slow exchange of potassium for sodium.

Ohm's law and the importance of relative ionic permeabilities

The size of the background currents at a given membrane potential can be expressed in terms of Ohm's law. This states that current (i) is proportional to potential difference (ΔV) and electrical conductance (g – the reciprocal of resistance): $i = g. \Delta V$. In the case of a cell membrane, conductance to a given ion at a given membrane potential is proportional to ionic permeability and concentration (see Appendix II for the full relation). For potassium ions the potential difference driving the current is the difference between the resting membrane potential V_m and the potassium equilibrium potential E_K, so the background potassium current i_K is, by Ohm's law:

$$i_K = g_K(V_m - E_K) \tag{3.2}$$

where g_K is the membrane's potassium conductance at membrane potential V_m. Similarly, the inward background current of sodium ions, i_b, is by Ohm's law:

$$i_b = g_{Na}(V_m - E_{Na}) \tag{3.3}$$

where E_{Na} is the sodium equilibrium potential ($+70\,mV$). If the resting potential is stable, the inward and outward currents must be equal, so equations (3.2) and (3.3) are equal (neglecting other minor currents). Combining them we get an approximate expression for the resting potential:

$$V_m = \frac{E_K + E_{Na} \cdot g_{Na}/g_K)}{(1 + g_{Na}/g_K)} \tag{3.4}$$

This is a simplified form of the more complex Goldman constant field equation (which takes account of chloride and calcium currents too), but it is ideal for our purpose here, which is to highlight the importance of the *ratio of sodium permeability to potassium permeability* in setting the membrane potential. The expression tells us that the resting potential is a potassium equilibrium potential ($-94\,mV$) modified by a fraction of the sodium equilibrium potential ($+70\,mV$). The fraction in question is one-tenth if the ratio of g_{Na} to g_K is 1:10. This simplified constant field equation therefore predicts that the resting potential should be $(-94 + 7)/1.1$, or $-79\,mV$, and this is close to the potential in many work cells.

A word of caution is necessary here. Ohm's law can only be applied to membrane currents in a rather restricted way. This is because the conductance g of membrane ion channels is *not* usually independent of the potential V_m, but changes with it. Consequently, the current–voltage relation is not usually linear: ohmic expressions like (3.2) and (3.3) are useful for telling us the current flowing at a given conductance and potential, but do not tell us the shape of the current–voltage relation. The conductance of the potassium channels responsible for resting potential decreases as the membrane is depolarized (see Figure 3.8), making it increasingly difficult for this outward K^+ current to flow during depolarization – a useful 'economy' measure that conserves intracellular K^+. This phenomenon is called *inward rectification*, and the potassium channels involved (inward rectifying K^+ channels) are just one of many varieties of K^+ channel (see later).

Function of sarcolemmal ion pumps

As explained above, the cell is in effect a chemical battery, and the chemical that powers the battery, potassium, is slowly but continuously leaking out of the cell. Unchecked, the concentrations of both potassium and sodium would eventually equilibrate across the cell membrane, leaving the battery flat. This is prevented, however, by active pumps in the sarcolemmal membrane, whose function is to preserve the chemical composition of the interior. A *sodium–potassium pump* simultaneously transports sodium ions out of the cell and potassium ions into the cell (see Figure 3.5). Moreover, the pump rate is enhanced by a rise in intracellular Na^+ or rise in extracellular K^+ concentration. The exchange of Na^+ for K^+ is not 1 for 1; three sodium ions are pumped out for every two potassium ions pumped in, and the pump is therefore electrogenic. It must be stressed, however, that this effect makes only a minor contribution to the membrane potential. This can be proved by blocking the $3Na^+$–$2K^+$ pump by ouabain. This causes only a small immediate decrease in membrane potential, because the chief factor generating the resting potential is the potassium concentration gradient, not the ion pump. Pumping is an active process and consumes metabolic energy in the form of ATP. The pump is itself an ATPase.

The sarcolemmal membrane also possesses transport proteins which can expel intracellular calcium ions that have entered the cell during the action potential (see below). The predominant kind of calcium transporter is a *sodium–calcium exchanger*, in which the passage of 3 extracellular sodium ions into the cell causes the expulsion of 1 intracellular Ca^{2+} ion. The entry of the excess Na^+ ion contributes to the inward current during the plateau of the action potential (see below). The $3Na^+$–Ca^{2+} exchange is not powered directly by ATP but is driven by the 'downhill' sodium concentration gradient, rather as a water-wheel is turned by a water gradient. It therefore depends indirectly on the Na^+–K^+ pump, since it is the Na^+–K^+ pump that sets up the sodium gradient. This point is important for understanding the effects of digoxin (Section 3.5). The sodium-driven calcium exchange accounts for about three-quarters of the calcium expulsion. In addition, the membrane possesses a few calcium pumps powered directly by ATP, accounting for about a quarter of the calcium expulsion at rest. Ca^{2+}–ATPase pumps are abundant in network SR. Together the calcium transporters maintain the intracellular Ca^{2+} at an extremely low concentration in resting myocytes, namely 10^{-7}M.

3.4 Action potential and ionic currents in myocytes

The action potential, which triggers contraction, is an abrupt reversal of the membrane potential to a positive value (see Figure 3.4). In a ventricular or atrial myocyte, it is normally initiated by the action potential of an adjacent cell, which draws charge passively from the resting membrane and thereby reduces its potential. (The process of passive discharge is explained later, in Chapter 4 and Figure 4.3. The very different action potential of sino-atrial node cells is also covered in Chapter 4.) When the potential reaches a threshold value between $-70\,mV$ and $-60\,mV$, the membrane's ionic permeability suddenly changes; the cell very rapidly depolarizes (loses its negative charge) and overshoots to a positive potential of $+20\,mV$ to $+30\,mV$. In human atrial myocytes and Purkinje fibres, both of which have a spike-and-dome shaped action potential, the membrane then immediately begins to repolarize. When it reaches zero to $-20\,mV$, however, it becomes relatively stable for a long period (200–400 ms). This stage is called the 'plateau', and it causes the cardiac action potential to last far longer than a nerve or skeletal muscle action potential (1–4 ms). In the ventricular myocyte of many species the action potential is more rectangular in shape; the plateau follows immediately after depolarization (i.e. at a positive potential), without much intervening partial repolarization (Figure 3.4). Finally the membrane repolarizes, though at only 1/1000th of the rate of depolarization, to regain its resting potential.

Action potentials differ somewhat in form between the various cardiac cells (see Figure 3.4). Atrial potentials last 150 ms and are triangular in many non-human species. Ventricular potentials are longer (400 ms) and more rectangular owing to a more distinct plateau at $+30\,mV$ to $0\,mV$; and Purkinje cells have the longest potentials, up to 450 ms, with a distinct initial spike followed by a long plateau at approximately $-20\,mV$.

Rapid depolarization and sodium ions

The action potential is generated by a sequence of changes in sarcolemmal permeability to Na^+, Ca^{2+} and K^+, which allows ionic currents to flow passively down their electrochemical gradients. The depolarization spike of the myocyte is caused by an extremely rapid increase in permeability to sodium ions. At the threshold potential, voltage-sensitive sodium channels (fast channels) open very quickly and increase the sodium conductance of the sarcolemma around 100 times (Figures 3.7 and 3.8). This allows a rapid flux of sodium ions into the myoctye (the first inward current, i_{Na}) and drives the potential towards the sodium equilibrium potential (E_{Na}, $+70\,mV$, see Table 3.1). The membrane potential does not quite reach E_{Na} because an outward potassium current is still flowing. The situation at the *overshoot* (peak positive potential) is in effect a mirror image of the resting situation, and for a sodium:potassium conductance ratio of 10:1 an overshoot potential of $+55\,mV$ is predicted by equation 3.4.

The overshoot is brief because the fast channels are self-inactivating. Their conductance is controlled by two different 'gates', which are probably charged intramembranous particles. The 'm' or activating gate opens quickly at threshold potential, producing the sudden rise in sodium permeability (Figure 3.9). The 'h' or inactivation gate begins to close at the same time as the m gate opens, but it moves less quickly; it inactivates the channel automatically after a few milliseconds. The membrane potential then begins to fall again, owing to an outward current of K^+ ions.

Plateau and calcium ions

Events up to this point are very similar to those in a nerve. Next, however, the myocyte displays its unique feature, the plateau. This is produced by a small but sustained inward current of positive ions, called the second inward current (i_{SI}). This lasts 200–400 ms and prevents the myocyte from repolarizing rapidly like a nerve. The current consists mainly of calcium ions flowing into the cell down their electrochemical gradient and is now often called i_{Ca} rather than i_{SI}. The calcium current is caused by a rise in sarcolemmal permeability to calcium (see Figure 3.8) which is due to the opening of channels selectively

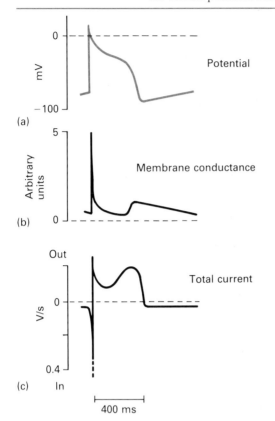

(a)

(b)

(c)

400 ms

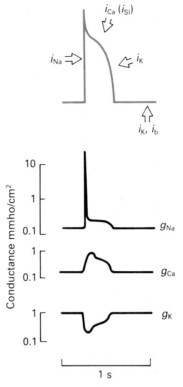

1 s

Figure 3.7 Changes in net electrical conductance of the myocyte cell membrane (b) during an action potential (a). This is a Purkinje cell with an unstable resting membrane potential. (c) Net electrical current, with inward current directed downwards and going off the scale during peak depolarization. (Weidmann's seminal observation of 1956, redrawn from Noble, D. (1979), see Further Reading, by permission)

Figure 3.8 Membrance conductance to individual cations during an action potential in a stable myocyte. The total membrane conductance shown in Figure 3.7(b) can be dissected into three main components, g_{Na}, g_{Ca} and g_K. The ionic currents which result from these conductances are marked on the action potential at the top. The plateau current, i_{SI}, is carried partly by calcium ions due to the rise in g_{Ca}, and partly by sodium ions due to the sodium–calcium exchange pump (see text). Using the voltage-clamp technique, extracellular ion substitution and blocking agents, it has been found that both g_{Ca} and g_K can be further subdivided. (Based on Noble, D. (1979) and (1984), see Further Reading, by permission)

permeable to calcium ions. These are voltage-operated channels (VOCs) which begin to activate slowly (relative to the fast Na^+ channels) when the cell depolarizes beyond $-35\,mV$ (i.e. during rapid depolarization). They stay open for a longer period than the fast Na^+ channels. The total conductance of the slow channels is much less than that of the fast sodium channels, and the inward Ca^{2+} current is therefore quite small, but it is sufficient, almost, to counterbalance the ever-present outward K^+ current. In this way i_{Ca} almost

stabilizes the potential at $0\,mV$ to $-20\,mV$. The net outward K^+ current is itself reduced during much of the plateau owing to a fall in the membrane permeability to potassium (see Figure 3.8). The fall in K^+ permeability can be viewed as an economy measure, minimizing the number of potassium and calcium ions exchanged during the long plateau and so

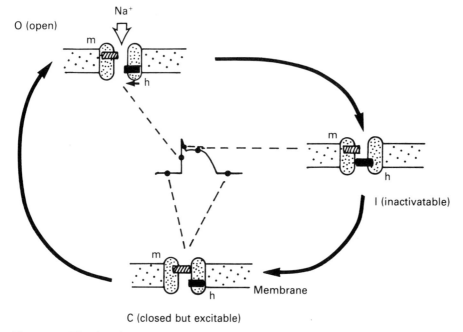

Figure 3.9 The closed–open–inactivated cycle of the fast Na$^+$ channel; sequence of positions of the m and h gates

reducing the eventual energy cost of the action potential.

The existence of the two distinct inward currents, i_{Na} and i_{Ca}, has been proved by the use of tetrodotoxin, which blocks only the fast, sodium channels. This is illustrated in Figure 3.10. Figure 3.10 also illustrates an important action of *adrenaline*, namely, it increases the size of the calcium current. This action contributes to the increase in contractile force produced by adrenaline. Conversely, drugs that block calcium channels, such as verapamil or nifedipine, attenuate the plateau and weaken the force of contraction.

The inward current during the late part of the plateau, when the calcium channels are beginning to inactivate, is due partly to sodium ions passing in through the sodium–calcium exchanger (i_{Na-Ca}). The exchanger's activity ($3Na^+$ transferred inwards for 1 cytoplasmic Ca^{2+} outwards) is high during the plateau, due to the rise in cytoplasmic Ca^{2+} (see 'Sodium–calcium exchanger', Appendix II). One obser-

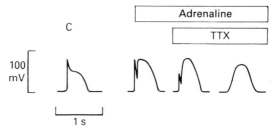

Figure 3.10 Effect of adrenaline (5.5 µM) and tetrodotoxin (TTX, 3 µM) on the action potential of calf Purkinje fibre. The control recording (C) shows a normal Purkinje action potential. Adrenaline enhances the plateau phase by increasing the inward calcium current. Tetrodotoxin, a poison from the Japanese puffer fish, abolishes the initial spike depolarization because it blocks the fast sodium channels. The remaining action potential is quite like that in the SA node (see Figure 3.4). (After Carmeliet, E. and Vereeke, J. (1969) *Pfluger's Archiv*, **313**, 303–315)

vation supporting this is that removal of sodium from the extracellular fluid shortens the plateau phase.

The long plateau is important for two reasons:

1. The cell is electrically inexcitable, or *'refractory'*, during the long period of depolarization (200–400 ms). Since active contraction lasts only 200–250 ms, contraction is weakening by the time the cell becomes repolarized and re-excitable. Consequently, the mechanical response of the myocardium is normally confined to a single twitch, as shown in Figure 3.11. A fused series of twitches, such as produce a sustained contraction in skeletal muscle, is not possible in myocardium. A sustained myocardial contraction would of course be fatal!
2. The cardiac action potential does more than just initiate contraction: the plateau phase also directly influences the *strength of contraction*, because the influx of calcium ions influences the size of the intracellular calcium store. Large plateau currents, such as those stimulated by adrenaline and noradrenaline (see Figure 3.10), are therefore associated with more forceful contractions.

Repolarization and potassium ions

The potassium conductance increases towards the end of the plateau phase (see Figure 3.8). As the calcium channels inactivate, the outward K^+ current begins to dominate, producing repolarization to resting potential.

When repolarization reaches about −50 mV, many of the fast Na^+ channels are reset from inactive to closed state (see Figure 3.9); that is to say, the inactivation gate reopens, although the activation gate is closed. Consequently the cell is now electrically excitable again. But since only a fraction of the channels have reset at this point, a large stimulus is needed and the resulting action potential is small. The period from −50 mV to full repolarization is therefore called the *relative refractory period*, in contrast to the preceding period of complete inexcitability (*absolute refractory period*); see Figure 3.11.

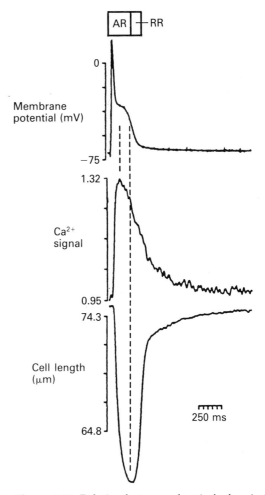

Figure 3.11 Relation between electrical, chemical and mechanical events in a single cardiac myocyte (rat). The myocyte was loaded with a fluorescent dye, indo-1; the fluorescence ratio at two different wavelengths is a measure of free sarcoplasmic Ca^{2+}. Note the time sequence of the peaks – electrical, chemical, mechanical. AR, absolute refractory period (extends to −50 mV repolarization). RR, relative refractory period (−50 mV to full repolarization). Rat myocytes have an unusually low plateau potential. (Records from Spurgeon *et al.* (1990) *American Journal of Physiology*, **258**, H574–H586)

The action potential is much shortened when the cell is hypoxic, as for example in *ischaemic heart disease*. This is because a special subtype of potassium channel, the

K_{ATP} channel, is abundant in cardiac myocytes. At normal ATP levels (about 5 mM) the open probability of these channels is low, but the open probability is much increased by a fall in ATP coupled with a rise in ADP and H^+ concentration, as in hypoxia. The resulting increase in K^+ conductance brings about early repolarization, leading to a short plateau and contributing to a weak beat. The effect of ischaemia is considered further in Section 7.8.

Quantity of ions exchanged per action potential

It must be stressed that all the ionic currents are small and the change in intracellular ion concentration resulting from an action potential is tiny. Students often assume, wrongly, that the 'rush' of sodium into the cell must raise intracellular Na^+ very substantially – but this is to mistake speed for quantity. In reality only about 40 million sodium ions enter a single myocyte during depolarization, and as the cell contains around 200 000 million sodium ions, the intracellular concentration increases by only 0.02%. For intracellular potassium, the change is only 0.001% (see Appendix II,

'Ion exchange'). The Na^+–K^+ and Na^+–Ca^{2+} transporters are therefore able to restore the chemical composition of the sarcoplasm with only a modest expenditure of metabolic energy. The ionic currents of the cardiac myocyte are summarized in Table 3.2. Ion channel properties are summarized in Table 4.2.

3.5 Excitation–contraction coupling and the calcium cycle

The link between electrical excitation and muscle contraction is provided by calcium ions. The arrival of an action potential causes the sarcoplasmic concentration of calcium ions to rise sharply, from 0.1 μM to around 2 μM in 10 ms or so. Some of the calcium then binds to troponin C to activate the contractile proteins (see Figure 3.3). The correlation between free intracellular calcium ions and contraction has been elegantly demonstrated by introducing a calcium-sensitive fluorescent dye into the myocyte (see Figure 3.11). The fluorescent signal, which depends on

Table 3.2 Ionic currents in a myocardial work cell

Current	Ion	Direction[*]	Function	Blocker
i_{Na}	Na^+	Inward	Rapid depolarization	Tetrodotoxin
i_{Ca} (i_{SI})	Ca^{2+}	Inward	1. Plateau maintenance 2. Excitation–contraction coupling	Mn^{2+} Verapamil Nifedipine
$i_{Na–Ca}$	$3Na^+$ in $1Ca^2$ out	Net inward current (Na–Ca exchanger)	Sustains late plateau and removes intracellular Ca^{2+}	–
i_K	K^+	Outward	1. Repolarization 2. Resting membrane potential	Ba^{2+} Tetraethyl ammonium 4-aminopyridine
i_b	Na^+ (mostly)	Inward	Inward background current keeping resting membrane potential below E_K	–

*'Inward' means from the extracellular to the intracellular compartment.

free Ca^{2+} in the cytoplasm, begins to rise immediately after depolarization, and is itself quickly followed by contraction.

To find the critical calcium concentration for contraction, Fabiato and Fabiato performed a classic experiment in 1975 which involved stripping the sarcolemma from the myocyte so that the intracellular calcium concentration would equilibrate with that in the bathing fluid. The 'skinned' cell was found to relax when the bathing fluid contained $0.1\,\mu M$ Ca^{2+}, contract slightly at $1\,\mu M$ Ca^{2+} and contract with maximum force above approximately $10\,\mu M$ Ca^{2+} (see Figure 7.4, Chapter 7). In the intact cell, the level of free calcium ions during excitation is in the range 1–$10\,\mu M$, and a typical concentration of, say $2\,\mu M$, produces only *partial* activation of the contractile proteins, i.e. it activates only a fraction of the potential crossbridges. If the free cytosolic calcium ion concentration is increased (e.g. by adrenaline), more cross-bridges are activated and contractile force increases.

How does the action potential produce a 20-fold rise in sarcoplasmic free Ca^{2+} concentration? As the right side of Figure 3.12 shows, the calcium ions arrive from at least two sources: the store of bound calcium in sarcoplasmic reticulum (the major source) and the plateau current, i_{Ca}.

Sarcoplasmic reticulum (SR): an internal source of calcium

The corbular and junctional SR contain a store of calcium ions linked to the protein calsequestrin. The SR membrane contains calcium-release channels, but these are in the closed state when the surrounding cytoplasmic Ca^{2+} concentration is low, i.e. during diastole. As the action potential travels into the cell along the T-tubule, the initial part of the plateau current, i_{Ca}, causes a

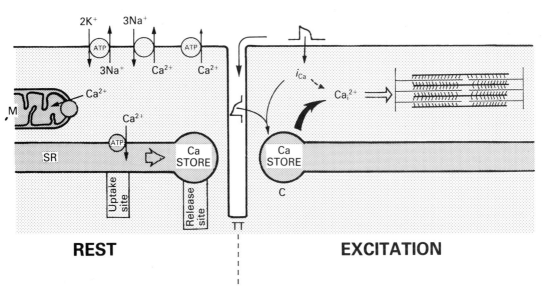

Figure 3.12 Sketch of the calcium cycle. Right side: Excitation. Transverse tubule (TT). Corbular and junctional sarcoplasmic reticulum (C) contain Ca^{2+}–calsequestrin. The plateau current (i_{Ca}) supplies additional calcium, as well as producing calcium-induced calcium release. Left side: Restoration of calcium levels. Calcium concentration is returned to baseline by sarcolemmal sodium–calcium exchange and by pumps in the network sarcoplasmic reticulum (SR). The mitochondrial store (M) may be important in the long-term buffering of the intracellular calcium

small rise in free intracellular Ca^{2+} concentration, within about 2 ms. This activates the SR calcium-release channels, leading to the release of a large quantity of stored calcium into the cytoplasm – a process known as *calcium-induced calcium release*. The escaping SR Ca^{2+} is exchanged for cytoplasmic K^+ and Mg^{2+}. The discharging of the SR store raises cytoplasmic Ca^{2+} concentration to a high level (e.g. 2 μM) within about 10 ms. The ions diffuse the micrometre or so into the sarcomere very rapidly, and the cell begins to develop tension (see Figures 3.11 and 3.12).

Stimulated by the raised sarcoplasmic calcium level, the SR then actively pumps calcium ions back into its interior, as shown on the left side of Figure 3.12. In combination with the sarcolemmal Na^+-Ca^{2+} exchanger, this reduces the calcium concentration in the sarcoplasm and terminates the contraction. About 80–90% of the released Ca^{2+} is taken back into the SR and 10–20% is expelled by the sarcolemmal transporters.

The SR uptake sites, namely the $Ca^{2+}-$ ATPase pumps, are located in the network part of the SR. The rate of uptake appears to be regulated by a protein, phospholamban, and the activity of phospholamban is regulated by adrenaline and noradrenaline, acting via an internal second messenger (Section 4.4). Uptake is followed by restocking of the calsequestrin stores in the corbular and junctional SR (*restitution*). Full restoration of the SR to its presystolic state takes a finite amount of time. As a result, if the interval between beats is suddenly reduced, as happens when an ectopic extrasystole occurs (Sections 5.8 and 7.8), the early beat is a weak one.

Plateau current: an external source of calcium

During the plateau the influx of extracellular calcium ions boosts the intracellular calcium content. The importance of extracellular calcium ions was discovered by Sidney Ringer in 1883, and as with many seminal discoveries chance played a part. It was the job of Ringer's assistant to prepare solutions of (apparently) sodium and potassium chlor-ide, and these maintained the beating of an isolated frog heart for many hours. When the 'same' solution was prepared in later experiments, however, using distilled water, the hearts quickly weakened and failed. Ringer discovered that, in the earlier work, his assistant had been using the local London tap water – which drains from limestone and chalk hills and has a considerable Ca^{2+} content.

Thus, extracellular calcium enhances the contractile force of the heart. This must be due to its influx during the plateau, because the force of myocardial contraction correlates with the size of this current; if, for example, the calcium current is increased by adrenaline, contractile force increases too. The way the calcium current influences contraction is, however, less direct than might be supposed, for the quantity of calcium entering the myocyte during a single action potential is only enough to raise the intracellular calcium concentration a little. The effect of the calcium current on contraction arises in two indirect ways. First, the arrival of the extracellular calcium ions in the sarcoplasm stimulates the release of far more calcium from the internal store ('calcium-induced calcium release'). It is estimated that about 80–90% of the systolic increase in cytoplasmic Ca^{2+} arises from the internal store and only about 10–20% directly from the plateau current (i_{Ca}). Secondly, the influx of extracellular calcium ions increases the amount of intracellular calcium available for re-uptake into the store, so, over several beats, the size of the calcium store and the strength of contraction can be increased. This focuses our attention on the question of what governs the size of the calcium store.

Size of the internal calcium store

The size of the intracellular store of calcium is important because it affects free Ca^{2+} concentration during systole and therefore contractile force. The size of the store depends on the balance between the influx of extracellular calcium ions during the plateau and their expulsion by the sarcolemmal pumps during diastole. The store, and with it the contractile force, depends therefore on (1) the extracellular Ca^{2+} concentration, (2) the size of the plateau current, which is increased by adrenaline and noradrenaline (see Figure 3.10), and (3) the relative duration of systole (the calcium influx phase) and diastole (the calcium efflux phase). This last point is considered further in Section 7.8.

There are also certain pharmacological agents that act on the SR membrane directly. *Caffeine* in high concentration increases the frequency of opening of the calcium-release channels in the SR and lowers the threshold for calcium-induced calcium release, which can lead to contracture (sustained contraction). At therapeutic levels, however, caffeine's chief action is to inhibit phosphodiesterase. This is an enzyme that normally breaks down the second messenger of β-adrenoceptors, cyclic adenosine monophosphate, cAMP. Caffeine thus elevates cAMP and has similar actions to the β-agonists adrenaline and noradrenaline: it increases contractile force and heart rate. *Ryanodine* by contrast can abolish the ability of SR to release calcium.

Action of digoxin

Digoxin is a cardiac glycoside produced by foxgloves, and it has been used for over two

centuries to treat heart failure because it enhances myocardial contractile force. It achieves this by increasing the level of intracellular calcium, as illustrated in Figure 3.13. Its immediate pharmacological action, however, is to slow down the sarcolemmal Na^+–K^+ pump, by inhibiting its ATPase activity. This produces a rise in intracellular sodium concentration and a fall in the sodium gradient across the cell membrane. Since the Na^+–Ca^{2+} exchanger is itself driven by the sodium gradient (see Figure 3.5), calcium expulsion is slowed and calcium accumulates in the cell.

3.6 Physiological regulation of contractile force

The degree to which the contractile machinery is 'switched on' is not fixed but can be altered by physiological mechanisms. During a quiet heart beat only a fraction of the potential actin–myosin crossbridges are activated, and this fraction can be increased to raise the force of contraction. The two principal mechanisms are (a) the length–tension relation and (b) chemically induced rises in the calcium store leading to higher sarcoplasmic Ca^{2+} concentrations in systole.

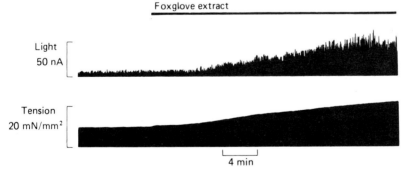

Figure 3.13 In 1785 William Withering reported that a folklore remedy based on an infusion of foxglove leaves (*Digitalis*) was beneficial in the treatment of 'dropsy' (cardiac failure). This experiment, to mark the bicentennial, shows how the extract increases both twitch force and the concentration of free intracellular calcium ions during contraction in ferret papillary muscle. The light emission from aequorin-injected muscle (top trace) is a function of calcium concentration. Aequorin is a protein from luminescent jellyfish and emits blue light in the presence of free Ca^{2+}. (From Allen, D. G., Eisner, D. A., Smith, G. L. and Wray, S. (1985) *Journal of Physiology*, **365**, 55P, by permission)

The most important agents doing this are the sympathetic neurotransmitter, noradrenaline and the circulating hormone adrenaline (the catecholamines).

Length–tension relation Figure 3.14 shows the effect of stretching a cardiac fibre. Increasing the diastolic length results in an immediate increase in the force of subsequent contractions, and this is accomplished without any rise in intracellular Ca^{2+} concentration. If the stretch is maintained, there is then a gradual further increase in force for several minutes, and this delayed increase is

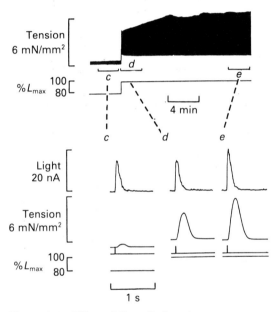

Figure 3.14 Effect of diastolic length on isometric tension developed by isolated papillary muscle from ferret heart. Upper trace shows that stretching the muscle from 80% of optimal length (L_{max}) at c to 100% at d produces an immediate rise in contractile force. This is followed by a slower, additional rise in force (e). Averaged records from periods c, d and e are shown below. The myocytes contained aequorin, which emits light when intracellular-free $[Ca^{2+}]$ rises. This shows that the immediate effect of length on tension (d) does not involve an increase in the systolic Ca^{2+} transient, whereas the delayed rise (e) does. (After Allen, D. G., Nichols, C. G. and Smith, G. L. (1988) *Journal of Physiology*, **406**, 359–370)

associated with a progressive rise in systolic Ca^{2+} level. The immediate rise in force upon stretching is the basis of *Starling's law of the heart*, which is described in Chapter 7. Its molecular mechanisms are covered later (Section 7.2), but briefly it is due partly to a change in overlap of the contractile filaments with stretch and, to a greater degree, to an increase in the sensitivity of the contractile apparatus to Ca^{2+} with stretch. The subsequent time-dependent increase in force and systolic Ca^{2+} level accounts for about 40% of the eventual response. The slow response is not well understood but might be related to stretch-sensitive ion channels in the cell membrane.

Inotropic effect of catecholamines Inotropic means strengthening. Noradrenaline and adrenaline increase the force of cardiac contraction by increasing the size of the sytolic Ca^{2+} transient. This is achieved by increasing the plateau calcium current (see Figure 3.10), leading to accumulation of a bigger store of Ca^{2+} in the sarcoplasmic reticulum. Uptake by the sarcoplasmic reticulum is also stimulated, so the Ca^{2+} transient declines faster, speeding relaxation too and helping preserve the diastolic filling period. Catecholamines also alter the heart rate and this effect, along with the biochemical pathways linking adrenergic receptors to ion channels, is described in Section 4.4.

To summarize, three mechanisms regulate contractile force: (1) the size of the systolic Ca^{2+} transient, which is affected by catecholamines among other things; (2) the affinity of the contractile proteins for Ca^{2+}, which depends on stretch; and (3) the degree of actin–myosin filament overlap, which also depends on stretch.

3.7 Summary

The resting membrane potential of the cardiac myocyte approximates to a K^+ equlibrium potential, modified by a small inward background current of Na^+. Ionic pumps maintain intracellular ionic composition but contribute only a little to the resting membrane potential. Contraction is initiated by an action potential. The initial, very rapid depolarization is due to a rapid inward current of Na^+. This is followed by a second inward current, carried by extracellular Ca^{2+}, which produces a prolonged depolarized plateau (200–400 ms). Contraction begins during this phase and the cell is absolutely refractory. Repolarization follows due to an outward current of K^+ ions.

The entry of relatively small amounts of Ca^{2+} into the cell during the early plateau triggers the release of a larger amount of Ca^{2+} from the sarcoplasmic reticulum (internal store). This raises intracellular free Ca^{2+} to around 2 μM. Some of the Ca^{2+} binds to troponin C on the thin (actin) filaments, leading to exposure of myosin binding sites on the actin. As a result, crossbridges (myosin heads) form between the thick and thin filaments. These 'row' the thick (myosin) filaments along, in between the thin filaments, producing shortening or tension.

The force generated depends on the fraction of the potential crossbridges that are actually activated. This is governed by two basic factors. (1) The longer the sarcomere in diastole, the greater the contractile force (the length–tension relation) – partly because stretch increases the degree of crossbridge activation by a given intracellular Ca^{2+} concentration, and partly because it changes the amount of filament overlap. Thus diastolic distension increases subsequent contractile force. (2) The higher the free intracellular Ca^{2+} during systole (in the range 1–10 μM), the stronger the contraction. Thus factors that raise the intracellular store of Ca^{2+} lead to stronger contractions. For example, adrenaline and noradrenaline increase the size of the plateau current, leading to a rise in internal stored Ca^{2+} and more forceful contractions in subsequent beats.

Further reading

Reviews and chapters

Bean, B. P. (1989) Classes of calcium channel in vertebrate cells. *Annual Reviews in Physiology*, **51**, 367–384

Brady, A. J. (1991) Mechanical properties of isolated cardiac myocytes. *Physiological Reviews*, **71**, 413–442

Coraboef, E. and Escande, E. (1990), Ionic currents in the human myocardium. *News in Physiological Sciences*, **5**, 28–31

Eisner, D. A. (1990) Intracellular sodium in cardiac muscle: effects on contraction. Wellcome Prize Lecture. *Experimental Physiology*, **75**, 437–457

Fabiato, A. (1989) Appraisal of the physiological relevance of two hypotheses for the mechanism of calcium release from the mammalian cardiac sarcoplasmic reticulum: calcium-induced release versus charge-coupled release. *Molecular and Cellular Biochemistry*, **89**, 135–140

Jewell, B. R. (1982) Activation of contraction in cardiac muscle. *Mayo Clinic Proceedings*, **57**, 6–13

Jongsma, H. J. and Gros, D. (1991) The cardiac connection (gap junction). *News in Physiological Sciences*, **6**, 34–40

Langer, G. A. (1992) Calcium and the heart: exchange at the tissue, cell and organelle levels. *FASEB Journal*, **6**, 893–902

Noble, D. (1979) *The Initiation of the Heart Beat*, Clarendon Press, Oxford

Noble, D. (1984) The surprising heart. *Journal of Physiology*, **353**, 1–50

Sommer, J. R. and Johnson, E. A. (1979) Ultrastructure of cardiac muscle. In *Handbook of Physiology, Cardiovascular System*, Vol. 1, *The Heart* (ed. R. M. Berne), American Physiological Society, Bethesda, pp. 113–186

Trautwein, W. and Hescheler, J. (1990) Regulation of cardiac L-type calcium current by phosphorylation and G proteins. *Annual Review of Physiology*, **52**, 257–274

Research papers

Joergensen, A. O. Broderick, R., Somlyo, A. P. and Somlyo, A. V. (1988) Two structurally distinct calcium storage sites in rat sarcoplasmic reticulum: an electron microprobe analysis study. *Circulation Research*, **63**, 1060–1069

O'Neill, S. C. and Eisner, D. A. (1990) A mechanism for the effects of caffeine on Ca^{2+} release during diastole and systole in isolated rat ventricular myocytes. *Journal of Physiology*, **430**, 519–536

Chapter 4
Initiation of heart beat and nervous control

4.1 Structure of pacemaker and conduction system	**4.4 Nervous control of heart rate**
4.2 Electrical activity of pacemaker	**4.5 Effects of some extracellular agents**
4.3 Transmission of excitation	**4.6 Summary**

Overview If a heart is excised from a cold-blooded animal and placed in a beaker containing an appropriate solution, the isolated heart continues to beat for a long period. This simple experiment proves that the heart beat is initiated from inside the heart itself; unlike skeletal muscle, extrinsic nerves are not necessary to initiate contraction. The heart beat is in fact initiated by a special electrical system situated within the walls of the heart, composed of modified muscle cells, not nervous tissue. The cardiac electrical system consists of (1) a group of cells forming the sino-atrial node or 'pacemaker' which discharge spontaneously at regular intervals, and (2) very elongated cells called conduction fibres that transmit the resulting electrical impulse quickly to the ventricular contractile cells. This triggers the ventricular cell's action potential, leading to contraction (Chapter 3). Although the firing of the pacemaker does not require any nervous input, the rate of firing can be changed by nerves innervating the heart, and this brings heart rate under nervous control.

4.1 Structure of pacemaker and conduction system

The sino-atrial node or pacemaker

The mammalian heart beat is initiated by the sino-atrial node (SA node), a strip of modified muscle roughly 20 mm long × 4 mm wide in man, located on the posterior wall of the right atrium close to the superior vena cava (Figure 4.1). The sino-atrial node is so-called because it evolved from the sinus venosus, an antechamber to the right atrium in lower vertebrates. The node is composed of small myocytes with only scanty myofibrils and an electrically unstable cell membrane. As a result of their unstable resting membrane potential, human nodal cells generate an action potential roughly once every second. This excites the adjacent atrial work cells and a wave of depolarization then spreads across the two atria, passing from cell to cell at a rate of approximately 1 m/s and initiating atrial systole.

Atrioventricular node

After passing down the atrial septum the electrical impulse reaches the atrioventricular node (AV node), which is a small mass of cells and connective tissue situated in the lower, posterior region of the atrial septum. The AV node marks the start of the only electrical connection across the annulus fibrosus, which otherwise completely insulates the atria from the ventricles. The impulse is delayed in the node for approximately 0.1 s (at resting heart rates), owing to the complex circuitry of the cells and their small diameter (2–3 μm), which reduces the conduction velocity to only 0.05 m/s. The resulting delay is important because it allows the atria sufficient time to contract before the ventricles are activated.

The main bundle (bundle of His) and its branches

A bundle of fast-conducting muscle fibres, called the bundle of His, next conveys the electrical impulse from the AV node across the annulus fibrosus into the fibrous upper part of the interventricular septum. Here the bundle turns forwards and runs along the crest of the muscular septum (see Figure 4.1), giving off the so-called 'left bundle branch', which really comprises two sets of fibres, one anterior and one posterior. These course down the left side of the septum to supply

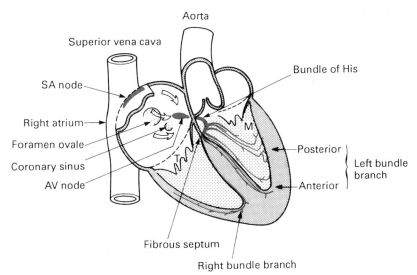

Figure 4.1 Diagram of the cardiac conduction system, with the heart cut obliquely in half. The posterior fibres of the left bundle branch are seen *en face*, running just within the septal wall, then curling round within the left ventricular wall. The broad arrows indicate preferential conduction routes through atrial muscle, called the anterior, middle and posterior internodal paths. Note the proximity of the valves (T, tricuspid; M, mitral) to the bundle of His; valvular lesions can affect the main bundle. The foramen ovale is the remnant of the fetal connection between right and left sides. The coronary sinus is the outlet of the main coronary vein

the left ventricle. The remaining bundle, the right bundle branch, runs down the right side of the septum and supplies the right ventricle. The bundle fibres are wide, fast-conducting myocytes arranged in a regular end-to-end fashion. They terminate in an extensive network of large fibres in the subendocardium which were described by the Hungarian histologist Purkinje in 1845. The Purkinje fibres are the widest cells in the heart and their large diameter (40–80 µm) endows them with a high conduction velocity (3–5 m/s). Their role is to distribute the electrical impulse rapidly to the endocardial work cells. From the endocardium the impulse spreads from work cell to work cell at approximately 0.5–1 m/s and excites the entire ventricular wall. The function of the conduction system is thus to excite the ventricular mass as near simultaneously as possible.

Dominance

There are other potential pacemaker sites in the heart besides the SA node: the SA node normally sets the heart rate simply because its cells have the fastest intrinsic rate of firing and thus 'get there first'. If the SA node is destroyed, cells in AV node or atrium take over as pacemaker because they have the next highest rate of firing. The cells of the bundle of His too are capable of spontaneous firing, albeit at the slower rate of 40 per min: and some Purkinje cells can generate their own rhythm too, though too slowly for an adequate cardiac output (15 beats per min). There is thus a gradient of intrinsic firing rates along the electrical system. The lower cells are normally excited from the SA node, however, before they have time to fire spontaneously, and this is called 'dominance'. The existence of an alternative, albeit slower pacemaker is revealed in a pathological condition called *'heart block'*, in which there is a blockage of the normal electrical connection across the annulus fibrosus. This prevents the SA node from dominating the bundle of His. Cells in the bundle then take over the pacemaker role, driving the ventricles at their own intrinsic rate of about 40

beats/min (see Section 5.8). This is too slow for many daily activities, however, and such patients usually benefit from insertion of an artificial pacemaker.

4.2 Electrical activity of pacemaker

The pacemaker potential

As pointed out earlier, myocytes can be divided into work cells with stable resting membrane potentials and pacemaker cells with unstable membrane potentials. The initial membrane potential of a SA node cell is only about −60 mV, and it decays spontaneously as illustrated in Figure 4.2. This slowly declining potential is called the pacemaker potential (or pre-potential). When the pacemaker potential reaches threshold (approximately −40 mV in nodal cells) it triggers an action potential, which sparks off the next heart beat. The *slope* of the pacemaker potential is very important, because it determines the time taken to reach the threshold value. Thus the slope governs heart rate; the steeper the slope the sooner threshold is reached and the shorter the time between beats. Since the pacemaker slope is steeper in SA node cells than elsewhere, the SA node has the fastest intrinsic firing rate and initiates each heart beat.

The decay of the pacemaker potential with time is caused by two factors. (1) There is a special 'pacemaker current'. This is a current of Na^+ ions flowing into the cell, which progressively depolarizes the cell. This inward current is often labelled i_f (the 'f' is for funny) and is distinct from the inward background current i_b described in Chapter 3. Caesium ions block this current and therefore slow the pacemaker rate. (2) The second mechanism is that membrane permeability to K^+ gradually falls; this is reflected in the fall in total electrical conductance of the membrane illustrated earlier in Figure 3.7. As a result, the depolarizing outward current i_K falls progressively, allowing inward currents (i_f and i_b) to dominate

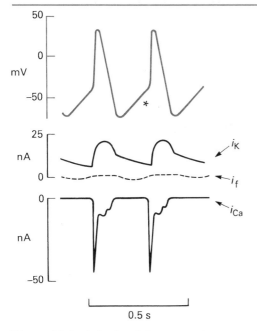

Figure 4.2 Ionic basis of the pacemaker potential and action potential in a sino-atrial cell. The slope of the pacemaker potential (asterisk) determines the interval between heart beats. Inward currents are shown as negative values, outward currents as positive values. The 'funny' inward current i_f produces depolarization of the pacemaker potential, and is carried by sodium ions (and some calcium ions in the late phase). The main inward current labelled i_{Ca} is due to calcium ions. (From Noble, D. (1984), see Further Reading, by permission)

increasingly. These currents are shown in Figure 4.2.

As the potential approaches −40 mV, some low-threshold voltage-operated channels permeable to calcium ions begin to open (T-type calcium channels). As a result, a small inward current of Ca^{2+} ions contributes to the final third of the pacemaker potential, accelerating the rate of depolarization and triggering the action potential.

The nodal action potential

The nodal action potential is slow-rising and small in amplitude, somewhat like the potential of a tetrodotoxin-blocked myocyte (see Figure 3.10). This is because the nodal cell lacks functional fast sodium channels; its action potential is generated solely by i_{Ca}, the slow inward current of calcium ions (see Table 4.1). This is true of both SA node and AV node cells. The action of calcium-channel blockers such as verapamil on nodal cells is therefore to reduce the size of the action potential, and also to reduce the rate of pacemaker depolarization.

4.3 Transmission of excitation

The spread of excitation from the SA node into the atria, conduction system and ventricles is mediated by local electrical currents acting ahead of the action potential. In the 'active' depolarized region, the exterior of the cell membrane is negatively charged with respect to the interior, while in the resting zone ahead it is positively charged (Figure 4.3). The two regions are connected by a conducting medium, the extracellular fluid, so positive charge flows from the outside of the resting membrane, depolarizing it. An intracellular current flows in the opposite direction along the cell axis via the gap junctions of the intercalated discs and depolarizes the inside of the membrane. The process is in fact the discharging of a capacitor, namely the lipid cell membrane. When the resting membrane has been depolarized to threshold it generates an action potential and the entire process moves on; and since the membrane to the rear is refractory, excitation progresses unidirectionally.

The *rate of conduction* is greater in wider cells such as Purkinje fibres because they have a lower axial resistance. It is also greater in cells with large, rapid-rising action potentials, because these create bigger propagating currents. Since nodal cells only have small, slow-rising action potentials and therefore small propagating currents, conduction is more easily blocked in nodal tissue.

Table 4.1 Main ionic currents in nodal pacemaker cells

Current	Ion	Direction	Function	Blocker
(i_{Na})	–	–	Absent	–
i_{Ca}	Ca^{2+}	Inward	1. Slow action potential 2. Last one-third of pacemaker potential	Mn^{2+} verapamil, nifedipine
i_K	K^+	Outward	1. Decay during pacemaker potential generates unstable resting membrane potential 2. Repolarization	
i_f*	Na^+ (mainly)	Inward	Supplies inward depolarizing current during pacemaker potential	Cs^+

*i_f is a 'funny' current.

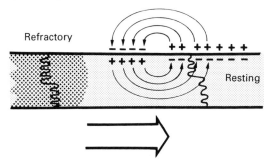

Refractory

Resting

Figure 4.3 The spread of excitation through myocardium by local currents acting ahead of the action potential. The external current flows through the extracellular fluid and the internal current through the sarcoplasm and intercalated junctions. This discharges the cell membrane, which behaves as a lipid capacitor.

4.4 Nervous control of heart rate

The heart rate of a resting adult human is 50–100 beats/min, while in small mammals it is faster (e.g. shrew, 600/min!) and in large mammals slower (e.g. elephant, 25/min). (The rate is in fact proportional to 1/mass$^{0.25}$.) The pacemaker is innervated by autonomic nerves and its intrinsic rate is continuously modified by activity in these nerves. Increased activity in the sympathetic

nerves innervating the SA node speeds up the heart rate (*tachycardia*), while increased activity of the parasympathetic nerves slows it down (*bradycardia*). Sympathetic and parasympathetic fibres also innervate the AV node, shortening or lengthening the transmission delay, respectively. Both sets of autonomic nerve are continuously active at rest but parasympathetic inhibition predominates: if both systems are blocked, the intrinsic heart rate turns out to be around 105 beats/min in a young adult. Physiological alterations of heart rate are usually due to reciprocal changes in autonomic nerve activity; for example, the tachycardia of exercise is induced by both an increase in sympathetic activity and a decrease in parasympathetic activity.

Pacemaker rate is also sensitive to *temperature*, and during a fever the heart rate increases by approximately 10 beats/min per °C. The temperature effect is put to practical use during open heart surgery, where cooling is used to slow the heart.

Action of cardiac parasympathetic fibres

The parasympathetic fibres to the heart arise in the vagal motor nuclei of the brainstem (Chapter 14). They are carried to the heart by the *vagus nerve*. The vagal fibres are preganglionic and they synapse with postganglionic parasympathetic neurons within the myocardium itself, mostly near the SA and AV nodes (Figure 4.4).

The parasympathetic postganglionic nerve terminals act by releasing a neurotransmitter substance called *acetylcholine*, which binds to receptor molecules in the cell membrane, the muscarinic receptors. (Acetylcholine was the first neurotransmitter to be identified, by Otto Loewi in 1921, and was actually discovered in fluid taken from a frog heart during vagal stimulation. The fluid was found to be capable of slowing an isolated frog heart.)

Vagal stimulation produces a virtually immediate bradycardia via two effects as shown in Figure 4.5: (1) the rate of upward drift of the pacemaker potential is slowed, and (2) the initial pacemaker potential becomes slightly more negative (hyperpolarization), though this is not sustained for long. The potential therefore takes longer to decay to threshold and the interval between beats

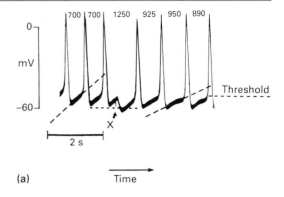

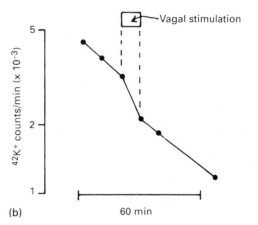

(b)   60 min

Figure 4.5 (a) Bradycardia induced by vagal stimulation in a kitten, and changes in pacemaker potential. The vagus nerve is stimulated briefly at point X. Note the brisk but poorly maintained hyperpolarization of the resting membrane and the reduced slope of the pacemaker potential (dashed lines). Numbers at top are beat interval in ms. (b) Change in radiolabelled potassium content of frog sinus venosus cells. Vagal stimulation increases the rate of efflux of K^+. [(a) After Jalife, J. and Moe, G. K. (1979) *Circulation Research*, **45**, 595–608; (b) From Hutter, O. F. (1961) *Nervous Inhibition* (ed. Florey), Pergamon Press, Oxford, by permission]

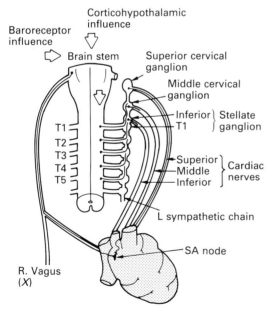

Figure 4.4 Diagram of innervation of the heart by sympathetic and parasympathetic nerves. The right sympathetic chain and nerves innervate mainly the SA node but are omitted for clarity, as is the left vagus

increases. Of the two effects, that on the slope of the pacemaker potential is more important and better sustained.

The actions of acetylcholine on the pacemaker potential are mediated via changes in ion channel states. The reduction in pacemaker *slope* is caused by a reduction in the depolarizing inward pacemaker current carried by Na^+ (i_f). The decrease in i_f appears to be due to a linkage between the muscarinic receptor and an inhibitory G protein (see Figure 4.7). The inhibitory G protein, G_i, reduces the activity of adenylate (or adenylyl) cyclase, leading to a fall in intracellular cyclic adenosine monophosphate (cAMP): cAMP normally contributes to the activation of the *if* channels. The *hyperpolarization* of the pacemaker potential is caused by opening of a particular subclass of K^+ channels called K_{ACh} channels, which are linked to the muscarinic receptor, again by a G protein, G_k. The resulting rise in K^+ conductance produces a bigger outward K^+ current and shifts the membrane towards the Nernst equilibrium potential for potassium, i.e. hyperpolarizes it.

Examples of vagal bradycardia in man include a slowing of the heart during each expiration (sinus arrhythmia, see Figure 5.9), slowing of the heart at the onset of fainting (see Chapter 16), and during diving (see Chapter 15). An extreme example of vagal bradycardia has even given rise to an everyday expression, 'playing possum'; to fool its attackers the possum feigns death by collapsing, with a profound bradycardia:

Quoth Fox to Brer Possum
"You're due in my antrum".
Old possum smiled; he had a hunch
His flaccid apnoe-a
And bradycardee-a
Would leave Fox in no mood for lunch.

Action of cardiac sympathetic fibres

The preganglionic sympathetic fibres to the heart arise from spinal cord segments T1 to T5. The short preganglionic fibres synapse in the paravertebral sympathetic ganglia (see Figure 4.4). The postganglionic fibres run along the surface of the great vessels to reach the heart. Unlike the parasympathetic fibres, sympathetic fibres richly innervate ventricular muscle as well as the atria and electrical system.

The sympathetic nerve terminals act by releasing the neurotransmitter *noradrenaline* ('norepinephrine' in the American literature). Noradrenaline binds to cell membrane receptors called β_1-adrenoreceptors, and over the course of several beats this leads to an increase in firing rate (Figure 4.6). The hormone adrenaline (epinephrine) acts similarly. Adrenaline and noradrenaline, known collectively as the catecholamines, not only increase the heart rate (their chronotropic action) but also increase the force of myocardial contraction (inotropic action).

The *chronotropic effect* of the catecholamines is mediated by an increase in the rate of rise of the pacemaker potential, which takes less time to reach threshold (Figure 4.6). The steeper rise is due to an increase in the inward current carried by Na^+ (i_f) and Ca^{2+} ions. If the heart is to function effectively at the higher rate, however, all the phases of the cardiac cycle must be shortened, and catecholamines have additional chronotropic effects which help achieve this. (1) They shorten the conduction delay in the AV node. (2) They increase the rate of relaxation of myocytes by stimulating the cisternal pumps to take up free cytosolic Ca^{2+} more rapidly. The resulting shortening of systole helps to preserve the diastolic period for refilling.

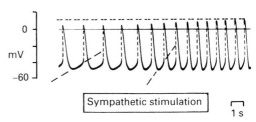

Figure 4.6 Effect of sympathetic stimulation on the pacemaker potential of the frog sinus venosus during the boxed interval. The dashed gradients highlight the increased slope of the pre-potential. The upper double-dashed line draws attention to the increased size of the action potentials, which is due to the enhancement of the inward calcium current by catecholamines. Note also the relatively slow onset of the tachycardia. (From Hutter, O. F. and Trautwein, W. (1956) *Journal of General Physiology*, **39**, 715–733, by permission)

The *inotropic (strengthening) effect* of the catecholamines is mediated by an increase in the inward calcium current during the plateau (see Figures 3.10 and 4.6). This enhances the intracellular calcium store over the course of several beats.

The *biochemical events* that link receptor activation to changes in ionic channels are an area of very active current research (see Appendix II, 'Second messengers') and some of the linkages are illustrated in Figure 4.7. The effects of β_1-adrenoreceptor activation are mediated by an intramembrane protein, the G_s-protein, which activates a membrane-bound enzyme, adenylate cyclase. The latter catalyses the formation of an intracellular

'second messenger', cyclic adenosine monophosphate (cAMP), which has several actions. (1) It appears to interact directly with the pacemaker current channels (i_f channels) to increase their open-state probability. This increases the pacemaker current, raising the depolarization rate and hence heart rate. (2) cAMP also activates an intracellular enzyme, protein kinase A, which, via phosphorylation, increases the number of functional calcium channels in the cell membrane (i_{Ca} channels). This increases the plateau current, leading to a gradual increase in the size of the Ca^{2+} store and therefore contractile force. (3) The second messenger chain also appears to increase the activity of phospholamban,

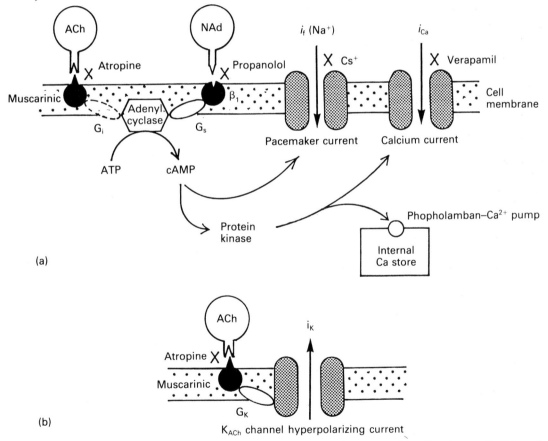

(a)

(b)

Figure 4.7 Mechanisms by which the autonomic neurotransmitters noradrenaline (sympathetic) and acetylcholine (parasympathetic) alter the rate and force of the heart beat. (a) Effect on pacemaker current (i_f) and on calcium current (i_{Ca}). G_s, stimulatory guanosine triphosphate-binding protein. G_i, inhibitory GTP-binding protein. (b) Effect of acetylcholine on potassium current

the protein associated with network SR responsible for regulating the activity of Ca^{2+}-ATPase pumps. As a result of the accelerated re-uptake of Ca^{2+} by the SR, the contraction period is shortened. The chain of biochemical events from β-adrenoceptor activation to biological response is quite long and relatively slow. This explains the slow time-courses of the on and off responses to sympathetic stimulation, which are clearly seen in Figure 4.6.

4.5 Effects of some extracellular agents

Severe extracellular electrolyte disturbances will in general be 'A Bad Thing' for cardiac function. As Ringer showed, hypocalcaemia reduces myocardial contractility, while extreme hypercalcaemia arrests the heart in systole. But it is probably hyperkalaemia (a raised concentration of extracellular potassium ions) that is most often a problem in clinical practice.

Hyperkalaemia

The normal potassium concentration in extracellular fluid is 3.5–5.5 mM and a level of only 7.5 mM K^+ can arrest the heart in diastole. Intermediate levels can cause a marked weakening of the heart beat. Chronic hyperkalaemia can arise gradually during renal failure, acidosis or potassium overloading or rapidly during haemolysis. Its direct effect is to reduce the resting membrane potential by lowering the potassium equilibrium potential (see Figure 3.6). The action potential is altered too, because gradual reductions in resting potential allow time for the inactivation gates (h gates) of fast Na^+ channels to close in Purkinje and work cells. At a resting potential of -70 mV, about half the 'h' gates are closed, while at -50 mV they are all closed. As a result the action potential has a sluggish rise and a small amplitude (see Figure 4.8). Small action potentials produce only small propagating currents, so the conduction of a small action

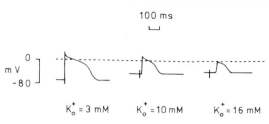

Figure 4.8 Effect of hyperkalaemia on the membrane potential of a Purkinje fibre (see text). The spike to the left of each action potential marks stimulation by an external impulse some distance away. Note the increasing conduction time, reduced resting potential, reduced action potential and slow rate of rise. (After Myerburg, R. J. and Lazzara, R. (1973) In *Complex Electrocardiography* (ed. E. Fisch), Davis Co., Philadelphia

potential is easily blocked, leading to arrhythmias and heart block. Moreover, the action potential becomes shorter, which reduces the total influx of Ca^{2+} ions and leads to a weakening of the heart beat.

Although hyperkalaemia itself weakens the heart beat, and can even arrest it, nevertheless the plasma K^+ concentration not infrequently doubles (8 mM) in severe exercise, without evident harm. (The K^+ is released from exercising skeletal muscle.) It appears that adrenaline and noradrenaline, whose levels can increase by up to $20\times$ in severe exercise, have a protective effect on the heart against the hyperkalaemia. This is probably due to the increased Ca^{2+} current into the cell induced by adrenaline and noradrenaline (see Figure 3.10).

Some drugs affecting cardiac electricity

The actions of many anti-arrhythmic drugs (e.g. quinidine, procainamide, lignocaine) are still ill-understood, but two classes of drug, β-adrenoreceptor blockers and calcium-channel blockers, are better understood. General β-antagonists like propranolol and oxprenolol, and selective β_1-antagonists like atenolol and metoprolol, block the β_1-adrenoreceptors on nodal and work cells. This interrupts the tonic sympathetic influence on the heart, reducing heart rate and contractile force.

Since this also reduces cardiac output and work, β-blockers are often used in the treatment of hypertension and angina (ischaemic heart pain due to cardiac work exceeding oxygen supply).

Calcium-channel blockers

Verapamil and nifedipine belong to a relatively new class of drug which act chiefly on high-threshold voltage-operated calcium channels involved in the plateau phase (L-type channels). These channels are partially blocked, impairing the slow inward current of Ca^{2+} ions. This reduces the duration of the action potential and produces a negative inotropic (weakening) effect. These calcium-channel blockers are used to treat certain arrhythmias.

4.6 Summary

The sino-atrial node initiates the heart beat and atrial contraction. The atrioventricular node delays transmission to the ventricle (allowing the atria to contract before the ventricles) and the bundle of His and Purkinje system then carry the electrical impulse rapidly to the ventricular muscle. The SA node membrane potential is unstable (the *pacemaker potential*). It decays with time due to an inward pacemaker current carried by Na^+ ions (and for its final one-third, Ca^{2+} ions), combined with a decaying potassium permeability. The rate of decay of potential determines the time taken to reach threshold and fire an action potential. The latter initiates the next heart beat. The nodal action potential is small and sluggish, and is generated solely by a slow inward current of Ca^{2+}.

Sympathetic fibre activity increases the rate of decay of the pacemaker potential and thereby increases heart rate (chronotropic effect). The main sympathetic neurotransmitter, noradrenaline, acts by increasing the inward pacemaker current. Sympathetic activity also increases the number of functional Ca^{2+} channels in the myocardium, leading to a more forceful contraction (inotropic effect). *Parasympathetic fibre activity* (vagal) reduces the rate of decay (slope) of the pacemaker potential, and also briefly hyperpolarizes the nodal cells. This reduces heart rate. The parasympathetic neurotransmitter, acetylcholine, acts by activating K_{ACh} channels and by reducing the inward pacemaker current. The principal ion channels governing the behaviour of heart cells are summarized in Table 4.2.

Further reading

Reviews and chapters

Brown, A. M. (1991) Ion channels as G protein effectors. *News in Physiological Sciences*, **6**, 158–161

Davies, M. J., Anderson, R. H. and Becker, A. E. (1983) *The Conduction System of the Heart*, Butterworths, London

DiFrancesco, D. (1993) Pacemaker mechanisms in cardiac tissue. *Annual Review of Physiology*, **55**, 451–467

Hirst, G. D. S., Edwards, F. R., Bramich, N. J. and Klem, M. F. (1991) Neural control of cardiac pacemaker potentials. *News in Physiological Sciences*, **6**, 185–190

Levy, M. N. and Martin, P. (1984) Parasympathetic control of heart. In *Nervous Control of Cardiovascular Function* (ed. W. C. Randall), Oxford University Press, New York, pp. 68–94

Noble, D. (1979) *The Initiation of the Heart Beat*, Clarendon Press, Oxford

Noble, D. (1984) The surprising heart. *Journal of Physiology*, **353**, 1–50

Robishaw, J. D. and Foster, K. A. (1989) Role of G proteins in the regulation of the cardiovascular system. *Annual Review of Physiology*, **51**, 229–244

Research papers

Choate, J. K., Edwards, F. R., Hirst, G. D. S. and O'Shea, J. E. (1993) Effects of sympathetic nerve stimulation on the sino-atrial node of the guinea-pig. *Journal of Physiology*, **471**, 707–727

Okazaki, O., Suda, N., Hongo, K., Konishi, M., Kurihara, S. (1990) Modulation of Ca^{2+} transients and contractile properties by β-adrenoceptor stimulation in ferret ventricular muscles. *Journal of Physiology*, **423**, 221–240

Table 4.2 Types of ion channel in cardiac work and/or nodal cells. To paraphrase Professor Noble in 'The surprising heart', the description of ionic currents in the preceding text 'may already have exhausted the reader, but it certainly does not exhaust the mechanisms that have been found'. This table attempts to categorize the most important of these for the benefit of the more advanced student; *first-year students should read no further and turn quickly to the next chapter!*

Channel and current	Properties and activator	Blocker	Role
Potassium			
Inward rectifier (i_{K1})	Activated by hyperpolarization. More permeable to inward than outward current	Ba^{2+}	Background K^+ current in myocyte. Few in SA node cell
Delayed rectifier (i_K)	Activated slowly on depolarization beyond $-40\,mV$	Ba^{2+}	Helps terminate action potential, supplying outward repolarization current. Gradual inactivation causes falling g_K during pacemaker potential
Muscarinic (i_{K-ACh})	Activated by ACh but some spontaneous opening too. Inwardly rectifying like i_{K1}	Ba^{2+} (partially) (Pertussis toxin blocks the linked G-protein)	Hyperpolarizing effect of ACh. Also contributes to background K^+ current
ATP-K (i_{K-ATP})	Closed by ATP (normally $5\,mM$). Opened by low ATP ($<0.1\,mM$), raised ADP, raised pH_i, cromakalim and pinacidil		In ischaemia, i_{K-ATP} terminates action potential early, reducing contractile force
Transient outward ($i_{t,o}$)	Activated by depolarization and rise in Ca_i^{2+}	4-aminopyridine	Affects shape of action potential, i.e. early repolarization spike when present
Sodium			
Fast-inactivating (i_{Na})	Voltage- and time-dependent opening	Tetrodotoxin, local anaesthetics	Spike of action potential. Few in SA node so no spike
Hyperpolarization-activated (i_f)	Opens slowly at potentials negative to $-45\,mV$. Carries mainly Na^+ at pacemaker potential	Cs^+	Depolarizing current of pacemaker. Increased by catecholamines. Reduced by acetylcholine
Background (i_b)	Passive background current		Attenuates resting membrane potential
(Na–Ca exchanger, i_{NaCa})	Not a channel but allows $3Na^+$ into cell for $1Ca^{2+}$ expelled. Activated by rise in Ca_i^{2+}		Supplies a net inward current (Na in > Ca out) that sustains latter part of plateau
(Na–K pump i_{NaK})	Not a channel but $3Na^+$ pumped out of cell for $2K^+$ in		

4.2   *(cot'd)*

Channel and current	Properties and activator	Blocker	Role
Calcium (VOCs)			
L-type (i_{Ca})	Voltage-operated channel of high threshold (positive to $-50\,mV$). 'L'ong-lasting, i.e. $>20\,ms$ before inactivates	Cd^{2+}, verapamil, nifedipine	Carries most of early plateau current and raises Ca_i^{2+} enough to trigger calcium-induced calcium release
T-type	Voltage-operated channel of low threshold (-30 to $-50\,mV$). 'T'ransient opening, i.e. fast inactivation	Ni^{2+}	May carry last third of pacemaker depolarizing current

Chapter 5
Electrocardiography and arrhythmias

5.1 Principle of electrocardiography

Electrocardiography is the process of recording the potential changes at the skin surface resulting from depolarization and repolarization of heart muscle; the record itself is called an electrocardiogram (ECG). The method was developed at the turn of the century by Willem Einthoven in Leiden, who invented the string galvanometer, and by Augustus Waller in London, whose demonstration to the Royal Society in 1909 provoked protests in Parliament (Figure 5.1). As explained in Chapter 4, the spread of excitation through the myocardium involves small currents flowing through the extracellular fluid (see Figure 4.3). These extracellular currents create slight potential differences at the body's surface because the extracellular fluid is a continuous conducting medium between the heart and skin. The minute differences in skin potential (approximately 1 mV) are picked up by metal contact electrodes, measured by a millivoltmeter and recorded on a moving paper strip to produce the ECG.

The size of the potential differences at the surface depends on the size of the cardiac extracellular current, which in turn depends on the mass of myocardium being activated. Since the mass of the conduction system is tiny its depolarization does not register on a surface ECG, though nodal

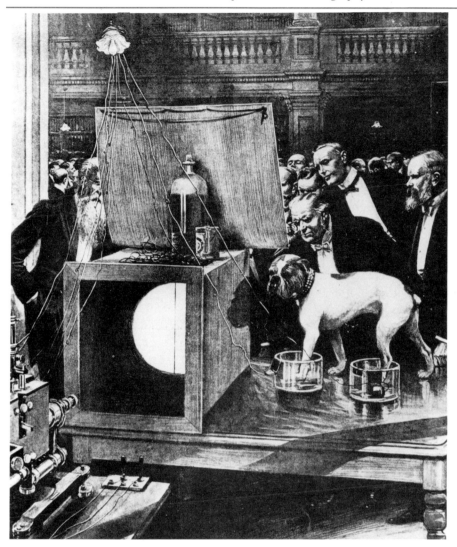

Figure 5.1 The electrocardiogram was demonstrated to the Royal Society by Waller's pet bulldog, Jimmie, in 1909. Jimmie has front and hind paws in pots of normal saline connected to a galvanometer. (From the Illustrated London News, May 22nd 1909.)

The Times newspaper of July 9, 1909 reported that Mr Ellis Griffith (MP for Anglesey) questioned the Secretary of State in Parliament over Waller's 'public experiment' on a dog with 'a leather strap with sharp nails secured around the neck, his feet being immersed in glass jars containing salts . . . connected by wires with galvanometers'. Had the Cruelty to Animals Act (1876) been contravened?

Mr. Gladstone: 'I understand the dog stood for some time in water to which sodium chloride had been added or in other words a little common salt. If my honourable friend has ever paddled in the sea he will understand the sensation. (Laughter) The dog – a finely developed bulldog – was neither tied nor muzzled. He wore a leather collar ornamented with brass studs. Had the experiment been painful the pain would no doubt have been immediately felt by those nearest the dog. (Laughter).'

Mr. MacNeill (Donegal South): 'Will the right honourable gentleman inform the person who furnished him with his jokes that there are members in this House who regard these experiments on dogs with abhorrence?' (Hear)

Mr. Gladstone: 'I certainly shall not. The jokes, poor as they are, are mine own.' (Laughter and cheers) (From Waller, A. D. (1910) *Physiology the Servant of Medicine*, Hodder and Stoughton, London)

and bundle activity can be recorded from an intracardiac electrode introduced by cardiac catheterization. With the usual surface ECG, however, only the activity of atrial and ventricular working muscle is detected.

5.2 Relation of ECG waves to cardiac action potentials

Figure 5.2 shows some typical human ECG recordings. There are three main deflections per cardiac cycle: the P wave, corresponding to atrial depolarization; the QRS complex,

corresponding to ventricular depolarization; and the T wave, corresponding to ventricular repolarization. The two regions where the trace returns to baseline (the isoelectric state) are called the PR interval and ST segment. These ECG features are compared with the underlying cardiac action potentials in Figure 5.3 and with the mechanical events of the cycle in Figure 2.3

P wave The first event of the cardiac cycle, SA node depolarization, does not register on the ECG because nodal mass is too tiny. The next event, depolarization of the atrial cell mass, produces the P wave, lasting approximately 0.08 s. The P wave coincides with the upstrokes of the atrial action potentials, not with contraction; atrial contraction follows during the PR interval.

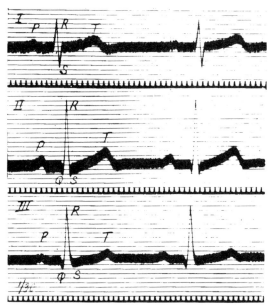

Figure 5.2 ECG of a young healthy adult recorded from Leads I, II and III. Ordinate divisions represent 0.1 mV, horizontal scale marks 1/30th second. (From Sir Thomas Lewis's classic textbook of 1920, *The Mechanism and Graphic Registration of the Heart Beat*, Shaw and Sons, London). Lewis's major contributions included the clinical application of the ECG, the recording of the jugular venous pulse and the discovery of the skin triple response (see Chapter 12). The thickness of the baseline is an interference artefact common with the early string galvanometers (cf. Figure 5.9a)

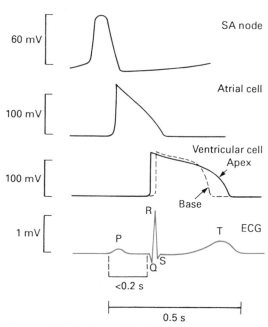

Figure 5.3 Timing of the ECG waves compared with intracellular recordings at different sites, including two sites in the ventricle (apex and base). Note that the ECG voltage scale is much smaller than that for the membrane potentials. Note also that the base (dashed line) repolarizes before the apex, which is why the T wave is upright

PR interval The interval between the beginning of the P wave and beginning of the QRS complex is always called the PR interval (even when it is, strictly speaking, a P–Q interval). It represents the time taken for excitation to spread over the atria and through the conduction system to reach the ventricular septum. Much of the PR interval is produced by the delay in conduction through the atrioventricular node, which allows time for atrial systole to develop. In a human ECG the total PR interval should not however exceed 0.2 s, and longer intervals indicate a defect in conduction through to the ventricle (see 'heart block', Figure 5.9c). The ECG is isoelectric during the PR interval despite the existence of a potential difference between atria (depolarized) and ventricles (polarized) because the insulating annulus fibrosus breaks the electrical circuit and no current flows. Atrial repolarization does not produce a detectable ECG signal, as can be seen in heart block (see Figure 5.9e). This is because atrial repolarization is too slow and diffuse to register.

QRS complex During ventricular excitation a large mass of muscle is activated almost synchronously and this produces a large deflection in the ECG, the QRS complex. The complex lasts 0.1 s or less, a longer period being suggestive of cardiac pathology such as a conduction block in one of the bundle branches. The Q wave is an initial downward spike, the R wave an upward spike, and the S wave a second downward spike: but all three components are not necessarily present in every record – the complex may have just an RS configuration as in Lead I of Figure 5.2, or just a QR configuration, as explained later.

ST segment This coincides with the plateau of the ventricular action potential, and rapid ejection occurs during this period. The first heart sound follows just after the S wave, and the second sound a little after the T wave (see Figure 2.3). Since the ventricle is uniformly depolarized, the ST segment is normally isoelectric. If, however, part of the myocardium is damaged by ischaemia (a poor blood supply, due usually to coronary artery disease) there is an apparent depression of the ST segment, a useful clinical sign illustrated in the first beat of Figure 5.9g. The electrical effect of ischaemia is to reduce the resting potential of the hypoxic myocytes, and since ventricular polarization is then non-uniform, a current, called the resting injury current, flows between the healthy myocytes and ischaemic cells. This shifts the baseline of the ECG (i.e. the T–P and P–R regions) and leaves the ST segment apparently depressed relative to the new baseline.

T wave, and why it is normally upright Ventricular repolarization produces a broad asymmetrical upright wave, the T wave. At first acquaintance it may seem odd that the T wave is upright when repolarization is a process of opposite sign to depolarization. The reason is that the myocytes of the base and epicardium have briefer action potentials than the myocytes of the apex and endocardium (see Figure 5.3). Repolarization therefore begins in the base and epicardium, followed by the apex and endocardium. Depolarization on the other hand spreads from apex and endocardium to base and epicardium (see Figure 5.4). Thus repolarization occurs in reverse sequence to depolarization, producing the upright T wave.

Myocardial ischaemia affects not only the ST segment but also the T wave, causing it to invert (see Figure 5.9g).

5.3 Standard limb leads

To understand the shape of the QRS complex we must consider: (1) the position of the recording electrodes relative to the heart, (2) the concept of the heart as an electrical dipole, and (3) the changes in dipole orientation during excitation. Taking the electrode positions first, the ECG is routinely recorded via three electrodes, one on each arm and one on the left leg. In addition, recordings are commonly made from electrodes on the chest

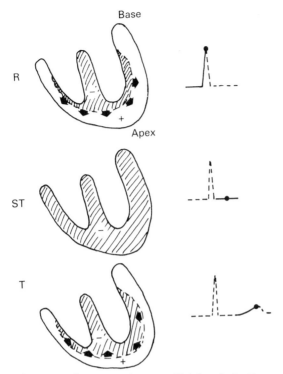

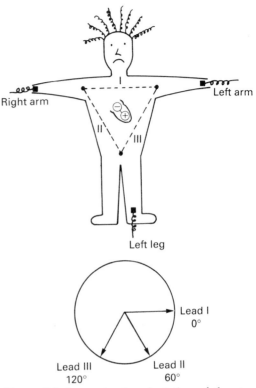

Figure 5.4 Sequence of myocardial depolarization and repolarization. The polarity is shown at three succeeding moments: partial depolarization (R wave), full depolarization (ST segment) and partial repolarization (T wave). Hatched regions are depolarized and the negative sign refers to the external charge. Arrows indicate the direction of advance of the change. Repolarization proceeds in reverse order to depolarization and therefore produces a net electrical difference (dipole) in the same direction as depolarization, creating an upright T wave

Figure 5.5 Approximate orientation of the standard bipolar limb leads relative to the horizontal (0°). Lead I, right arm – left arm; Lead II, right arm – left leg; Lead III, left arm – left leg

wall (the six unipolar precordial leads) but these will not be described here, since our primary concern is with general principles rather than detailed clinical practice. The three limb electrodes can be connected across a voltmeter in three different combinations, called the bipolar limb leads (Figure 5.5). They are:

Right arm – left arm = LEAD I
Right arm – left leg = LEAD II
Left arm – left leg = LEAD III

Since the limbs act as volume conductors to the trunk, the electrodes form a triangle around the heart, called Einthoven's triangle. The three leads in effect view the heart from three different angles in the frontal plane. Lead I forms the top of the triangle, oriented horizontally across the chest, and this angle is taken as zero. Lead II is oriented more vertically, at roughly 60° to Lead I, and Lead III at roughly 120°. The electronics are arranged so that an upward deflection occurs when the positive pole of a potential difference is directed towards the left arm (Lead I) or left leg (Leads II and III). We must therefore consider next the overall polarity of the heart during excitation.

5.4 Cardiac dipole

At any one instant during the spread of excitation through the ventricle, there exists a resting zone with a diffuse cloud of positive extracellular charges and an excited region with a diffuse cloud of negative extracellular charges (Figure 5.6a). Just as a diffuse mass can be represented by a centre of gravity, so a diffuse charge can be represented as a single charge at its electrical centre or pole. During the spread of excitation, the heart has two such poles, one negative and one positive; it is an electrical dipole.

A dipole is surrounded by positive and negative potential fields, which grow weaker with increasing distance. The potential differences can be measured by a voltmeter aligned across the two poles. If, however, the voltmeter is placed exactly at right angles to the dipole it will register no difference in potential (Figure 5.6b). This extreme case highlights a crucial point: the potential difference actually recorded depends on the orientation of the recording electrodes relative to the dipole. This is because a dipole is a vector quantity having direction as well as magnitude. The symbol for a vector is an arrow whose length represents vector size and whose direction represents the vector's angle. Like a force vector, the cardiac vector can be resolved into two components at right angles and it is the magnitude of the component directed at the recording lead which is actually registered (Figure 5.6c). This brings us to the question of the orientation of the cardiac dipole.

5.5 Vector sequence

The size and orientation of the cardiac dipole in the frontal plane changes continuously as excitation spreads through the ventricles. (For simplicity, only orientations in the frontal plane are described here, but as the ventricles are three-dimensional bodies lying in an oblique, rotated position, the dipole rarely lies purely in the frontal plane.) The

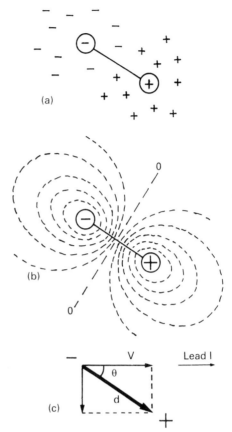

Figure 5.6 Properties of a dipole. (a) Representation of two diffuse groups of opposite charges by a dipole (two points of electrical charge of opposite sign, e.g. the terminals of a battery). (b) Equipotential lines around an electrical dipole. The zero potential run across the middle of the dipole. The potential is inversely proportional to the square of the distance and current flows at right angles to the potential contour. (c) Resolution of a cardiac dipole vector (thick arrow, d) into two components at right angles (thin arrows). The length of the arrow is proportional to vector magnitude, d. The voltage difference (V) detected by Lead I depends on angle θ since V equals d $\times$ cosine θ

first region to depolarize is the left side of the interventricular septum, activated by the left bundle branch (Figure 5.7). This creates a small dipole directed to the right, about 120° to the horizontal. Next, the remaining

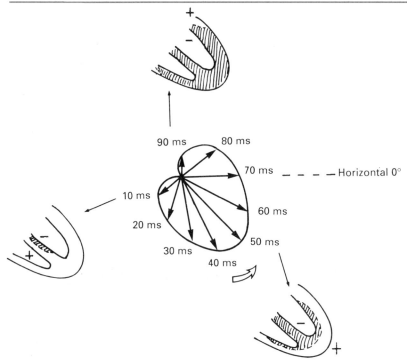

Figure 5.7 Change of the cardiac dipole with time in milliseconds during excitation of the ventricles. Bold arrows show size and direction of the vector in the frontal plane at successive instants in time as depolarization spreads through the ventricles. Hatched areas represent depolarized myocardium, which carries a negative external charge. The vector waxes and wanes, and also rotates in an anti-clockwise direction as depolarization proceeds. The electrical axis (see text) is about 70° here

septum and most of the endocardium depolarize. The epicardium is still polarized and the bulky left ventricle predominates, creating a large dipole directed to the left, about 60° to the horizontal. The last region to be excited is the base of the ventricles close to the annulus fibrosus, so the final dipole is small and directed upwards. As Figure 5.7 shows, this sequence of ventricular activation causes the cardiac vector to swing round in an anticlockwise direction, and to wax and wane in size over approximately 90 ms.

5.6 Why the QRS complex is complex

From the lead positions and vector sequence it is possible to understand why the QRS wave contains negative waves and why the QRS complex differs from lead to lead. As a simple example let us consider the ventricular dipole at three instants: the beginning, middle and end of excitation, as 'seen' by Leads I and III. In the particular case illustrated in Figure 5.8, the small initial dipole at approximately 120° (the little arrow) is directed obliquely away from Lead I. Resolving the vector, we find a small component directed at 180°, which is in the opposite direction to Lead I (0°), so Lead I records a small negative deflection or Q wave. At the same instant Lead III (120°) records a positive deflection – the beginning of an R wave, with no preceding Q wave. After 50 ms the dipole has a large component directed at Lead I, which records a large upward deflection, the R wave. Lead III is at right angles to the dipole at this instant, and

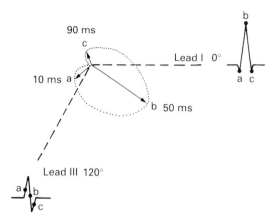

Figure 5.8 Illustration of how the dipole sequence gives rise to different QRS complexes in different leads. The dipole is drawn at three instants (a,b,c) and the component of the vector detected by Leads I and III at these instants is marked on the ECG

so records zero potential difference. By 90 ms the dipole has swung round to $-100°$ in the case illustrated, causing small negative deflections in both Leads I and III, i.e. S waves. Thus the same event produced a QRS complex in Lead I but an RS complex in Lead III. It must be emphasized that *there are many variations from the pattern illustrated owing to variations in cardiac orientation in three dimensions*. The above analysis for teaching purposes is limited to two dimensions.

5.7 Electrical axis of the heart

The direction of the largest dipole is called the electrical axis of the heart, and in Figure 5.8 this is about $60°$ below the horizontal. The electrical axis can be estimated roughly by comparing the size of the R wave in Leads I, II and III. If for example the largest R wave is in Lead II, the electrical axis is closer to $60°$ than to $0°$ or $120°$. Conversely the lead with the smallest QRS complex and R and S waves of nearly equal height lies roughly at

right angles to the electrical axis. The normal range for the electrical axis is very wide, from $-30°$ to $+110°$. It depends partly on the anatomical orientation of the heart in the chest, being more vertical in a tall person with a narrow thorax. It also becomes more vertical during each inspiration as the pericardium is pulled down by the descending diaphragm (see Figure 5.9a). The axis depends, too, on the relative thickness of the walls of the right and left ventricles. Hypertrophy of the left ventricle shifts the electrical axis to the left (left axis deviation) while hypertrophy of the right ventricle produces right axis deviation.

5.8 Palpitations: benign or bad?

The ECG is an invaluable aid to the diagnosis of many cardiac disorders, such as myocardial ischaemia, ventricular hypertrophy and especially irregular rhythms (arrhythmias).

Sinus arrhythmia This is one form of arrhythmia that is perfectly normal. It is a physiological slowing of the SA node's rate of firing during expiration, i.e. bradycardia during expiration, tachycardia during inspiration. It is especially marked in children and young adults. In the medical student of Figure 5.9(a), for example, the rate slowed from 92 to 52 beats/min during expiration. Sinus arrhythmia is caused by a phasic rise in vagal activity during expiration. This is partly a reflex initiated by lung stretch receptors, but it persists even when ventilation is paralysed in anaesthetized animals, so there is an innate central (brainstem) periodicity too (Chapter 14). The tachycardia during inspiration helps counteract the effect on left ventricular output of a concomitant fall in left ventricular stroke volume. The latter is due to reduced left-side filling pressure as the lung vascular bed is expanded by inspiration (Chapter 7). Other arrhythmias are pathological and arise from various different mechanisms, as follows.

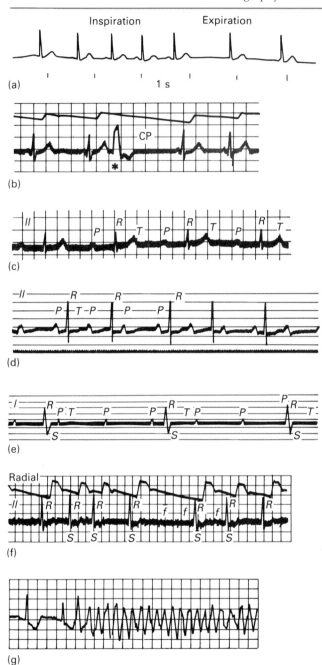

(a)

(b)

(c)

(d)

(e)

(f)

(g)

Figure 5.9 A cornucopia of arrhythmias. (a) Sinus arrhythmia in a healthy 19-year-old medical student. (b) The first example of an extrasystole (ventricular ectopic, asterisk) recorded by Einthoven. (CP, compensatory pause). The upper trace is a radial pulse. (c–e) Progressive stages of heart block. (c) First-degree block. (d) Second-degree block. (e) Third-degree block. (f) Atrial fibrillation. (g) Ventricular fibrillation. (Records c–f are from Lewis' classic book, *The Mechanism and Graphic Registration of the Heart Beat*, Shaw, London, 1920)

Ectopics An aberrant group of cells at a site other than the SA node may occasionally fire before the SA node, initiating a premature or extra systole. This is called an ectopic beat. If the ectopic site is in the ventricle, as in Figure 5.9(b), the resulting QRS wave looks abnormal; it is broad and ill synchronized because excitation has not followed the normal route through the Purkinje system. It also fails to pump much blood, as can be seen from the blood pressure trace in the figure. Since the ventricle is then in its refractory period, the next normal impulse from the SA node fails to excite it. There is therefore a long interval between the ectopic beat and the next normal one – a *'compensatory pause'*. The patient often notices this, commenting that 'My heart keeps missing a beat'.

Heart block Owing to ischaemic heart disease or other causes, the main bundle or one of the bundle branches may fail to conduct. Three degrees of main bundle block, of increasing severity, can be recognized from the characteristic ECG patterns. *First-degree heart block* is a lengthening of the PR interval (to 0.45 s in Figure 5.9c) due to slowing of conduction between the AV node and ventricle muscle mass. *Second-degree heart block* involves intermittent failure of excitation to pass from atria to ventricles. In Figure 5.9(d), for example, there are four labelled P waves but only three corresponding QRS complexes. In *third-degree heart block*, excitation fails totally to pass from atria to ventricles, so the atria and ventricles beat entirely independently of each other. In Figure 5.9(e) the atria (P waves) are beating at 72 per min, driven by the SA node, but the ventricles are beating at 30 per min, driven by a pacemaker in the bundle of His or Purkinje system that has now escaped from domination by the SA node. The patient may experience sudden faints (Stokes–Adams attacks) and will need an artificial pacemaker.

Circus mechanisms Sometimes an abnormal conduction circuit develops in the myocardium that allows a wave of excitation

to travel in a never-ending circle or *circus*; as cells emerge from their refractory period, they are immediately re-excited by *re-entry* of the excitation wave. A classic example is the unforgettably-named Wolff-Parkinson–White syndrome. This is characterized by episodes of *paroxysmal tachycardia*, experienced by the patient as 'palpitations', where the heart beats at over 200 min^{-1}. The syndrome is caused by an anomalous electrical connection across the annulus fibrosus called the bundle of Kent. This allows the ventricular wave of excitation to re-enter the atria and re-excite the AV node prematurely.

Drugs like quinidine and procainamide prolong the refractory period, which renders re-entry more difficult and terminates some circus arrhythmias. The calcium blocker verapamil shortens the action potential and upsets the timing of re-entry, so it too terminates some circus arrhythmias.

Atrial fibrillation A circus mechanism may also underlie fibrillation. This is an uncoordinated, repetitive excitation that results in a writhing movement of the wall, incapable of expelling blood. Fibrillation in the atria is a relatively benign condition, quite common in the elderly and compatible with a sedentary life. Irregular oscillations replace the normal P wave (see 'f' waves in Figure 5.9f). Excitation is transmitted irregularly to the ventricles, resulting in a highly characteristic and easily diagnosed radial pulse, which is 'irregularly irregular' in timing and variable in amplitude (upper trace, Figure 5.9f).

Ventricular fibrillation This a fatal sequel to myocardial ischaemia, anaesthetic overdosage and electrocution. In Figure 5.9(g), the preceding *ischaemia* is evident from two characteristic ECG features – ST segment depression and T wave inversion, which are seen clearly in the first two beats of the record. After the second sinus beat a ventricular ectopic occurs during the latter half of the T wave, a period known as the *vulnerable period*. The ventricle is vulnerable at this moment because some of its cells have repolarized while others are still in their refractory period, so circus pathways can be triggered. This initiates a series of rapid uncoordinated excitations, producing ineffective rippling motions. There is no cardiac output and death follows within minutes. 'Cardioversion' by a DC electric shock to the chest wall sometimes succeeds in restoring sinus rhythm.

Calcium store overload and arrhythmias
Proneness to ventricular fibrillation following ischaemia varies considerably between different animal species and has been found to correlate with increased sympathetic drive to the ischaemic heart. Ischaemia raises intracellular calcium content because as ATP levels fall the rate of extrusion of intracellular calcium declines; at the same time sympathetic activity raises i_{Ca}, the plateau calcium current into the cell. The resulting overload of the intracellular calcium store has been implicated in arrhythmogenesis. The overloaded store discharges partially during diastole, raising cytoplasmic

Ca^{2+}. This stimulates the $3Na^+ - 1Ca^{2+}$ exchange pump and the net inward current of Na^+ causes an *afterpotential* (Figure 5.10). If big enough, the afterpotential can trigger an arrhythmia. Thus calcium-channel blockers like verapamil can substantially reduce the risk of sudden death after myocardial infarction, provided that heart failure (which verapamil exacerbates) is absent.

5.9 Summary

The electrocardiogram records small potential differences across the chest (about 1 mV) that arise from electrical depolarization and repolarization of the heart. The *P wave* is due to atrial depolarization, the *QRS complex* to ventricular depolarization, and the *T wave* to ventricular repolarization. The *PR interval* is largely due to the delay in transmission through the atrioventricular node and should not exceed 0.2 s in man. The delay allows atrial systole to precede ventricular systole. The isoelectric *ST segment* corresponds to the long plateau of the cardiac action potential. The T wave is upright because repolarization occurs in reverse sequence to depolarization, i.e. the last region to depolarize is the first to repolarize.

The shape of the QRS complex for a given beat is different in Leads I (right arm–left arm), II (right arm–left leg) and III (left arm–left leg) because each lead 'views' the electrical potential from a different angle. In the frontal plane these are roughly $0°$ to the horizontal (I), $60°$ (II) and $120°$ (III), forming Einthoven's triangle. The complex's triple composition, namely Q wave–R wave–S wave, stems from the changing size and direction of the cardiac dipole as excitation spreads first along the interventricular septum, then out through the apex and main muscle mass, and finally to the base of the ventricle. The dipole is dominated by the larger mass of the left ventricle and, viewed in the frontal plane, rotates

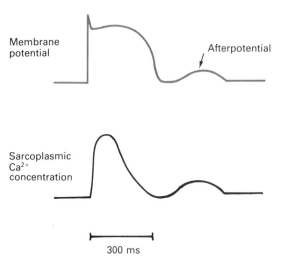

Figure 5.10 Afterpotential (upper trace) arising from partial discharge of overloaded internal calcium store into sarcoplasm (lower trace), stimulating the $3Na^+ - 1Ca^{2+}$ exchange pump

anti-clockwise, waxing and waning as it does so. The largest dipole usually develops between $0°$ and $90°$ and its angle is called the electrical axis of the heart.

The ECG is invaluable for the diagnosis of cardiac arrhythmias, such as ectopic beats, heart block, supraventricular tachycardias, atrial fibrillation and ventricular fibrillation. The principal mechanisms underlying arrhythmias are thought to be conduction impairment, circus (re-entrant circuits) and afterpotentials due to calcium store overload.

Further reading

Billman, G. E. (1992) Cellular mechanisms for ventricular fibrillation. *News in Physiological Science*, **7**, 254–259

Noble, D. (1979) *The Initiation of the Heart Beat*, 2nd edn, Clarendon Press, Oxford

Rowlands, D. J. (1986) The electrocardiogram. In *Oxford Textbook of Medicine* (eds D. J. Weatherall, J. G. G. Leddingham and D. A. Warrell), Oxford University Press, London, pp. 13.23–13.41.

Schamroth, L. (1980) *The Disorders of Cardiac Rhythm*, 2nd edn, Blackwell Scientific Publications, Oxford

Scher, A. M. and Spach, M. S. (1979) Cardiac depolarization repolarization and the electrocardiogram. In *Handbook of Physiology, Cardiovascular System*, Vol. 1, *The Heart* (ed R. M. Berne), American Physiological Society, Bethesda, pp. 357–392

Chapter 6
Assessment of cardiac output

Cardiac output is defined as the volume of blood ejected by one ventricle in one minute: it equals the stroke volume multiplied by heart rate. In human subjects the output can be measured by a variety of methods, which either measure the cardiac output as a whole (the Fick principle and the dilution methods) or measure stroke volume and heart rate separately (Doppler and radionuclide methods). The output can also be assessed indirectly by echocardiography, and at the bedside by examining a subject's peripheral pulse. In anaesthetized animals, direct methods requiring surgery can also be employed, such as the placing of an electromagnetic flowmeter around the aorta. We will concentrate here, however, on the methods which are currently most important in medicine, beginning with the 'gold-standard' method based on Fick's principle.

6.1 Fick's principle and the measurement of cardiac output

Adolf Fick pointed out in 1870 that the rate at which the circulation takes up oxygen from the lungs must equal the change in oxygen concentration in the pulmonary blood multiplied by the pulmonary blood flow. Since the pulmonary blood flow is of course the output of the right ventricle, this offers a way of determining the cardiac output. The reasoning behind the method is illustrated in illustrated in Figure 6.1(a). The amount of oxygen carried into the lungs in venous blood per minute is the blood flow ($\dot{Q}$) times venous oxygen concentration (C_v):

O_2 in venous blood entering the lungs per minute $= \dot{Q} . C_v$

Similarly, the amount of oxygen carried out of the lungs per minute in the blood equals blood flow times arterial oxygen concentration ($\dot{Q} . C_a$):

O_2 in arterial blood leaving the lungs per minute $= \dot{Q} . C_a$

The amount of oxygen taken up by the blood during its passage through the lungs there-

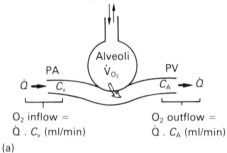

Rate of O$_2$ uptake (ml/min)

Alveoli
$\dot{V}_{O_2}$
PA
PV
$\dot{Q} \rightarrow C_v$ $C_A \rightarrow \dot{Q}$

O$_2$ inflow = $\dot{Q} . C_v$ (ml/min)   O$_2$ outflow = $\dot{Q} . C_A$ (ml/min)

(a)

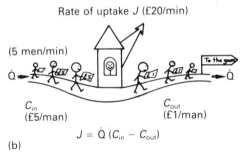

Rate of uptake J (£20/min)

(5 men/min)

$\dot{Q} \rightarrow$ To the game $\rightarrow \dot{Q}$

C_{in} (£5/man) C_{out} (£1/man)

$J = \dot{Q} (C_{in} - C_{out})$

(b)

Figure 6.1 Fick's principle applied to the measurement of pulmonary blood flow (a). PA, pulmonary artery; PV, pulmonary veins. Fick's principle is quite general and could be applied, for example, to measure crowd flow at a football ground (b). Here the flux of material (money) is in the opposite direction as with CO$_2$ in the lung. If £20 per min is taken and each man emerges poorer by £4, the crowd flow is five men/min. Analogous physiological situations include the passage of carbon dioxide from blood into the alveolar gas, and glucose from blood into muscle.

fore equals $\dot{Q} . C_a - \dot{Q} . C_v$ over one minute. In a steady state, this oxygen uptake must equal the loss of oxygen from the alveolar gas in the lungs over one minute ($\dot{V}_{O_2}$): oxygen consumption by the alveolar cells can be neglected. We can therefore write:

alveolar oxygen removed per min = blood oxygen gained per min

$\dot{V}_{O_2} = (\dot{Q} . C_a) - (\dot{Q} . C_v)$

or in terms of the arteriovenous concentration difference $C_a - C_v$:

$$\dot{V}_{O_2} = \dot{Q} . (C_a - C_v)$$

This is Fick's expression, and it tells us that the rate of oxygen uptake from alveolar gas (ml/min) equals pulmonary blood flow (litres/min) times the arteriovenous difference in oxygen concentration (ml/litre). Since pulmonary blood flow is actually the output of the right ventricle, we can replace $\dot{Q}$ by cardiac output and write:

Cardiac output (l/min) =

$$\frac{\text{Oxygen uptake rate (ml/min)}}{\text{Arterial } O_2 \text{ conc.} - \text{Venous } O_2 \text{ conc. (ml/litre)}}$$

A resting man, for example, absorbs around 250 ml/min of oxygen from the alveolar gas ($\dot{V}_{O_2}$). Arterial blood contains 195 ml per litre of oxygen, while mixed venous blood in the pulmonary artery contains 145 ml per litre of oxygen. Each litre of blood therefore takes up 50 ml of oxygen, i.e. ($C_a - C_v$) = 50 ml/litre. To take up 250 ml oxygen, 5 litres of blood are required (i.e. 250/50). As this uptake takes 1 min, the pulmonary blood flow must be 5 litres/min.

Practical aspects

Fick's theoretical method became practicable in man in the 1940s, when progress in cardiac catheterization allowed mixed venous blood to be sampled from the right ventricle. Samples from peripheral veins are unsuitable for this purpose because their oxygen concentration varies; it is 170 ml/litre in renal venous blood, but only 70 ml/litre in coronary venous blood. Venous blood only becomes fully mixed and uniform in the right ventricle outflow tract and pulmonary artery. The problem of obtaining a sample of fully mixed venous blood was solved by the German physician Werner Forssman, who in 1929 passed a ureteric catheter through his own arm vein and into the right heart, watching its progress on an X-ray screen. (This brave act founded human cardiac catheterization, won Forssman the disapproval of his head of department and, later, the Nobel prize.)

The Fick method is now as follows. The subject's resting oxygen consumption is measured over 5–10 min by spirometry, or by collection of expired air in a Douglas bag. During this period an arterial blood sample is taken from the brachial, radial or femoral artery, and a mixed venous sample is taken from the pulmonary artery or right ventricle outflow tract by a cardiac catheter, introduced through the antecubital vein. The oxygen content of each blood sample is measured and the cardiac output calculated as above.

Limitations of the method

Fick's method is the yardstick by which new methods are usually judged but it has its limitations. It is slow, and beat-by-beat changes in stroke volume cannot be followed. The method is only valid in the steady state, so the transient early response to exercise cannot be measured. The method is invasive, and cannot be used during severe exercise because the cardiac catheter may provoke arrhythmias in a violently beating heart. An indirect version, in which catheterization is avoided and C_v estimated by analysis of rebreathed gas, is rarely used today–except in orbiting spacecraft, where it has provided useful data!

The Fick principle generalized

The Fick principle is quite general and applies to any perfused organ in which material or heat is exchanged at a steady rate. In general terms the flux J of material or heat between the fluid and the perfused organ equals the fluid flow ($\dot{Q}$) multiplied by the concentration change between the inlet (C_{in}) and outlet (C_{out}):

$$J = \dot{Q}(C_{out} - C_{in})$$

As Figure 6.1(b) shows, Fick's principle applies even to the influx of money at the turnstile of a football ground. In physiology, Fick's principle is widely used to work out the rate at which an organ consumes nutrients like glucose or fatty acids, from measurements of blood flow and the arteriovenous concentration difference for the nutrient.

6.2 Indicator dilution and thermal dilution methods

Indicator dilution method

In Hamilton's indicator dilution method, a known mass of a foreign substance (the indicator) is injected rapidly into a central vein or into the right heart. The indicator must be confined to the bloodstream and easy to assay, for example the dye indocyanine green, or albumin labelled with radioiodine. The bolus of indicator becomes diluted in the returning venous blood, passes through the heart and lungs and is ejected into the systemic arteries (see Figure 6.2(a)). Samples of arterial blood are taken at frequent intervals from the radial or femoral artery, and the concentration of the indicator in the arterial plasma is plotted against time. For simplicity, let us at first suppose that the concentration of indicator in the ejected bolus is uniform, as in Figure 6.2(b). The concentration against time plot tells us: (1) the time t needed for the bolus to pass a given point, and (2) the average concentration of indicator in the bolus over that period. Concentration, C, is by definition the injected mass, m, divided by the volume of plasma, V, in which the indicator became distributed: $C = m/V$. Therefore:

$$V = m/C$$

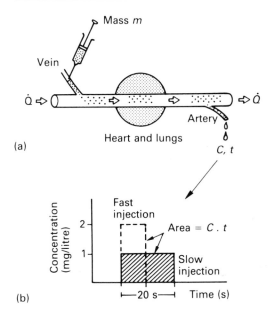

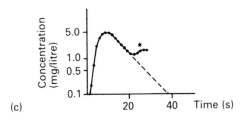

(a)

(b)

(c)

Figure 6.2 Hamilton's dye-dilution method. (a) Arterial concentration C depends on the mass of indicator injected (m) and the volume of blood in which it became diluted. (b) Idealized plot of arterial concentration against time. Although the shape of the plot depends on injection rate, the area $C \times t$ (20 mg s per litre) does not; the increase in concentration produced by a fast injection is offset by the shorter duration of the bolus. If the injected mass of dye is 2 mg, the cardiac output of plasma is $2/20 = 0.1$ litres/s, or 6 litres/min. For a haematocrit of 0.4, the cardiac output of blood is 10 litres/min. (c) The grim reality. True shape of the concentration curve, with concentration plotted on a logarithmic scale to linearize the decay and allow extrapolation past the recirculation hump (asterisk). Area under the extrapolated curve is used to calculate the cardiac output. (After Asmussen, E. and Nielsen, M. (1953) *Acta Physiologica Scandinavica*, **27**, 217)

For example, if 2 mg of indicator produces a mean plasma concentration of 1 mg/litre, the volume of distribution must be 2 litres. If this volume takes t seconds to pass a fixed point, the left ventricle pumps plasma along at rate V/t (2 litres in 20 s in Figure 6.2(b), or 6 litres/min). In other words the cardiac output of plasma can be calculated as:

Cardiac output of plasma =

$$\frac{V}{t} = \frac{\text{Mass of indicator } m}{\text{Mean concentration } C \times t}$$

The output of blood is then easily calculated, being the output of plasma divided by $1 -$ haematocrit (the haematocrit is the fraction of blood consisting of cells). Notice that the denominator $C.t$ in the above expression is the area under the plot of concentration against time. Thus:

Cardiac output of plasma =

$$\frac{\text{Mass of indicator}}{\text{Area under } C - t \text{ curve}}$$

In reality the $C-t$ plot is not a square wave; it is a curve which rises to a peak and decays exponentially (Figure 6.2c), but the above expression still applies. The exponential decay is caused by the ventricle ejecting only a fraction of its content with each systole, leaving some indicator behind. Indicator-free venous blood returning to the heart during each diastole dilutes the residual indicator, and this in turn is only partially ejected in the next systole, and so on. After about 15 s, however, the decay curve is disrupted by a 'recirculation hump'. This is caused by blood of high indicator concentration returning to the heart after completing one transit of the myocardial circulation (the shortest route back). To apply the above dilution equation, we must find the area under a $C-t$ curve uncomplicated by recirculation, and this is done by extrapolating the early part of the decay curve, before the recirculation hump. A semi-logarithmic plot facilitates the extrapolation, because it converts the exponential decay into a straight line; the latter is then extrapolated to a negligible concentration (conventionally 1% of the peak value) as in Figure 6.2c. The area under the corrected $C-t$ curve is computed and used to calculate cardiac output.

Pros and cons

The results agree with Fick's direct method to ±5%. The dilution method has an improved time resolution (30 s, cf. >5 min for Fick's method) and can be used in exercise, since ventricular catheterization is not required. The error involved in extrapolating the decay curve is, however, a drawback. In diseased hearts, where the initial part of the decay curve may be short and distorted, this can be a serious limitation.

Thermal dilution method

This variant of the dilution method is widely used in cardiac departments. Instead of a foreign chemical, temperature is used as the indicator. A known volume of cold saline is injected quickly into the right atrium, right ventricle or pulmonary artery, and the dilution of the cold saline by warm blood is recorded by a thermistor-tipped catheter (Swan–Ganz catheter) in the more distal pulmonary artery. Cardiac output can then be calculated from the area under the temperature–time plot and the amount of heat (i.e. cold) injected. The major advantage is that the recirculation problem is circumvented because the saline warms up to body temperature long before it returns to the right side. Another advantage is that the ejection fraction can be calculated from the step rise in temperature that follows each refilling of the heart by warm blood. One problem is heat transfer across the walls of the right ventricle and pulmonary artery, which can cause over-estimation of the distribution volume and therefore cardiac output; a computed correction is usually made for this.

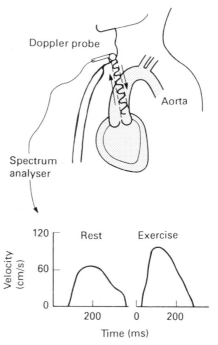

Figure 6.3 Transaortic pulsed Doppler method for measuring the mean velocity of blood across the aorta at each instant of systole. The area under the curve (velocity × time, i.e. distance) represents the average distance the blood advances along the aorta per stroke (stroke distance). Stroke volume is stroke distance × cross-sectional area of the aorta. Recordings at rest and during bicycle ergometer exercise at 75 W. (From Innes, J. A., Simon, T. D., Murphy, K. and Guz, A. (1988) *Quarterly Journal of Experimental Physiology*, **73**, 323–341, by permission)

6.3 Pulsed Doppler method

This is a relatively new and increasingly popular method in which a pulse of ultrasound is directed down the ascending aorta from a transmitter crystal at the suprasternal notch. Some of the ultrasound is reflected back by the red cells, and this is collected and analysed. Since the cells have a high velocity, the frequency of the returning sound waves is different from that of the transmitted signal; this is the Doppler effect, analogous to the change in pitch of a car siren as it speeds past.

The average blood velocity across the aorta at each instant is computed from the spectrum of frequencies in the returning signal, and the velocity is plotted against time as in Figure 6.3. To convert the time-averaged velocity (cm/s) to flow (cm^3/s) the diameter of the aorta must be measured by echocardiography (see Section 2.5) and the cross-sectional area, πr^2, then multiplied by mean velocity. The result, aortic flow, represents cardiac output minus coronary blood flow. Although the Doppler method has calibration and 'noise' problems, it has the enormous advantages of non-invasiveness and speed, and can record each individual ejection.

6.4 Examination of the peripheral pulse

The oldest, fastest, cheapest and easiest method of assessing cardiac output, albeit subjectively, is to lay a finger on the radial pulse. Heart rate can be measured and the finger also senses whether the pulse is 'strong' or 'weak', a strong pulse being associated with a large stroke volume (e.g. exercise) and a weak pulse associated with a low stroke volume (e.g. haemorrhage). What the finger actually detects is the expansion of the artery as pressure rises during systole. The rise in pressure, or 'pulse pressure', equals systolic pressure minus diastolic pressure, and this is easily measured with a sphygmomanometer (see Section 8.4). The relation between pulse pressure and stroke volume is illustrated in Figure 6.4. Most of the stroke volume (70–80% at rest) is temporarily accommodated in the elastic arteries, owing to the resistance of the arteriolar system to runoff. The distension of the elastic arteries raises the blood pressure and the amount by which pressure rises depends partly on the stroke volume and partly on the distensibility of the arterial system. Distensibility or 'compliance' is defined as change in volume per unit change in pressure:

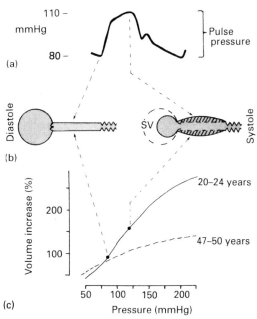

Figure 6.4 Relation of the pulse pressure to stroke volume. (a) Aortic pressure wave. (b) Left ventricle, elastic arterial system and resistance vessels during diastole and systole. SV is stroke volume. (c) Pressure–volume curve of the human thoracic aorta. The volume at diastolic pressure is expressed as 100% here. Note the decline in distensibility with age. Note also the flattening of the pressure–volume curve at high pressures, which indicates that compliance (distensibility) is decreasing. Consequently, a rise in mean pressure would increase the pulse pressure even if stroke volume remained the same ((a) After McDonald, D. A. (1974) *Blood Flow in Arteries*, Edward Arnold, London; and (c) after Hallock and Benson (1937) *Journal of Clinical Investigation*, **16**, 597)

Compliance = Increase in volume/Increase in pressure

Rearranging this, we can see how pulse pressure relates to stroke volume:

Pulse pressure =

$$\frac{\text{Stroke volume (minus Initial runoff)}}{\text{Compliance}}$$

In a young adult, arterial compliance is around 2 ml per mmHg at normal pressures. The compliance is not, however, a constant and is affected by three factors. (1) High arterial pressures and volumes reduce arterial compliance. This is evident from the curvature of the arterial pressure–volume relation in Figure 6.4. (2) High ejection velocities reduce compliance because the artery wall is a viscoelastic material (see Appendix II) and needs time to expand. During exercise the pulse pressure increases proportionately more than stroke volume because there is less time available for viscous relaxation in the wall. (3) Advancing age is associated with arteriosclerosis, a hardening of the artery walls, which reduces compliance and leads to large pulse pressures in the elderly.

Because arterial compliance is so variable, and also because the percentage runoff during early systole varies with peripheral resistance, the pulse pressure offers only an indirect assessment of stroke volume. Nevertheless, within its limitations the peripheral pulse provides an exceedingly convenient indication of changes in cardiac output in an individual patient from day to day.

6.5 Radionuclide ventriculography and other methods

Radionuclide ventriculography An intravenous injection of a radionuclide is given and the number of counts emanating from the ventricles is monitored by a precordial gamma camera. The radionuclide is commonly a compound of technetium that binds to red cells. The difference between the radioactive content of the ventricles in diastole and in systole allows calculation of ejection fraction and stroke volume.

Echocardiography (see Section 2.5 and Figure 7.20) The end-diastolic and end-systolic diameters of the ventricle can be estimated using echocardiography. These measurements can be converted into stroke volume if some assumptions are made about chamber shape.

Electromagnetic flowmeter This technique is used only in animal experiments, because it is necessary to place a curved magnet with its poles directly on either side of the aorta or pulmonary artery. Since blood is an electrical conductor, the flowing blood induces an electrical potential as it cuts the magnetic field. The measured potential is proportional to blood velocity (cm/s). The internal diameter of the vessel must be known to convert mean velocity to flow. Being small, this device can be left inside a conscious animal, transmitting a signal by telemetry (radiowaves), and in this way much has been learned about the regulation of stroke volume of unfettered exercising animals – the subject of the next chapter.

6.6 Summary

The 'gold-standard' method for measuring human cardiac output has been the *Fick principle*, namely, rate of uptake of solute = flow × concentration difference between incoming and outgoing fluid. Applied to the lungs, rate of oxygen uptake is measured by spirometry or expired air collection. The oxygen content of incoming venous blood is measured in a mixed venous blood sample, taken from the right ventricle by cardiac catheterization. Outgoing blood is sampled from a systemic artery. Pulmonary blood flow (i.e. right ventricular output) can then be calculated.

The *indicator or thermal dilution method* offers better time resolution. A small bolus of dye or cold saline is injected quickly into the right ventricle or pulmonary artery, and at a point downstream the concentration (or temperature as appropriate)-versus-time profile is recorded. From the mass of indicator injected (m) and the average measured concentration (C) the volume of blood in which the indicator has distributed is calculated ($V = m/C$). The time taken for this volume of blood to pass the sampling point gives the cardiac output.

More recent, high-technology methods include *pulsed Doppler ultrasound* measurement of aortic flow velocity. When coupled with an ultrasound measurement of aortic diameter, this enables aortic flow to be calculated as mean velocity × cross-sectional area. In *radionuclide ventriculography*, stroke volume is calculated by comparing the radioactive counts present in the ventricle during end-diastole and end-systole; then, cardiac output = heart rate × stroke volume.

The commonest, lowest technology method for assessing cardiac output, albeit qualitatively, is used at the clinic and bedside – counting the pulse and measuring blood pressure by sphygmomanometry. The pulse pressure, namely systolic pressure minus diastolic pressure, is proportional to stroke volume, although additional factors complicate this relation such as non-linear aortic compliance, runoff and rate of ejection.

Further reading

Hamilton, W. F. (1962) Measurement of the cardiac output. In *Handbook of Physiology, Cardiovascular System Circulation I* (eds W. F. Hamilton and P. Dow), American Physiological Society, Washington D.C., pp. 551–571

Loeppky, J. A., Greene, E. R., Hoekenga, D. E., Caprihan, A. and Luft, U. C. (1981) Beat-by-beat stroke volume assessment by pulsed Doppler in upright and supine exercise. *Journal of Applied Physiology*, **50**, 1173–1182

Schelbert, H. R., Verba, J. W., Johnson, A. D. *et al.* (1978) Non-traumatic determination of left ventricular ejection fraction by radionuclide angiography. *Circulation*, **51**, 902–909

Chapter 7
Control of stroke volume and cardiac output

7.1 Overview

Cardiac output ranges from 4 litres/min to 7 litres/min in a human adult at rest. The output correlates with the body surface area, which is about $1.8\,m^2$ in a 70 kg adult, and the resting cardiac output per unit surface area (the cardiac index) averages 3 litres/min per m^2. In everyday life the output is continually changing in response to circumstances. Moving from the lying position to standing reduces cardiac output by approximately 20%, while sleep reduces it by approximately 10%. A heavy meal, excitement or fear can increase the output by 20–30%. Pregnancy gradually raises the output by 40%. Heavy exercise causes the greatest increase, by as much as four times in untrained students and six times in Olympic athletes (see Chapter 15). Diseased hearts, on the other hand, have a much more restricted range of outputs, as Table 7.1 shows.

Table 7.1 Output of human heart (litres/min ± standard deviation)

	Rest	Exercise
Normal adult	6.0(±1.3)	17.5(±6.0)
Coronary artery disease	5.7(±1.5)*	11.3(±4.3)

*The output of the diseased heart was within the normal range at rest but became inadequate during exercise on a bicycle ergometer. Subjects were exercised to 85% of maximum heart rate or to onset of angina; $n = 30$ (normal) and $n = 20$ (diseased). After Rerych, S. K., Scholz, P. M., Newman, G. E. *et al.* (1978) *Annals of Surgery*, **187**, 449–458

Heart rate. Cardiac output is the product of heart rate and stroke volume and is usually altered by changes in both. In exercise, heart rate and stroke volume both increase. In other circumstances they can change in opposite directions. After a haemorrhage, for example, heart rate increases while stroke volume decreases (see Chapter 16). Autonomic control of heart rate was described in Chapter 4. This chapter concentrates on the control of stroke volume, and its coordination with heart rate and vascular factors to determine the cardiac output.

Stroke volume is regulated primarily by two opposing factors: the energy with which the myocytes contract and the arterial pressure against which they have to expel the blood (Figure 7.1). A highly energetic contraction produces a large stroke volume, other things being equal, while a high arterial pressure opposes ejection and reduces the stroke volume, other things again being equal.

The *energy of contraction* of the myocyte is a variable, regulated quantity, and can be increased by two processes. (1) Stretching the cells during diastole enhances their subsequent contractile energy; and since the stretch of the relaxed ventricle depends on the pressure distending it, contractile energy is regulated indirectly by the ventricular end-

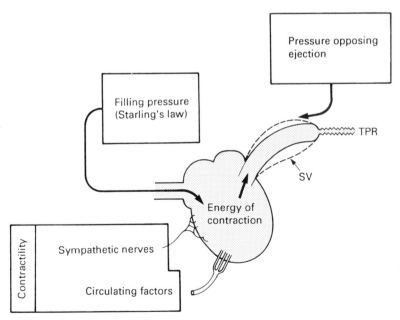

Figure 7.1 Diagram of principal factors regulating stroke volume (SV). The heart and lungs are shown as a single unit. TPR is total peripheral resistance, which influences arterial pressure

diastolic pressure. This is known as Starling's law of the heart. (2) The innate strength with which a myocyte contracts from a given initial stretch, or 'contractility', can be increased by nervous, hormonal and chemical influences, for example noradrenaline.

The *arterial pressure* opposing ejection has a negative effect on stroke volume. This is because the immediate effect of active tension is not to produce ejection but to raise intraventricular pressure during the isovolumetric phase of the cardiac cycle (see Section 2.2). Ejection cannot begin until ventricular pressure exceeds arterial pressure, and this consumes a substantial part of the energy available per contraction. If arterial pressure is raised, more of the contractile energy is consumed in raising the pressure in the isovolumetric phase and less remains for ejection. Since arterial pressure depends partly on total peripheral resistance (TPR), any rise in TPR tends to diminish the stroke volume.

Stroke volume is thus governed by three factors: (1) *stretch* during diastole, which depends on ventricular end-diastolic pressure, (2) *contractility*, which is modulated by sympathetic nerve activity and other chemical influences, and (3) *arterial pressure*, which opposes ejection and is influenced by TPR (see Figure 7.1). Each factor is next considered in more detail, beginning with the effect of stretch.

7.2 Contractile properties of isolated cardiac muscle

It is helpful to see how the contraction of an isolated strip of myocardium is affected by stretch and load before dealing with the intact heart. Papillary muscle is convenient for this purpose because its fibres run a fairly straight course.

Isometric contraction

To study the effect of stretch, the relaxed muscle is stretched to a known length by

means of a small weight or preload, and is then stimulated electrically (Figure 7.2). If the muscle is anchored between two rigid points, excitation cannot cause shortening; it produces tension (force) alone which can be measured by a force transducer. Contraction at constant length is called an isometric contraction, and is roughly analogous to isovolumetric contraction *in vivo*. The active tension generated during an isometric contraction is found to increase steeply with initial length, as shown by the length–tension relations in Figures 7.2(i) and 7.3. This demonstrates that *stretching the relaxed myocardium enhances its subsequent contractile energy*.

Isotonic contraction

To study the ability of muscle to shorten, one end of the muscle is left free to move but is compelled to lift a weight, so that it shortens under a constant tension. This is called an isotonic contraction and the weight is called the 'afterload'. (In intact ventricles, the afterload is related to arterial pressure and ventricular radius, as explained later.) If the afterload is increased, both the velocity of contraction and the amount of shortening are reduced (see Figure 7.2(ii) and (iii)). If, however, the resting papillary muscle is stretched by raising the preload, and the isotonic contraction repeated, the muscle now contracts with a greater velocity and achieves a greater shortening (see the red curves). These observations again demonstrate that the energy of contraction of isolated myocardium is a function of the resting fibre length.

The sarcomere length–tension relation

When a relaxed muscle is stretched the length of the basic contractile unit, the sarcomere, increases and this raises its contractile energy (Figure 7.3). Studies of sarcomere length by laser diffraction show that maximum contractile energy develops at

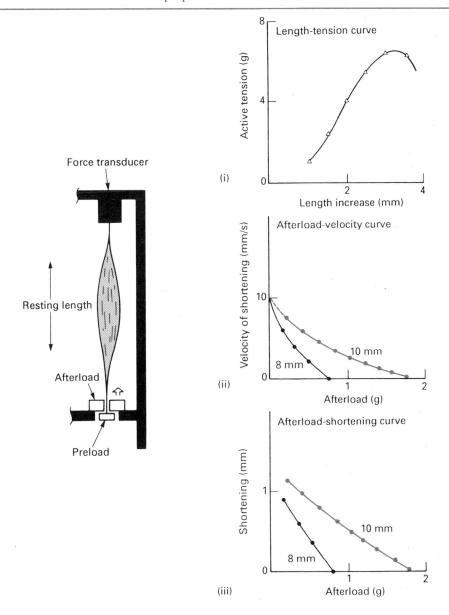

Figure 7.2 Contractile properties of myocardial muscle. Left: Simplified arrangement to study contraction of isolated cat papillary muscle. In isotonic contractions, the weight labelled 'afterload' is picked up as soon as shortening begins. The weight labelled 'preload' sets the resting length. If the preload is clamped in place, contraction becomes isometric. Right: Three fundamental relations: (i) isometric contraction at increasing lengths, (ii) and (iii) isotonic contractions beginning from two different resting lengths (8 mm and 10 mm). Contractile force, velocity and shortening are all increased by stretching the relaxed muscle. (After Sonnenblick, E. H. (1962) *American Journal of Physiology*, **202**, 931–939)

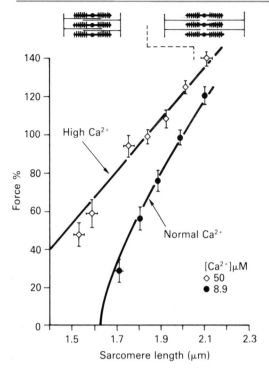

Figure 7.3 Effect of resting sarcomere length on contractile force of 'skinned' myocardium (rat trabecular muscle, *in vitro*). The sarcolemma has been permeabilized by a detergent and the muscle strip exposed to a physiological Ca^{2+} concentration (8.9 μM) or a saturating one that produces maximal contracture at each length (50 μM). Active force is expressed as a percentage of that developed at 2.1 μm length in a reference solution of 4.5 μM Ca^{2+}. The lower curve closely resembles that of intact, unskinned cardiac muscle. Sketches at top show change in resting actin–actin overlap with stretch. (From Kentish J. C., ter Keurs, H. E. D. J., Ricciardi, L., Bucx, J. J. J. and Noble, M. I. M. (1986) *Circulation Research*, **58** 755–768, by permission)

sarcomere lengths of 2.2–2.3 μm. The sarcomere length in intact hearts at normal end-diastolic pressures (0–9 mmHg) is below this optimal value, so the intact ventricle normally operates on the ascending limb of the length–tension curve. Beyond 2.2–2.3 μm, contractile force decays, but it is very difficult to stretch sarcomeres beyond this point, even *in vitro*, because they become very stiff: it is

therefore most unlikely that sarcomere lengths above 2.3 μm are ever produced in intact hearts during life.

Mechanisms underlying the length–tension relation

It was pointed out in Section 3.6 that stretching a cardiac fibre causes an immediate rise in contractile force (about 60% of the eventual rise), followed by a slower rise over many minutes. The delayed response is due to a rise in the systolic Ca^{2+} transient, but the immediate response involved no change in the size of the Ca^{2+} transient.

The question arises, then, 'How does an increase in sarcomere length cause an immediate rise in active tension?' Part of the explanation is that at sarcomere lengths below 2.0 μm, the opposing actin filaments overlap each other or buckle (being 1μm long each) and this interferes with the formation of actin–myosin crossbridges and hence with force generation (see Figure 7.3 top). Also, at <1.6μm the myosin filaments 'hit' the Z lines. When these various mechanical interferences are reduced by stretching the sarcomere, contractile force increases.

The same rod interferences operate in skeletal muscle, yet the length–tension curve of cardiac muscle is much steeper than that of skeletal muscle. This shows that some additional factor is at work in the myocardium. To investigate this, 'skinned' preparations have been employed in which the sarcolemma is either removed mechanically or permeabilized chemically, so that intracellular calcium ion concentration equilibrates with that in the bathing solution. The upper curve of Figure 7.3 shows the length–tension relation for skinned fibres when *all* the potential crossbridges at each sarcomere length are activated by a high Ca^{2+} bath (50 μM). A physiological concentration of cytoplasmic calcium (8.9 μM) evidently activates only a fraction of the crossbridges, so tension is reduced (lower curve). The lower curve closely resembles that for intact, unskinned fibres. The curve for partially activated fibres is much steeper than that for fully activated fibres and gradually approaches the full activation curve as sarcomere length is increased. This indicates that the fraction of potential crossbridges that are activated by physiological concentrations of Ca^{2+} increases with stretch ('length-dependent activation').

Length-dependent activation is due to an increase in the sensitivity of the contractile proteins to calcium with stretch. This is shown by the results in Figure 7.4. The curve relating active tension to Ca^{2+} concentration in skinned myocytes is shifted to the left when sarcomere length is increased, so there is a substantial reduction in the calcium concentration needed to produce 50% of maximal tension. This phenomenon is known as the 'length-dependence of calcium sensitivity'. How the sensitivity to Ca^{2+} is increased by stretch is still under investigation, but there is growing evidence that troponin C may be the length-sensor. Cardi-

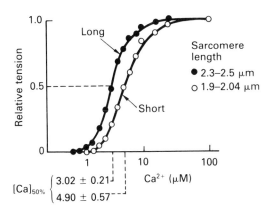

Figure 7.4 Sensitivity of contractile apparatus to calcium ion concentration. The graph shows the effect of bath Ca^{2+} concentration on the isometric force developed by chemically skinned rat ventricular muscle, at two different resting sarcomere lengths. Active tension is expressed as a fraction of the maximum tension at each sarcomere length. The figures below the graph show that the Ca^{2+} concentration required to produce 50% of the maximum response was reduced by stretch. (From Hibberd, M. G. and Jewell, B. R. (1982) *Journal of Physiology*, **329**, 527–540, by permission)

ac and skeletal muscle have different forms of troponin C, and substitution of the 'wrong' troponin C into a muscle cell alters its length–tension relation.

We can now turn from isolated muscle to the intact heart and consider the role of the length–tension relation in regulating stroke volume.

7.3 Starling's law of the heart

The length–tension relation in *intact* hearts was investigated by the German physiologist Otto Frank. In 1895 he studied the effect of diastolic stretch on the contraction of the frog ventricle. The aorta was ligated so that contraction was isovolumetric (i.e. roughly analogous to the isometric state) and fluid was injected into the chamber to stretch the wall. As shown in Figure 7.5, distension during diastole caused the development of a greater pressure during systole, indicating that the energy of contraction depended on diastolic distension.

Ernest Starling and his co-workers in London followed this up using the ejecting mammalian heart, and showed that diastolic stretch influences stroke volume. In Starling's classic experiments (see Figure 7.6) the isolated heart and lungs of a dog were perfused with warm oxygenated blood from a venous reservoir. The height of the reservoir above the heart controlled central venous pressure (CVP). CVP is the pressure in the great veins at their point of entry into the right atrium, and the pressure distending the right ventricle, right ventricular end-diastolic pressure (RVEDP), is almost equal to the CVP. (Similarly, pulmonary vein pressure governs left ventricle end-diastolic pressure, LVEDP. A general term for all these pressures is *'filling pressure'*.) The aortic pressure opposing outflow from the left ventricle was held constant by a variable resistance called a Starling resistor, and the combined stroke volumes of the two ventricles were recorded by a bell cardiometer. Being isolated and denervated, the

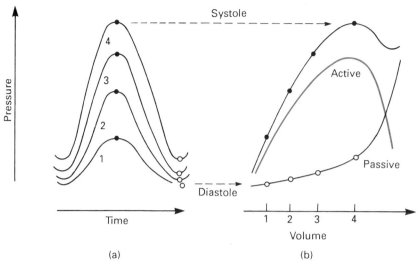

Figure 7.5 Effect of diastolic volume on energy of contraction, as measured by systolic pressure in an isovolumetric frog ventricle (aorta ligated). (a) Active pressure generated between diastole (open circles) and systole (closed circles) increases as ventricular volume is raised from 1 to 4 (arbitrary units). (b) Effect of volume plotted out. Bottom curve shows passive pressure–volume relation: note the increasing stiffness as the ventricle is distended. Top curve shows systolic pressure as function of diastolic volume. Red curve shows pressure generated actively, i.e. systolic pressure minus diastolic pressure. (After Otto Frank's seminal experiment of 1895)

heart–lung preparation was free of extrinsic nervous or hormonal influences. The major findings with the heart–lung preparation are as follows.

Active response to central venous pressure

When CVP is increased, ventricular end-diastolic pressure rises, and this increases the end-diastolic volume. The stretched ventricle at once develops a greater contractile energy, which results in the ejection of a greater stroke volume, as shown in Figure 7.7. Although a rise in CVP initially affects only the right side of the heart, the left ventricular stroke volume increases too within a few beats. This is because the increased right ventricular output raises the pressure in the pulmonary vessels, which in turn raises the filling pressure for the left ventricle.

The ventricular function curve

If filling pressure is raised in a series of steps, a curve can be plotted showing how

stroke volume increases with filling pressure. This is called a ventricular function curve, or *Starling curve* (see Figure 7.8). Stroke volume increases as a curvilinear function of filling pressure between zero and 10 mmHg, forming the 'ascending limb' of the Starling curve. In the human left ventricle *in situ*, the curve almost reaches a plateau above 10 mmHg filling pressure (see Figure 7.8b). During standing and sitting, the filling pressure for the left ventricle (left ventricular end-diastolic pressure, LVEDP) is 4–5 mmHg, and the heart is on the ascending limb of the curve, while in a supine subject (LVEDP 8–9 mmHg) the heart operates close to the plateau. In isolated dog hearts, the curve peaks at about 20 mmHg and then falls off (see Figure 7.8a), but human hearts *in vivo* probably never reach this 'descending limb'. Stroke volume declines in the over-distended preparation partly because the distended atrioventricular valves begin to leak and partly because the reduced curvature of the cardiac wall impairs the

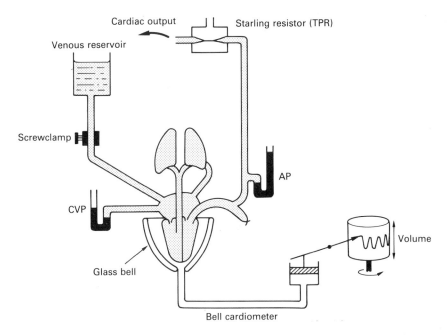

Figure 7.6 Isolated dog heart–lung preparation of Starling. The height of the venous reservoir and the screwclamp regulated central venous pressure (CVP). CVP and arterial pressure (AP) were measured by manometers and AP was held constant by a variable resistance equivalent to the total peripheral resistance (TPR). Ventricular volume was measured by Henderson's bell cardiometer (an inverted glass bell) which is attached to the atrioventricular groove by a rubber diaphragm. Beat-by-beat volume changes were recorded on a rotating smoked drum. (After Knowlton, F. P. and Starling, E. H. (1912) *Journal of Physiology*, **44**, 206–219)

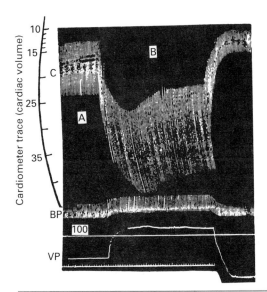

Figure 7.7 Volume of the ventricles recorded beat-by-beat by a cardiometer in the isolated heart–lung preparation; note the the inverted volume scale (ml): diastolic volume is at the bottom of the volume excursion, systolic volume is at the top. Stroke volume is represented by the distance from top to bottom of the trace. There was a 64% rise in stroke volume upon raising central venous pressure (VP) from 9 cmH$_2$O (period A) to 14 cmH$_2$O (period B), while arterial pressure is kept almost constant. There is a modest reduction in ventricular distension without any fall in stroke volume following the increase in work load, indicating a small rise in contractility (the *Anrep effect*). (From the original smoked-drum recordings of Patterson, S. W., Piper, H., Starling, E. H. (1914) *Journal of Physiology*, **48**, 465–511, by permission)

conversion of active tension into pressure (Laplace's law, see later).

The shape of the Starling curve is similar for the right and left ventricles except that the left ventricle has slightly higher filling pressures (see Figure 7.8 and Table 2.1). This is because the left ventricle has thicker, less distensible walls, and LVEDP has to be 4–5 mmHg higher than right ventricular end-diastolic pressure (RVEDP) to produce an equivalent stretch and output.

A bewildering variety of plots are called 'ventricular function curves' in the literature. This is because any graph whose ordinate is stroke volume or any other measure of contractile energy, and whose abscissa is filling pressure or any other index of resting fibre length, is a ventricular function curve. The curve therefore appears in many guises. For the *abscissa*, CVP is often chosen because human CVP is easily measured by catheterization and is an important regulator of average fibre length; however, its relation to fibre length is indirect and non-linear. Other indices of stretch include RVEDP, LVEDP, ventricular end-diastolic volume measured by two-plane cineangiography or radionuclide angiography, and ventricular diameter measured by echocardiography. All of these are indirect indices of resting fibre length. For the *ordinate*, stroke volume can serve as an index of contractile energy if mean arterial pressure is held constant, as in the heart–lung preparation. However, it obviously takes more energy to eject blood at a high pressure than at a low pressure, and the product of stroke volume and mean arterial pressure (the stroke work) is a better energy index (see Section 7.4).

The results shown in Figure 7.8 establish that *the greater the stretch of the ventricle in diastole, the greater the stroke work achieved in systole.* As Patterson, Piper and Starling concluded in 1914, 'The energy of contraction of a cardiac muscle fibre, like that of a skeletal muscle fibre, is proportional to the initial fibre length at rest'. This deduction, now honoured as Starling's law of the heart, has been amply confirmed by the direct studies illustrated in Figures 7.2 and 7.3.

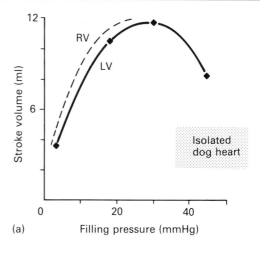

(a)

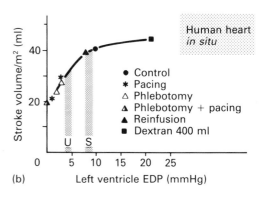

(b)

Figure 7.8 The ventricular function curve. (a) Effect of filling pressure on the stroke volume of an isolated dog heart pumping against a constant arterial pressure. The solid line shows Starling's data for left ventricular stroke volume (LV) and left atrial pressure. Dashed line is right ventricle. (b) Human ventricular function curve. Left ventricular end-diastolic pressure was varied *in vivo* by phlebotomy (venous bleeding) and other manoeuvres, and the effect on stroke volume per unit body surface area observed (stroke index). Normal range of human LVEDP in supine position (S) and upright position (U) are shown. Human ventricle *in situ* reaches a virtual plateau above 10 mmHg. A similar curve is obtained if stroke work is plotted. (From Parker, J. D. and Case, R. B. (1979), see Further Reading, by permission)

7.4 Stroke work and the pressure–volume loop

The energy expended in systole results partly in heat formation and partly in external mechanical work. The latter takes the form of an increase in the pressure and volume of blood in the arterial system. Mechanical work equals 1 newton force displaced over 1 metre. This definition needs to be modified slightly for a fluid because, in a fluid, force metre. This definition needs to be modified slightly for a fluid, because, in a fluid, force is applied not by a point but by a surface, such as the ventricle wall. The active force exerted on the blood by the ventricle in systole equals the rise in pressure ΔP times the wall area A (since pressure is by definition force per unit area). If the wall moves an average distance L, a volume (ΔV) equal to $L \times A$ is displaced into the aorta (Figure 7.9). Thus the work performed per beat, the stroke work (W), is:

$$W = F \times L = (\Delta P \times A) \times L = \Delta P \times (A \times L) = \Delta P \times \Delta V$$

In other words, stroke work equals the rise in

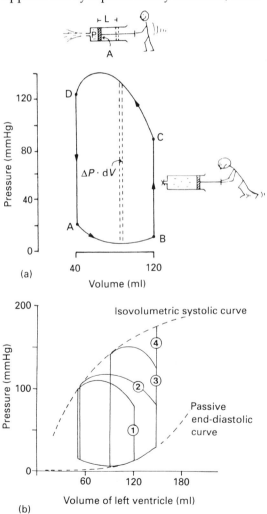

(a)

(b)

Figure 7.9 (a) Pressure–volume cycle of the human left ventricle. A, opening of mitral valve; AB, filling phase; B, closure of mitral valve at onset of systole; BC, isovolumetric contraction; C, opening of aortic valve; CD ejection phase; D, closure of aortic valve; DA, isovolumetric relaxation. The *mechanical work* performed equals the sum of all the *P.dV* strips within the loop, i.e. *total loop area*. The sketches indicate how the isovolumetric phase produces no external work despite a large energy expenditure by the myocardial manikin. (b) Factors influencing the pressure–volume cycle. The lower border is set by the passive pressure–volume curve of the relaxed ventricle. The upper boundary is set by the systolic pressure that would be produced in a purely isovolumetric contraction from a given end-diastolic volume; this line represents the Frank–Starling mechanism. Loop 1 represents a control state. Loop 2 shows the effect of increasing the end-diastolic volume; stroke volume increases, provided arterial pressure is held steady. If arterial pressure is then raised (loop 3), stroke volume decreases, provided end-diastolic volume is held steady. Line 4 depicts a purely isovolumetric contraction

ventricular blood pressure × volume ejected (stroke volume).

Ventricular blood pressure varies throughout the ejection phase, so to evaluate stroke work properly it is necessary to return to the plot of ventricular pressure against volume described in Section 2.3. This is reproduced in Figure 7.9(a). During isovolumetric contraction (line BC) the heart is 'working' very hard in the everyday sense of the word (consuming metabolic energy and oxygen to generate force), but since no blood is transported out of the system, the ventricle accomplishes no external work. This phase can be likened to a man trying to push over a house; he accomplishes no external work but consumes a lot of oxygen in the process. At point C the aortic valve opens; the height of line BC is set by the diastolic arterial pressure. In the ejection phase (CD), external work is accomplished. Since the total *stroke work* is the sum of the pressure gain × displaced volume at each instant ($\int \Delta P \cdot dV$), it equals the *total area within the pressure–volume loop*.

Figure 7.9(b) shows how the Frank–Starling mechanism affects the pressure–volume loop. The loop is confined within two lines. The lower confine is the end-diastolic pressure–volume curve as explained above; each contraction begins from this line. The upper confine is the curve relating systolic pressure to end-diastolic volume in a purely isovolumetric contraction (see Figure 7.5b). This line depicts the contractile energy available due to the Frank–Starling mechanism. If ejection were prevented, ventricular pressure would just reach this upper confine. Loop 1 represents a normal cycle, in which ejection occurs. The aortic valve closes when the end-systolic pressure and volume reach the upper confining line. In loop 2, the end-diastolic volume has been raised, increasing the contractile energy by the Frank–Starling mechanism. Stroke volume increases, provided that the arterial pressure opposing ejection is prevented from rising. If, however, the arterial pressure is raised, as in loop 3, more of the available energy goes into raising ventricular pressure and stroke volume decreases. If ejection is prevented totally, as

in line 4, stroke volume and stroke work are zero but maximum systolic pressure is generated.

7.5 Control of ventricular filling and central venous pressure

Because of the Frank–Starling mechanism, any factor that affects end-diastolic volume also affects cardiac output. End-diastolic volume (EDV) depends primarily on the distensibility of the ventricle and on the transmural pressure distending it. Ventricular distensibility decreases with stretch (rather like the distensibility of a bicycle tyre), so EDV becomes less and less sensitive to diastolic pressure above approximately 10 mmHg. This can be seen in Figure 7.9(b). Transmural pressure is the internal pressure minus the external pressure (intrathoracic pressure).

Pressure outside the heart

Intrathoracic pressure falls from about $-5\,cmH_2O$ at the end of expiration to $-10\ cmH_2O$ at the end of inspiration. Inspiration thus produces a suction effect around the heart and central veins, enhancing right ventricular filling. Conversely, when intrathoracic pressure becomes positive, as for example during a forced expiration (Valsalva manoeuvre; see Chapter 15), ventricular filling is reduced. Pressure outside the ventricle also becomes positive in patients with constrictive pericarditis and pericardial effusions, impairing filling and output.

Pressure inside: control of central venous pressure (CVP)

End-diastolic pressure in the right ventricle is nearly equal to central venous pressure, so the latter plays a key role in regulating stroke volume. Central venous pressure is set by the interplay of a number of factors:

1. *Blood volume*. About two-thirds of the entire blood volume is located in the venous system, so the greater the blood volume, the greater the average venous pressure. Conversely, haemorrhage or dehydration reduces the blood volume and lowers CVP, unless compensated for by venoconstriction.

2. *Gravity*. Gravity, venous tone and the muscle pump together govern the *distribution* of venous blood between peripheral veins and thoracic veins. In a standing man, gravity redistributes around 500 ml of blood from the intrathoracic vessels into the veins of the lower limbs (venous 'pooling'). This reduces the CVP, and stroke volume declines. Conversely, lying down redistributes venous blood from the lower limbs into the thoracic vessels, and stroke volume increases.

3. *Peripheral venous tone*. The veins of the skin, kidneys and splanchnic system are innervated by sympathetic nerves that cause venoconstriction. The nervous system can thus control the proportion of blood in the peripheral veins and thereby influence CVP. Venoconstriction occurs during exercise, stress, deep respiration, haemorrhage, shock and cardiac failure. Conversely, venodilatation occurs in skin vessels under hot conditions for reasons of temperature regulation, and incidentally lowers the CVP.

4. *The muscle pump*. Rhythmic exercise repeatedly compresses the deep veins of the limbs and displaces venous blood centrally. This can enhance CVP and stroke volume during dynamic exercise. At the opposite extreme, guardsmen standing at attention for long periods in hot weather have an embarrassing propensity to faint, partly because their muscle pump is inactive. Combined with gravitational venous pooling and heat-induced venodilatation, this reduces the CVP and stroke volume, leading to cerebral hypoperfusion.

5. *Respiration*. During inspiration, intrathoracic pressure becomes more negative and intra-abdominal pressure more positive. This increases the venous pressure gradient from abdomen to thorax and promotes filling of the central veins.

6. *Cardiac output*. The pumping action of the heart transfers blood from the venous system into the arterial system, and this not only raises arterial pressure but also simultaneously lowers the central venous pressure (Figure 7.10). If uncorrected, the fall in CVP and rise in arterial pressure then act as a brake on output. This important negative effect is considered further in Section 7.9.

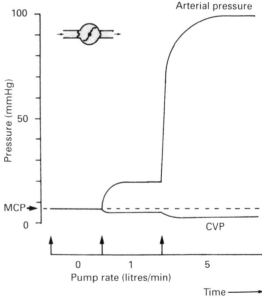

Figure 7.10 Effect of a pump on input and output pressure: volume transfer lowers the input pressure, as well as raising output pressure. At zero pumping rate, the central venous pressure (CVP) and arterial pressure would be equal (mean circulatory pressure, MCP). When volume transfer rate is increased, CVP changes, though not as much as arterial pressure because veins are an order of magnitude more compliant than arteries. (From Bern, R. M. and Levy, M. N. (1981) *Cardiovascular Physiology*, C. V. Mosby Co., St. Louis, by permission)

7.6 Operation of Starling's law in man

The Frank–Starling mechanism has many important effects, of which the most vital is to *balance the outputs of the right and left ventricle*. It also contributes to an increase in stroke volume during upright exercise if CVP rises (see Chapter 15). It mediates postural hypotension (a fall in cardiac output and blood pressure leading to dizziness following a fall in CVP in the upright posture) and it mediates the arterial hypotension that follows haemorrhage (see Chapter 16). It also causes a fall in stroke volume during the Valsalva manoeuvre (forced expiration, see Chapter 15).

To expand on the single most important role, it is vital that right ventricular output equals left ventricular output, except transiently for a few beats. A mere 1% imbalance between the outputs, such as a right ventricular output of 5.05 litres/min and a left output of 5.00 litres/min would, if sustained, raise the pulmonary blood volume from its normal level of 0.6 litres to 2.1 litres in half-an-hour, causing pulmonary congestion and oedema. In heavy exercise, with outputs around 25 litres/min, a sustained imbalance would be catastrophic within minutes. The Frank–Starling mechanism, however, preserves a balance between the two outputs. If right ventricular output transiently exceeds that from the left ventricle, pulmonary blood volume increases slightly and raises pressure in the pulmonary veins, which constitutes the left ventricle filling pressure. This distends the left ventricle and, by the length–tension mechanism, raises left ventricular output. The opposite happens if left ventricular output transiently exceeds right output. The two outputs are thus kept equal in the long term. Common situations that provoke a transient imbalance include standing up, where the right output drops below the left output for a few beats (see 'Gravity' above), and inspiration, where right output transiently exceeds left output owing to the operation of the respiratory pump and the fall in pulmonary vascular resistance as the lungs expand.

Caution: 'venous return' in the intact circulation

'Venous return' is the flow of blood into the right side of the heart, and it is driven by the pressure drop between the capillaries and central veins. In the intact circulation, venous return must equal the cardiac output in the steady state because the circulation is a closed system of tubes: any inequality can only be transient. In general, it is best to avoid the notion that venous return 'controls' cardiac output, because this is a circular (literally) and unhelpful viewpoint. In the steady state, venous return *is* the cardiac output, simply observed in veins rather than arteries. Venous return is thus directly dependent on cardiac output. Central venous pressure by contrast is an independent variable (it can be adjusted by venous tone) and can regulate the stroke volume. Venous return 'controls' cardiac output only in the sense that transient inequalities between the two alter the CVP.

Guyton's graphical analysis of output control

The pivotal role of CVP is illustrated by a plot devised by Guyton. His 'cardiac output curve' (Figure 7.11) shows how CVP raises the output by the Frank–Starling mechanism, provided that heart rate and arterial pressure are unchanged. The direct hydraulic effect of CVP is, by contrast, to oppose venous return, because a high CVP reduces the pressure gradient driving blood from the capillaries into the great veins. This effect is shown as a 'venous return curve' in Guyton's plot. If flow ceased altogether, pressures would in principle equilibrate throughout the circulation to produce a 'mean circulatory pressure' (approximately 7 mmHg), so the venous return curve is shown falling to zero flow at approximately 7 mmHg. Since the axes for the output curve and return curve are the same, the two curves can be plotted on the same graph. Cardiac output and venous return must be equal when the circulation is in a steady state and this happens at only

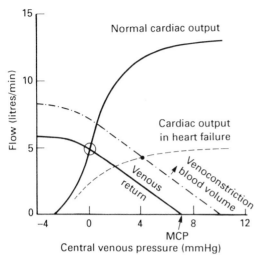

Figure 7.11 Guyton's analysis of the circulation. The cardiac output–CVP relation follows Starling's law of the heart, at constant heart rate. The venous return curve reflects blood flow from the peripheral vasculature into the central veins (see text). MCP is mean circulatory pressure at zero flow. The normal operating point is where the two lines cross, i.e. output equals return (open circle). The output curve can be shifted upwards by increased contractility (not shown) and downwards by impaired contractility, as in heart failure (dashed curve). The venous return curve is shifted upwards if MCP is increased by venoconstriction or increased plasma volume; or downwards if MCP is reduced by hypovolaemia. (After Guyton, A. C., Jones, C. E. and Coleman, T. G. (1973) *Circulatory Physiology: Cardiac Output and its Regulation*, Saunders, Philadelphia)

one point – the point of intersection of the two curves, where CVP creates the same output and return.

Guyton's graphical method can also be used to analyse altered states, as illustrated in Figure 7.11. In cardiac failure the myocardium is weak, so the output curve is depressed. Mean circulatory pressure (MCP) is raised, however, due to venoconstriction and fluid retention, and this raises the venous return curve. The new steady state (filled circle) occurs at a cardiac output that is only slightly subnormal, but the CVP is greatly raised – a characteristic feature of right ventricular failure (Chapter 16).

Laplace's law and wall tension

The *radius* of the heart has a physical effect on the conversion of a given muscle tension in the wall into pressure within the chamber, and this becomes important clinically when the heart is highly distended, as in heart failure. In any hollow chamber it is the radius that relates wall tension to internal pressure, as pointed out in 1806 by a French mathematician, the Marquis de Laplace – in a treatise on celestial mechanics! Laplace's law states that the pressure P within a sphere is proportional to the wall tension and is inversely proportional to the internal radius, r:

$$P = \frac{2T}{r} \tag{7.1}$$

'Tension' is defined as stress, S, times wall thickness, w. Stress is the force per unit cross-sectional area of wall. Laplace's law can also be written, therefore, as

$$P = \frac{2Sw}{r} \tag{7.2}$$

The involvement of radius is readily understood by considering the wall's curvature. As radius increases, curvature is reduced, so a smaller component of the wall tension is angled towards the cavity, generating less pressure (Figure 7.12). Thus, the curvature of the ventricle wall determines how effectively the active wall tension is converted into intraventricular pressure. Since the Frank–Starling mechanism requires some increase in chamber size, it also involves a small fall in mechanical efficiency. This becomes a dominating effect in grossly dilated, failing hearts and contributes to their low outputs (Chapter 16).

Laplace's law can be rearranged to give $S = Pr/2w$, and this helps us to understand what governs the *afterload* on myocytes in an intact heart. The afterload is the stress, S, during systole, and from the statement $S = Pr/2w$ we see that it depends not only on arterial pressure but also on chamber radius and wall thickness. Since both pressure and radius decline in the later stages of ejection, there is a gradual reduction in

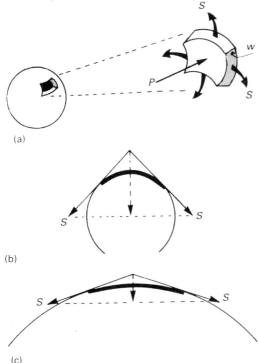

(a)

(b)

(c)

Figure 7.12 Relation between wall stress (*S*), pressure (*P*) and curvature of a hollow sphere; stress is force per unit cross-sectional area of wall. (a) Depicts a hollow sphere, such as a tennis ball, with an 'exploded' segment showing the two circumferential wall stresses. (b) Shows, in two dimensions, how the wall stresses (tangential arrows) give rise to an inward stress equal and opposite to pressure. Arrow length is proportional to stress magnitude. The thick line represents a muscle segment exerting tension. (c) Shows how an increase in radius reduces curvature, which in turn reduces the inward component of the wall stress. w, Wall thickness.

afterload, which facilitates late ejection. Any contraction in which afterload changes is not a truly isotonic one, and is called auxotonic.

Summary of Starling's law of the heart

Few summaries of the operation of Starling's law in man could be more memorable than Professor Alan Burton's rhyme, 'What goes in, must come out':

The great Dr. Starling, in his Law of the Heart
Said the output was greater if, right at the start,
The cardiac fibers were stretched a bit more,
So their force of contraction would be more than before.
Thus the larger the volume in diastole
The greater the output was likely to be.

If the right heart keeps pumping more blood than the left,
The lung circuit's congested; the systemic – bereft.
Since no-one is healthy with pulmo-congestion,
The Law of Doc. Starling's a splendid suggestion.
The balance of outputs is made automatic
And blood-volume partition becomes steady-static.

When Guardsmen stand still and blood pools in their feet
Frank–Starling mechanics no longer seem neat.
The shift in blood volume impairs C-V-P,
Which shortens the fibers in diastole.
Contractions grow weaker and stroke volume drops
Depressing blood pressure, and down the Guard flops.

But when the heart reaches a much larger size,
This leads to heart failure, and often, demise.
The relevant law is not Starling's, alas,
But the classical law of Lecompte de Laplace.
Your patient is dying in decompensation,
So reduce his blood volume or call his relation.

(From *Physiology and Biophysics of the Circulation* (1972), Year Book Medical Publishers, Chicago, by courtesy of the publishers. With apologies to Alan Burton's spirit for the addition of verse 3.)

7.7 Effects of arterial pressure on stroke volume

Arterial pressure affects the output of the heart both directly and indirectly.

Direct effect: the pump function curve

As stated in Section 7.1, a high arterial pressure directly opposes ejection. One of the basic properties of any pump, for example a laboratory roller pump, is that the outflow goes down when the pressure at the outlet is raised (Figure 7.13, dotted line). This relation is called a 'pump function curve' and its intercepts characterize the power of the pump. The cardiac pump obeys the same rule; the direct effect of a high arterial pressure is to depress the stroke volume by increasing the proportion of the available energy that is consumed in the isovolumetric contraction phase. This is illustrated by pressure–volume loop 3 in Figure 7.9. Because arterial pressure depends partly on the resistance of the peripheral circulation, stroke volume is influenced by vascular resistance. Thus, the stroke volume of failing hearts can be improved by treatment with peripheral vasodilator drugs.

Secondary effects of arterial pressure on stroke volume

If ventricular end-diastolic volume is not artificially held constant, there is a further change after arterial pressure is raised. The initial decrease in ejection allows ventricular diastolic volume to increase, since input continues unabated for the next few beats. This enhances contractile energy by the Frank–Starling mechanism and helps to restore stroke volume within a few beats. This is beautifully illustrated by Starling's experiment, reproduced in Figure 7.14. Another way of putting this is to say that the Frank–Starling mechanism displaces the pump function curve upwards (Figure 7.13, dashed line).

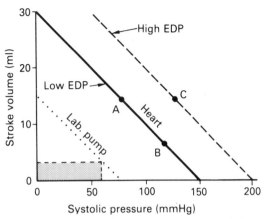

Figure 7.13 Pump function curves. Dotted line: output of a laboratory roller pump *versus* outflow pressure. Volume × pressure (area of shaded rectangle) is stroke work. Solid line: left ventricular stroke volume as a function of pressure opposing ejection in the isolated dog heart, with end-diastolic pressure (EDP) held constant. Raising the ejection pressure reduces the stroke volume from A to B. Dashed line: if EDP is raised, the Frank–Starling mechanism shifts the pump function line to a higher energy level and stroke volume is restored (C) as in Starling's experiment of Figure 7.14. The increased pressure intercept at zero output corresponds to the increase isovolumetric pressure with distension in Frank's experiment (see Figure 7.5). (After Elzinga, G. and Westerhof, N. (1979) *Circulation Research*, **32**, 178–186, and Weber, K. T., Janicki, J. S. and Hefner, L. L. (1976) *American Journal of Physiology*, **231**, 337–343)

In hearts *in situ* a third factor, the baroreceptor reflex, comes into play and leads to a fall in stroke volume. The baroreceptor reflex is described fully in Chapter 14, but in brief it is a nervous reflex triggered by a rise in arterial pressure. The reflex reduces the activity of the cardiac sympathetic nerves, diminishing the heart rate and contractility (Figure 7.15). In the intact heart *in situ* the effect of arterial pressure on stroke volume thus depends on the interplay of three effects (direct opposition, ventricular distension and altered sympathetic drive) and the outcome depends on their balance in the specific situation.

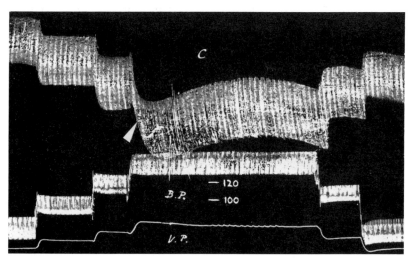

Figure 7.14 Changes in ventricular volume (top) and stroke volume (distance from top to bottom of upper trace) upon raising the arterial blood pressure (*B.P.*) opposing ejection via an artificial resistance device. Starling isolated heart–lung preparation; other details as in Figure 7.7. A high arterial pressure depresses stroke volume initially (white arrowhead) in accordance with the pump function relation. Continuing venous inflow leads, however, to a rise in venous filling pressure (*V.P.*) and ventricular distension. This raises contractile energy and restores stroke volume. There is later a small reduction in distension without any fall in stroke volume, indicating that increased work loads produce a small rise in contractility (Anrep effect). (Smoked-drum recording from Patterson, S. W., Piper, H. and Starling, E. H. (1914) *Journal of Physiology*, **48**, 465–511, by permission)

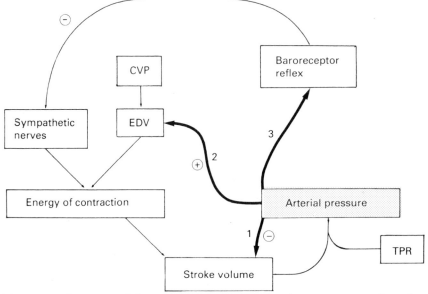

Figure 7.15 Summary of three effects of a rise in arterial pressure on stroke volume. Effect 1: increased afterload reduces stroke volume. Effect 2: a compensatory rise in stroke volume is mediated by increased ventricular distension. Effect 3: a fall in stroke volume is mediated by a reflex reduction in contractility. CVP, central venous pressure; EDV, end-diastolic volume; TPR, total peripheral resistance

7.8 Regulation of contractile force by extrinsic factors

Meaning of 'contractility' and inotropic state

Contractile energy is affected by chemical influences outside the myocyte (extrinsic regulation) as well as by resting fibre length (intrinsic regulation). *A change in contractile energy that is **not** due to changes in fibre length is called a change in contractility.* This definition of contractility specifically excludes the Frank–Starling mechanism.

The term 'inotropic state' is synonymous with contractility. The most important natural inotropic (strengthening) agent is noradrenaline, the neurotransmitter released from sympathetic nerve terminals within the myocardium. Other important physiological inotropic factors include circulating adrenaline, angiotensin II and extracellular Ca^{2+} ions.

Effect of a positive inotropic agent, noradrenaline

Noradrenaline is released from sympathetic nerve terminals in the ventricle wall and binds to β_1-receptors on the myocytes. This activates the G_s protein–cAMP–protein kinase A –Ca^{2+} channel phosphorylation sequence (see Section 4.4 and Figure 4.7). This leads to an increase in the inward calcium current during the plateau of the action potential, which in turn builds up the intracellular calcium store. Aequorin emission studies show that more free Ca^{2+} is then liberated from the store during depolarization, increasing the proportion of crossbridges activated and generating a greater contractile force. In addition, the Ca^{2+} uptake pumps of the sarcoplasmic reticulum are accelerated, via phosphorylation of phospholamban, resulting in a shorter systole. The effect of noradrenaline is therefore to stimulate a more forceful and shorter systole. This has the following

effects on ventricular pressure and volume.

Ventricular pressure rises more rapidly in the isovolumetric phase (Figure 7.16a) and a higher arterial pressure is produced. The maximum rate of rise of pressure, dP/dt_{max}, can be measured with a transducer-tipped cardiac catheter and may, with caution, be used as an index of myocardial contractility. The need for caution arises from the fact that dP/dt_{max} is affected also by initial fibre length and hence end-diastolic volume (see Figure 7.5).

Ejection fraction increases, because both the velocity of contraction and the shortening are enhanced by noradrenaline. Ejection fraction is often used clinically as an indirect index of contractility. The enhanced transfer of blood out of the central veins into the arterial system lowers the filling pressure, so heart size is reduced in diastole as well as systole (Figure 7.16b).

Stroke volume increases transiently as ejection fraction rises but is then limited by the concomitant fall in end-diastolic pressure and rise in arterial pressure. If these counter-productive pressure changes are prevented by experimental intervention (as at signal B in figure 7.16b) or by peripheral vascular adjustments (as happens in exercise), a substantial increase in stroke volume occurs.

The duration of systole grows briefer, which helps to preserve diastolic filling time. The shorter ejection time does not significantly curtail stroke volume because the velocity of shortening is increased.

The net effect of noradrenaline then is to increase arterial pressure and ejection fraction and to reduce ejection time, EDP and heart size. Stroke volume increases substantially only if the resulting changes in arterial pressure and EDP are offset by peripheral circulatory adjustments.

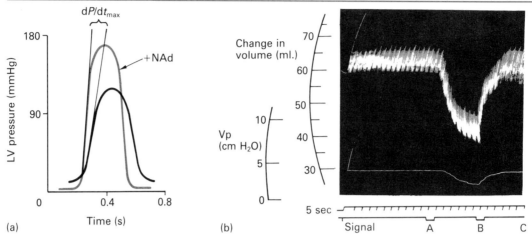

Figure 7.16 Effect of sympathetic stimulation or noradrenaline on cardiac performance. (a) Left ventricular pressure wave shows increased rate of climb (dP/dt_{max}), increased peak pressure, reduced EDP and reduced duration. (b) Combined stroke volume recorded by a cardiometer with heart rate held constant. The left cardiac sympathetic nerves were stimulated continuously from point A onwards. An increase in ejection fraction caused right atrial pressure (Vp) and cardiac volume to fall, and the Frank–Starling mechanism then largely prevented any rise in stroke volume. Enhanced contractility is evident from the maintenance of a normal stroke volume despite a smaller end-diastolic volume. At B the filling pressure was artificially restored to its previous level, allowing the effect of contractility on stroke volume to be fully expressed. (From Linden, R. J. (1968) *Anaesthesia*, **23**, 566–584, by permission)

Sympathetic innervation and the family of ventricular function curves

The anatomy of the cardiac sympathetic nerves was described in Chapter 4. The left nerves supply mainly atrial and ventricular muscle, while the right nerves supply the pacemaker and conduction system. The sympathetic firing rate increases in response to exercise, orthostasis (standing up), stress and haemorrhage, raising the ejection fraction in these conditions.

Sympathetic stimulation augments the contractile energy produced at a given end-diastolic length. The effect of this is to shift the entire ventricular function curve upwards and make it steeper (Figure 7.17). Sarnoff showed in the 1960s that this shift occurs in graded fashion so that the heart has not just one Starling curve but an entire 'family' of curves, depending on the intensity of stimulation. A change in stroke work can be produced either by movement along one Starling curve (involving a change in filling pressure and contractile energy but not contractility), or by movement from one curve to another curve (involving a change in contractility). *In vivo*, both processes usually operate simultaneously because both the inotropic drive and filling pressure are altered by challenges like exercise and postural change.

Figure 7.18(a) illustrates the effect of sympathetic activity on the pressure–volume loop. The upper confine of the loop is the pressure generated by isovolumetric contraction from a given diastolic volume. An increase in contractility causes the upper confine to steepen and shift upwards. This allows ejection pressure and ejection fraction to increase. The increased ejection fraction reduces the end-diastolic volume, however, and this in turn limits the growth in stroke volume (as in the experiment of Figure 7.16b). Stroke work (i.e. loop area) increases. During hard dynamic exercise not only is contractility increased but also the end-diastolic volume is increased by venoconstriction and the muscle pump, resulting in a much larger

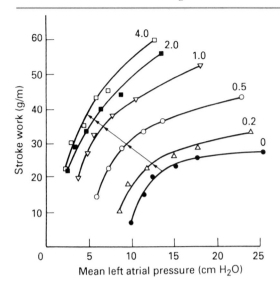

Figure 7.17 Effect of graded cardiac sympathetic nerve activity on ventricular function curve (isolated canine heart–lung). Sympathetic stimulation at frequencies 0 to 4 per s generate a 'family' of curves of increasing contractility. (From Sarnoff, S. J. and Mitchell, J. H. (1962) *Handbook of Physiology, Cardiovascular System,* Vol. 1, *Circulation,* American Physiological Society, Baltimore, pp. 489–532, by permission)

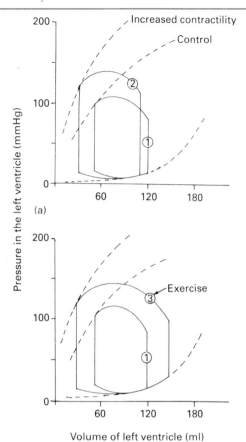

Figure 7.18 Schematic pressure–volume loops for human left ventricle when myocardial contractility is increased. The upper dashed confine is the relation between systolic pressure and end-diastolic volume for a purely isovolumetric contraction (Frank–Starling mechanism). (a) Loop 1 represents a basal state. Loop 2 represents a state of increased contractility. Ejection fraction is increased, so end-diastolic volume falls unless actively regulated. Loop area (stroke work) is increased. (b) During exercise (loop 3), contractility is raised by sympathetic activity and end-diastolic volume is raised by peripheral circulatory adjustments (venoconstriction, muscle pump). The increase in stroke volume is now much greater

rise in stroke volume and stroke work, as shown in Figure 7.18(b).

Note on the parasympathetic innervation of myocardium. The vagal nerves innervate the conduction system and atrial muscle, but the ventricular muscle is not well innervated, except in diving mammals. In man, vagal innervation of the ventricle is mainly confined to the endocardial zone, where the Purkinje fibres lie, and is very sparse in the rest of the ventricular myocardium. The vagal neurotransmitter, acetylcholine, binds to muscarinic receptors and exerts a negative inotropic effect (weakening) on atrial contractility. This is mediated by an inhibitory G_i protein and fall in intracellular cAMP (see Figure 4.7). Since few parasympathetic fibres innervate the human ventricle, it is thought that their effect on human stroke volume is slight. In the dog, maximal vagal stimulation reduces ventricular contractility by 15–25%, but this is associated with a reduction in

noradrenaline level in the coronary venous blood. It seems that, in the dog, the vagal fibres terminate close to sympathetic endings and can inhibit the release of noradrenaline from these endings. Conversely, the sympathetic fibres can release the neuropeptides neuropeptide Y and galanin, which inhibit the release of ACh by vagal fibres. In the SA node, this facilitates an increase in heart rate.

Circulating inotropic factors

The human adrenal medulla secretes the hormones adrenaline and noradrenaline (the *catecholamines*) in the ratio of approximately 4:1. Their concentrations can increase up to 20 times in maximal exercise. Adrenaline has similar effects on the heart to noradrenaline, but at physiological levels its cardiac effects are small compared with those of the cardiac sympathetic nerves. β-agonists like isoprenaline and dopamine have similar inotropic and chronotropic effects to the catecholamines.

Angiotensin, a circulating hormone (see Section 12.6), has a positive inotropic action. It acts partly by enhancing the plateau Ca^{2+} current and, to a greater degree, by neuromodulation; it acts upon the sympathetic terminals to facilitate the release of noradrenaline (see Figure 12.12). Angiotensin levels, like those of circulating adrenaline and noradrenaline, increase in exercise.

Calcium ions and certain *drugs* are again positive inotropic agents but unlike the catecholamines, calcium ions do not shorten systole. Studies with intracellular aequorin show that extracellular Ca^{2+} and the drugs digoxin, caffeine and theophylline all act by raising the concentration of free sarcoplasmic Ca^{2+} ions during excitation (see Figure 3.13); this rise is due to an increased store of calcium in the sarcoplasmic reticulum. In the longer term, *thyroxine* too exerts a positive inotropic effect.

Negative inotropic factors, including ischaemic disease

There are also negative inotropic agents that reduce contractility. They include hyper-

kalaemia, acidosis, hypoxia, acetylcholine and cholinergic agonists, β-receptor antagonists such as propranolol and practolol, calcium-channel blockers like verapamil and nifedipine, barbiturates and many anaesthetics.

Ischaemia of myocardium is, medically, a particularly important negative inotropic influence. Myocardial ischaemia is associated with hypoxia and intracellular acidosis, both of which depress contractility. Consequently, coronary artery disease commonly leads to impaired contractility and exercise limitation (see Table 7.1). Hypoxia acts by raising intracellular inorganic phosphate concentration, which interferes with the binding of Ca^{2+} to troponin C. Hypoxia also raises intracellular H^+ concentration. Acidosis markedly reduces the sensitivity of the myofibrils to Ca^{2+}, probably by interfering with the Ca^{2+} – troponin binding process.

Contractility is also severely impaired in chronic cardiac failure of non-coronary origin, as described in Chapter 16.

Inotropic effect of beat frequency (the interval–tension relation)

The American physiologist Bowditch noted in 1871 that the force of beating of a frog heart increases markedly when the interval between beats is reduced. The same phenomenon occurs in isolated cardiac muscle stimulated electrically, and is not due to noradrenaline release.

The Bowditch rate effect is illustrated in Figure 7.19(a). Upon reducing the frequency of electrical stimulation, the first beat is stronger than usual but subsequent beats grow progressively weaker in a 'staircase' pattern, until a new steady state is reached. When stimulation rate is increased, the first beat is weaker than the preceding ones, then the strength of the contraction increases progressively. The Bowditch rate effect is caused by changes in the size of the systolic Ca^{2+} transient, as the lower record in Figure 7.19(a) shows. The rise in Ca^{2+} with heart rate appears to be caused by a rise in intracellular Na^+ (due to the increased number of depolarization spikes per minute), which slows the expulsion of intracellular Ca^{2+} by the sarcolemmal Na^+–Ca^{2+} exchanger.

As noted above, the first beat after an interval reduction is weaker rather than stronger. Similarly, when a premature depolarization occurs in the human heart due to an ectopic beat, the resulting systole is weaker than normal and the beat after the compensatory pause is stronger than usual (Figure 7.19b). The latter effect is called *post-extrasystolic potentiation* and the patient often notices it: 'My heart gives a jump, Doctor'. In intact hearts, an increased filling time contributes to post-extrasystolic potentiation, but this cannot explain the same phenomenon in muscle strips. Several possible explanations are under investigation. Restitution of the releasable Ca^{2+} store may be slow, so that a premature stimulus finds the sarcoplasmic reticulum store only partially releasable; or the release mechanism itself may still be slow to recover from inactivation after the previous release; or the Ca^{2+} pump of the sarcoplasmic reticulum may still be sufficiently active in a premature beat to attenuate the rise in free cytoplasmic $[Ca^{2+}]$.

The effects of interval on the mammalian heart *in vivo* are rather modest and probably contribute only a little to the enhanced contractility during exercise. In the example in Figure 7.19(a), changes in heart rate far in excess of those that occur physiologically were used, to explore the mechanisms involved. It is worth emphasizing that cardiac sympathetic nerve activity is the dominant factor regulating contractility *in vivo*.

7.9 Coordinated control of cardiac output

Minimal effect of an uncoordinated stimulus

Up to this point, each factor affecting stroke volume and heart rate has been presented essentially in isolation, but in the intact

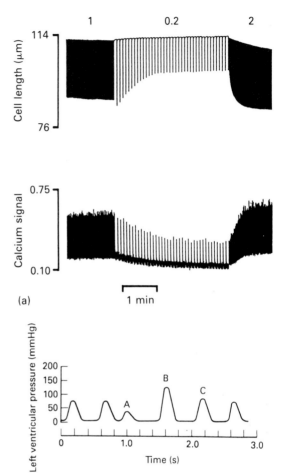

Figure 7.19 Effect of interval between beats on contractility. (a) Twitches of isolated rat ventricular myocyte stimulated at 1, 0.2 and 2 beats/s. Calcium signal is from intracellular fluorescent dye Fura-2. (b) In an isovolumetrically beating canine left ventricle a premature systole (beat A) is feeble but the beat after the compensatory pause (beat B) is stronger than usual (*post-extrasystolic potentiation*). ((a) from Frampton, J. E., Orchard, C. H. and Boyett, M. R. (1991), *Journal of Physiology*, **437**, 351–375, by permission; (b) from Berne, R. M. and Levy, M. N. (1981) *Cardiovascular Physiology*, Mosby Co., St. Louis, by permission)

animal it is usual for several factors to change simultaneously in a coordinated fashion so as to produce an effective regulation of the output. It is illuminating to see how truly ineffective a single uncoordinated drive to output can be. If, for example, the heart rate alone is 'turned up' in a patient with an artificially paced heart, the cardiac output increases remarkably little because stroke volume falls. The reasons for the decrease in stroke volume are that: (1) any increase in pumping transfers blood from the input (venous) side to the output (arterial) side at a faster rate, lowering end-diastolic pressure and raising arterial pressure (see Figure 7.10), both of which impair stroke volume, and (2) an increase in artificial pacing rate shortens diastole but not systole, and this curtails the filling time. These effects are so marked that the cardiac output of a resting subject actually declines at high pacing rates. Thus a change in a single drive to output is remarkably ineffective; a *coordinated cooperative change in all the controlling factors is needed to alter output substantially*. This is well illustrated by the cardiac response during physical exercise, described next.

Coordinated response to exercise

Cardiac output increases by approximately 6 litres/min for every extra litre of oxygen consumed per min in the human adult. The changes in heart rate and stroke volume have been studied by echocardiography and aortic Doppler flowmetry in man, and by implanted electromagnetic flowmeters around the aorta in dogs. These techniques reveal that cardiac output can be increased by various combinations of tachycardia and increased stroke volume, the precise combination depending on exercise intensity, posture and perhaps species. In the dog, changes in heart rate predominate during light exercise and stroke volume hardly alters; but during maximal exercise the stroke volume increases too. In man, tachycardia is again the major factor increasing the

output, with heart rate increasing in proportion to oxygen consumption and reaching a maximum of about 180–200 beats/min. In upright exercise, the stroke volume can increase substantially too, by 50–100% (see Table 7.2 and Figures 7.20 and 15.4). In the supine position however, where stroke volume is already high at rest, changes in stroke volume are slight.

The changes in rate and stroke volume are coordinated as follows:

1. At the onset of exercise, cardiac sympathetic nerve activity increases and vagal activity decreases. This increases the heart rate and shortens both systole and diastole. Augmented atrial contractility helps to offset the effect of the reduced filling time by increasing the atrial contribution to ventricular filling.

2. Ventricular contractility is increased by cardiac sympathetic activity and to a lesser degree by the secretions of the adrenal medulla. This increases the ejection fraction and stroke volume, as can be seen in the echocardiogram of Figure 7.20. The positive inotropic influences, namely local sympathetic drive, increased plasma adrenaline and noradrenaline (up to $20\times$) and angiotensin, more than counteract the negative inotropic actions of the hyperkalaemia and lactic acidosis that also accompany severe exercise.

3. Sympathetic vasomotor nerves induce venoconstriction in the splanchnic circulation, and the skeletal muscle pump compresses veins in the limbs. This shifts blood into the central veins and prevents CVP from falling as cardiac pumping increases. CVP may even increase by a mmHg or so in man during upright exercise, raising the end-diastolic volume and enabling the Frank–Starling mechanism to contribute to the increase in stroke volume (Figure 7.20).

4. Vasodilatation in the exercising skeletal muscle reduces the peripheral vascular resistance, which minimizes any rise in arterial pressure – indeed arterial pressure can fall a little at the start of light

Table 7.2 Typical cardiac response to upright exercise in a non-athlete

	Rest	*Hard exercise*
Oxygen consumption (litres/min)	0.25	3.0
Cardiac output (litres/min)	4.8	21.6
Heart rate (beats/min)	60.0	180.0
Stroke volume (ml)	80.0	120.0
End-diastolic volume (ml)	120.0	140.0
Residual volume (end-systolic)	40.0	20.0
Ejection fraction	0.67	0.86
Cycle time (s)	1.0	0.33
Duration of systole (s)	0.35	0.2
Duration of diastole (s)	0.65	0.13

(After Braunwald, E. and Ross, J. (1979), see Further Reading, and Rerych, S. K., Scholz, P. M., Newman, G. E. *et al.* (1978) *Annals of Surgery*, **187**, 449–458)

exercise. This prevents impairment of the stroke volume by large rises in arterial pressure.

The increased cardiac output of exercise thus involves a coordinated interaction between changes within the heart (rate and contractility) and outside it (CVP and systemic vascular resistance).

Transplanted and artificially paced hearts

Cardiac transplantation involves denervation but this has less functional effect than one might imagine. Racing greyhounds with denervated hearts are almost as fast as normal animals, with only a 5% reduction in track speed. In the denervated heart there is no instant tachycardia on commencing exercise but cardiac output does nevertheless increase. There is a brisk increase in stroke volume, which is caused by a rise in end-diastolic pressure as the leg muscle pump becomes active, and by a fall in arterial pressure as the skeletal muscle

arterioles dilate. This is followed by a rise in heart rate and contractility over 1–2 min as the adrenal glands secrete catecholamines into the plasma. Circulating levels of adrenaline and noradrenaline can increase by up to 20 times in intense exercise, and circulating angiotension rises too. It is only when the adrenergic back-up system is blocked by a β-antagonist that the track performance of the denervated greyhound deteriorates substantially (Chapter 15 and Figure 15.6).

Patients with an artificial pacemaker, as well as greyhounds, benefit from the reduplication of cardiac control systems. Even at fixed pacing rates, moderate increases in stroke volume can be produced by increased muscle pumping, peripheral vasodilatation and adrenaline-enhanced contractility during exercise. These changes may not make for Olympic records, but more importantly they allow thousands of people to walk in the park, do the shopping and generally lead a full life.

7.10 Cardiac energetics and metabolism

Pressure work and kinetic work

Some of the energy expended in systole is 'useful' in the sense that it performs work on an external system, the arteries, while the remainder of the energy appears as heat. The external, mechanical work takes the form of an increase in the volume, pressure and velocity of blood in the arterial system. The mechanical work involved in displacing a pressurized volume of blood is the product of stroke volume and mean pressure rise (see Section 7.4), and it equals the area within the ventricular pressure–volume loop ($\Delta P.\Delta V$). This *pressure work* can be estimated roughly as follows. If the left ventricle raises the pressure by 100 mmHg ($1.33 \times 10^4 \, \text{N/m}^2$) and ejects 75 cm^3 blood ($0.75 \times 10^{-4} \, \text{m}^3$), it performs very nearly 1 Nm or 1 joule of mechanical work, and the external system gains 1 joule of potential energy (pressure energy).

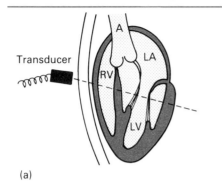

(a)

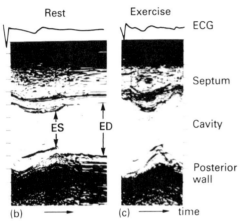

(b)   (c) ⟶ time

Figure 7.20 (a) Ultrasound beam directed across ventricle, in sagittal section. Echocardiograms of human left ventricle during rest (b) and upright exercise (c). Resting end-diastolic dimension (ED) *increased* on average by 2 mm and end-systolic dimension (ES) *fell* by 5 mm. The change in dimension upon contraction serves as an index of stroke volume and increased by 24% during exercise. (From Amon, K. W. and Crawford, M. H. (1979) *Journal of Clinical Ultrasound*, **7**, 373–376, by permission)

In estimating cardiac work, we ought also to take account of the fact that the heart imparts velocity to the blood during ejection, as well as pressure. It therefore imparts *kinetic energy* (KE, energy of motion) as well as potential energy. Kinetic energy depends on velocity v and mass m, and work is required to provide it. The total mechanical work of the heart, W_T is therefore:

$$W_T = \Delta P . \Delta V + KE = \Delta P . \Delta V + mv^2/2$$

Under resting conditions, where 0.08 kg of blood is ejected at a mean velocity of only 0.5 m/s, the kinetic energy works out at 0.01 kg m^2 s^{-2} or 0.01 J. For the left ventricle, this is merely 1% of the external work at basal outputs, and can be neglected. For the right ventricle on the other hand, kinetic energy constitutes approximately 5% of the mechanical work because the blood velocity in the pulmonary artery is almost the same as in the aorta, whereas the pressure rise (and hence pressure work) is only about 20% as great. During heavy exercise, the ejection velocity increases greatly in both the pulmonary artery and aorta (to approximately 2.5 m/s), while pressure increases only slightly. Even in the left ventricle, kinetic energy then accounts for up to 14% of the total external work, and in the right ventricle the figure can reach 50%.

The *power* of the heart is its rate of working, i.e. stroke work × heart rate. Cardiac power ranges from approximately 1.2 W (J/s) at rest to around 8 W in heavy exercise, which is about a fiftieth the power of a small electric lawn mower.

Cardiac efficiency during exercise, emotional stress and cardiac dilatation

The gross mechanical efficiency of any machine is the external work achieved per unit of energy expended. Cardiac efficiency is rather low at resting outputs, being only 5–10%. Even if allowance is made for the 'baseline' energy costs of cell maintenance and ionic pumping, which account for 25% of the oxygen consumption at basal outputs, the net efficiency is only a little better. The reason for the low efficiency is that the generation of tension during isovolumetric contraction has a high energy cost, yet accomplishes no external work. Myocardial oxygen consumption is in fact dominated by internal work rather than external work, and correlates better with active tension multiplied by the time for which it is maintained (the *tension–time* index) than with stroke work. This may seem odd, until one recalls that the oxygen consumption of a tug-of-war team depends mainly on the huge tension they exert, rather than on the external work involved in shifting the opposition a metre or so.

During dynamic exercise the gross efficiency can improve to around 15% because stroke volume increases relatively more than arterial pressure, producing more external work without much increase in the energy-expensive isovolumetric phase. This is an important point in relation to patients with cardiac disease, allowing them to indulge in gentle exercise such as walking. The opposite side of the coin, however, is that a high blood pressure, whether acute or chronic, raises myocardial oxygen demand and reduces efficiency. An angry emotional scene, which causes a large rise in blood pressure, will raise the tension–time index and increase myocardial oxygen demand sharply – the very thing to be avoided by patients with coronary artery insufficiency. As the celebrated eighteenth-century anatomist John Hunter observed in relation to his own ischaemic heart, 'My life is at the mercy of any rascal who chooses to annoy me'; and the couch on which Hunter expired after a stormy committee meeting can still be seen in the library at St. George's Medical School in London.

Another clinically important aspect of mechanical efficiency involves cardiac dilatation. Dilatation can be gross during chronic heart failure (see Figure 16.7) owing to a chronically raised filling pressure. Laplace's law (Section 7.6; $P = 2Sw/r$) shows that in order to maintain a normal systolic pressure, P, a heart of enlarged radius, r, has to exert a greater contractile force, Sw. This entails a rise in oxygen consumption and a fall in efficiency – the very things a failing heart can least afford. Excessive cardiac dilatation is thus dangerous in heart failure, and it is important to reduce the dilatation by diuretic therapy.

Myocardial oxygen consumption and metabolic substrates

Myocardial metabolism is normally aerobic. The immediate energy source for the actin–myosin machinery is ATP, which is synthesized by oxidative phosphorylation in the abundant mitochondria. The small store of ATP is backed up by a bigger reserve of high-energy phosphate bonds in the form of creatine phosphate. There is also a small store of oxygen as oxymyoglobin. Even so, the delivery of oxygen by coronary vessels must keep pace with demand because the heart, unlike skeletal muscle, cannot stop for a prolonged rest. At basal outputs, myocardial oxygen consumption is approximately 10 ml/min per 100 g. This represents a high proportion of the oxygen delivered by the coronary blood, and about 65–75% of the coronary blood oxygen is normally extracted. The additional oxygen needed at increased work loads is obtained chiefly by increasing the coronary blood flow (see Chapter 13).

The metabolic substrates of myocardium have been determined by chemical analysis of coronary sinus blood, collected by cardiac catheterization. It appears that myocardium is something of an opportunist, increasing its utilization of whatever substrate is currently most abundant in the bloodstream – for example glucose after a carbohydrate meal or ketone bodies in uncontrolled diabetes. Generally, however, free fatty acids supply 65–70% of the energy requirement (or more during endurance exercise) and the remaining 30–35% is supplied roughly equally by glucose and lactate. Myocardium, unlike skeletel muscle, can oxidize lactate, and this is a useful asset during hard exercise when blood lactate rises at the same time as myocardial energy demand. If myocardium becomes hypoxic, however, there is a switch to the anaerobic production of lactate, leading to local acidosis and impaired contractility.

The oxidation of lactate involves lactic dehydrogenase of a type specific to heart (LDH-H4). When heart muscle dies after a coronary thrombosis, LDH-H4 and other intracellular enzymes, such as creatine phosphokinase and aspartate aminotransferase, escape into the circulation. Their detection in plasma is a valuable diagnostic test for myocardial infarction.

7.11 Summary

Cardiac output can be varied by changes in stroke volume as well as heart rate. Stroke volume can be raised by increasing the force of contraction of the myocardium *and/or* by lowering the arterial blood pressure opposing ejection. The force of ventricular contraction can be raised by (1) stretching the myocytes in diastole (length–tension relation, Chapter 3) and (2) extrinsic stimulation by sympathetic nerves, circulating catecholamines and inotropic drugs.

1. The degree of distension of the relaxed ventricle is determined by diastolic filling pressure, i.e. central venous pressure (CVP, right side) and pulmonary venous pressure (left side). Diastolic fibre length influences contractile energy, partly because it affects actin–actin overlap and, to a greater extent, because the sensitivity of the contractile machinery to free intracellular Ca^{2+} is length-dependent. Raising the filling pressure and end-diastolic volume therefore increases contractile energy and stroke work (stroke volume × pressure rise). This is known as *Starling's law of the heart*. The single most important function of Starling's law is to equalize the stroke volumes of the right and left ventricles over several beats. Central venous pressure, a key determinant of stroke work, is influenced by blood volume, posture, peripheral venous tone, the muscle pump and respiration. An excessive rise in CVP is undesirable, however, because distension reduces the curvature of the wall and hence impairs its mechanical effectiveness (*Laplace's law*).

2. The endogenous positive inotropic agents, noradrenaline (sympathetic neurotransmitter) and adrenaline (circulating hormone), activate myocyte β-adrenoceptors. This leads to production of a second messenger, cAMP, and an increase in the slow inward current of Ca^{2+} (plateau current) during the action potential. Over several beats this raises the intracellular Ca^{2+} store, which in turn raises free $[Ca_i^{2+}]$ in systole and produce a stronger contraction. A rise in contractile force that is *not* due to a change in diastolic length (i.e. not due to operation of Starling's law) is called a rise in *contractility*. Increased contractility raises the ejection fraction to >2/3, reduces end-systolic volume, increases rate of ejection and relaxation, and shortens systole. Since a greater stroke work is obtained from a given filling pressure, a rise in contractility shifts the entire Starling curve upwards (plot of stroke work versus filling pressure).

Other positive inotropic influences include other β-adrenoceptor agonists (e.g. isoprenaline), extracellular Ca^{2+}, digoxin and increased beat frequency (Bowditch effect). Medically important *negative inotropic (weakening) influences* include acidosis and hypoxia, which impair contractility in ischaemic heart disease.

An increase in cardiac output, such as occurs during exercise, requires *coordinated* control of both the heart and the systemic vasculature. Stimulating the heart alone (e.g. by cardiac sympathetic nerve stimulation) raises arterial pressure and lowers filling pressure, both of which tend to oppose an increase in stroke volume. In exercise, vasodilatation in the active muscle minimizes the rise in arterial pressure, and peripheral venoconstriction and the muscle pump maintain or slightly raise the filling pressures. In upright exercise, stroke volume can double, partly due to increased end-diastolic volume (effect of raised filling pressure) and partly due to reduced end-systolic volume (increased ejection fraction as a result of increased contractility).

The gross efficiency of the heart is at best 15%. Much of the contractile energy goes into raising pressure rather than ejection, so lowering a patient's blood pressure can improve the stroke volume in heart failure. The metabolic energy source is variable but is generally two-thirds to three-quarters free fatty acid and the rest glucose and lactate.

Further reading

Reviews and chapters

Allen, D. G. and Kentish, J. C. (1985) The cellular basis of the length-tension relation in cardiac muscle. *Journal of Molecular and Cellular Cardiology*, **17**, 821–840

Brady, A. J. (1991) Mechanical properties of isolated cardiac myocytes. *Physiological Reviews*, **71**, 413–427

Braunwald, E. and Ross, J. (1979) Control of cardiac performance. In *Handbook of Physiology, Cardiovascular System*, Vol. 1, *The Heart* (ed. R. M. Berne), American Physiological Society, Bethesda, pp. 533–579

Chapman, C. B. and Mitchell, J. H. (1965) *Starling on the Heart*, Dawsons, London

Drake-Holland, A. J. and Noble, M. I. M. (1983) *Cardiac Metabolism*, Wiley, Chichester

Jewell, B. R. (1982) Activation of contraction in cardiac muscle. *Mayo Clinic Proceedings*, **57**, 6–13

Noble, M. I. M. (1979) *The Cardiac Cycle*, Blackwell, Oxford

Rüegg, J. C. (1987) Dependence of cardiac contractility on myofibrillar calcium sensitivity. *News in Physiological Sciences*, **2**, 179–182

Sagawa, K., Maughan, L., Suga, H. and Sunagawa, K. (1988) *Cardiac Contraction and the Pressure-Volume Relationship*, Oxford University Press, New York

te Keurs, H. E. D. J. and Noble, M. I. M. (1988) *Starling's Law of the Heart Revisited*, Kluwer Academic, Dordrecht

Research papers

Banner, N. R., Guz, A., Heaton, R., Innes, J. A., Murphy, K. and Jacoub, M. (1988) Ventilatory and circulatory responses at the onset of exercise in man following heart or heart-lung transplantation. *Journal of Physiology*, **399**, 437–449

Gulati, J., Sonnenblick, E. and Babu, A. (1990) The role of troponin C in the length dependence of Ca^{2+}-sensitive force of mammalian skeletal and cardiac muscles. *Journal of Physiology*, **441**, 305–324

Orchard, C. H., Hamilton, D. L., Astles, P., McCall, E. and Jewell, B. R. (1991) The effect of acidosis on the relationship between Ca^{2+} and force in isolated ferret cardiac muscle. *Journal of Physiology*, **436**, 559–578

Toska, K. and Eriksen, M. (1993) Respiration-synchronous fluctuations in stroke volume, heart rate and arterial pressure in humans. *Journal of Physiology*, **472**, 501–512

Chapter 8

Haemodynamics: pressure, flow and resistance

8.1 Hydraulic principles

Darcy's law

The science of haemodynamics concerns the relation between blood flow, pressure and hydraulic resistance. The simplest guide to this is *Darcy's law of flow*, the hydraulic equivalent of Ohm's law of electricity. By studying the flow of water through the gravel beds of the fountains of Dijon, Darcy showed in 1856 that flow in the steady state ($\dot{Q}$) is linearly proportional to the pressure difference between two points ($P_1 - P_2$):

$$\dot{Q} = K.(P_1 - P_2) = \frac{(P_1 - P_2)}{R} \qquad (8.1a)$$

where K is a proportionality coefficient called hydraulic conductance. The reciprocal of hydraulic conductance is hydraulic resistance R, and this arises from internal friction within the moving liquid.

Darcy's law can be applied to channels of any geometry including the branching network of blood vessels. For the systemic circulation, the flow is the cardiac output (CO), the driving pressure is mean arterial pressure minus central venous pressure ($P_a - \text{CVP}$), and resistance is the total peripheral resistance (TPR). Therefore we can write Darcy's law in the form:

$$\text{CO} = \frac{(P_a - \text{CVP})}{\text{TPR}} \qquad (8.1b)$$

Since CVP is nearly zero (atmospheric pressure) the expression can be simplified to $\text{CO} = P_a/\text{TPR}$, or alternatively $P_a = \text{CO} \times \text{TPR}$. The latter expression has been tested experimentally by driving blood through the aorta and peripheral circulation at various rates from an artificial pump. Provided that active changes in peripheral resistance are blocked pharmacologically, the arterial pressure is virtually a linear function of the flow, and the extrapolated line passes close to the origin. (The slight positive pressure upon extrapolating to zero flow is considered in Section 8.6.) The slope of the pressure–flow plot represents the systemic peripheral resistance, which is typically approximately 1 mmHg per ml/s in human adults (1 peripheral resistance unit or PRU).

Darcy's law concerns *flow*, the units of which are volume/time, and this must be distinguished from fluid *velocity* (distance/time). Mean velocity is flow divided by the total cross-sectional area of the channels. Since the latter increases as blood enters the branching microvascular network, velocity decreases progressively (see Figure 1.6). Total flow by contrast is unaltered and equals the cardiac output.

Bernoulli and total mechanical energy of fluid

Pressure, with which Darcy's law is concerned, is only one of three forms of mechanical energy affecting blood flow. The other two are potential energy and kinetic energy. A more general law taking account of this was introduced by Bernoulli, an 18th century Swiss physician who was also a professor of mathematics by the age of 25. *Bernoulli's theory* states that flow between point A and point B in the steady state is proportional to the difference in the fluid's mechanical energy between A and B, mechanical energy being the sum of pressure energy, potential energy and kinetic energy. *Pressure energy* equals pressure × volume (PV), as explained in Section 7.4. *Potential energy* is the capacity of a mass to do work in a gravitational field by virtue of its vertical height above a reference level, such as the heart. The potential energy equals fluid mass (density ρ × volume V)

× height (h) × gravitational force (g). *Kinetic energy* is the energy that a moving mass possesses due to its momentum. Kinetic energy increases in proportion to velocity squared (v^2) and equals $\rho V \cdot v^2/2$. Adding the three energies together we have:

Mechanical energy per unit volume =

$$P + \rho gh + \rho v^2/2 \qquad (8.2)$$

The experiment shown in Figure 8.1 demonstrates the interconvertibility of pressure energy and kinetic energy, and proves that flow occurs down a gradient of total energy rather than pressure alone.

While Darcy's law is often sufficient for our needs in vascular physiology, the more general Bernoulli theory has been introduced

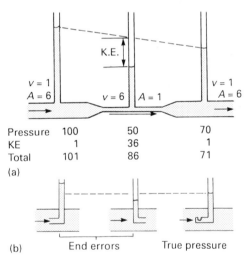

Figure 8.1 Some basic hydraulic considerations. (a) Flow is driven by the gradient of total mechanical energy. When the cross-sectional area A narrows, velocity (v) increases, converting pressure energy into kinetic energy (KE). When the tube widens, kinetic energy is converted back into pressure energy. Flow from the narrow to broad segment is contrary to the pressure gradient but down the total energy gradient. (b) Kinetic energy error in pressure measurement with an open-ended catheter pointing upstream or downstream. (From Burton, A. C. (1972) *Physiology and Biophysics of the Circulation*, Year Book Medical Publishers, Chicago, by permission)

here to clarify some aspects of haemodynamics which might otherwise seem puzzling. For example, mean arterial pressure is typically 95 mmHg above atmospheric pressure in the aorta and 180 mmHg above atmospheric pressure in the foot during standing (Section 8.4), yet blood flows from aorta to foot against a pressure gradient and apparently in defiance of Darcy's law. The explanation is of course that in the upright posture the aortic blood possesses more gravitational *potential energy* than blood in the foot, in fact about 90 mmHg more, so that the total energy of aortic blood is 185 mmHg relative to the foot, and there is in fact a net energy gradient of 5 mmHg driving flow from the aorta into the foot.

Kinetic energy accounts for only 1% of the fluid energy in the aorta in a resting subject, and 5% in the pulmonary artery, rising to 14% and 50%, respectively, at maximal cardiac output (Section 7.10). In the great veins, the kinetic energy forms a greater proportion of the fluid energy because the blood velocity is similar to that in the aorta while blood pressure is much lower: kinetic energy accounts for 12% of the fluid energy in the vena cava at rest and for most of it at maximal flows. On reaching the relaxed ventricle, the returning blood's kinetic energy falls virtually to zero, so there is a kinetic energy gradient from vein to ventricle, and this aids ventricular filling. Put another way, the momentum of the returning blood contributes to ventricular expansion. Kinetic energy can also be an important consideration when measuring pressure: the measuring catheter should face neither upstream (collecting kinetic energy and therefore overestimating pressure) nor downstream (which has the reverse effect), but should be directed laterally (see Figure 8.1).

It should be noted that the above laws describe flow that does not vary with time. If flow is pulsatile, as in arteries, the laws can still be applied to the mean flow, if this is not varying with time. To describe an oscillating flow instant by instant, however, is a more complex matter (Section 8.4).

8.2 Nature of flow in blood vessels

Three different patterns of flow occur in the circulation: laminar flow, turbulent flow and single-file flow (see Figures 8.2 and 8.3). Laminar flow occurs in normal arteries, arterioles, venules and veins, turbulent flow in the ventricles, and single-file flow in capillaries.

Laminar flow along a cylindrical tube

In laminar flow, the liquid follows smooth, parallel streamlines. If the flow is along a cylindrical tube the liquid behaves like a set of thin concentric shells (the laminae), which slide past each other during flow. The lamina in direct contact with the vessel wall is fixed there by molecular cohesive forces (the 'zero-slip' condition) and has zero velocity. The adjacent lamina slides slowly past the non-slip lamina. The next (third) lamina slides past the second lamina, and since the second lamina is itself moving, the third lamina has a higher velocity relative to the tube wall – and so on until maximum velocity is reached at the centre of the tube. The high velocity of red cells in the central stream and the slow velocity of marginal red cells are plainly visible when a small blood vessel *in vivo* is viewed through a microscope.

For a simple fluid like water, the transverse velocity profile is a parabola (Figure 8.2). It takes some distance from the tube entrance, however, to establish the parabola, several tube diameters in fact. In the entrance region the velocity profile is almost flat, i.e. a broad core of fluid flows at almost uniform velocity. This situation exists in the ascending aorta and this facilitates the estimation of aortic flow by the Doppler method (Section 6.3).

With a particulate suspension like blood, the velocity profile is more blunted than a parabola (Figure 8.2, red line). Also the shearing of lamina against lamina causes

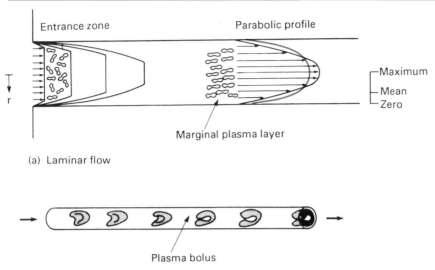

(a) Laminar flow

(b) Single-file flow

Figure 8.2 Blood flow patterns in a large vessel (a) and capillary (b). In (a), arrow length indicates the velocity (v) of each lamina. For a Newtonian fluid in fully-developed laminar flow, velocity is a parabolic function of radial position (r): $v = v_{max}(1 - r^2/R^2)$ where R is tube radius. Mean velocity is $v_{max}/2$. The profile is blunter for a non-Newtonian fluid like blood (red line). The gradient of the velocity curve is called the 'shear rate'. (b) In capillaries the red cells deform into parachute/slipper configurations (left) and folded shapes (right). (After Chien, S., Usami, S. and Skalak, R. (1984) see Further Reading)

the red cells to tend to orientate themselves parallel to the direction of flow at high shear rates. *Shear rate* is an important factor in haemodynamics: it is the change in fluid velocity per unit distance across the tube, i.e. the slope of the velocity profile in Figure 8.2(a). Another effect of shear is that the cells are displaced a little towards the central axis ('*axial flow*'), leaving a thin cell-deficient layer of plasma at the margins. The *marginal layer* is only 2–4 μm thick, but it is important in arterioles, where it helps to ease the blood along (Section 8.5).

Turbulence in the circulation

If the pressure drop along a rigid tube is progressively raised, a point is reached where flow no longer rises linearly with driving pressure, as in Darcy's law, but increases only as the square-root of pressure (see Figure 8.3). This is caused by a transition

from smooth laminar flow to turbulent flow, in which swirling cross-currents dissipate part of the pressure energy as heat. The conditions which create turbulence were explored in 1883 by the engineer Sir Osborne Reynolds, who visualized turbulence by injecting dye into water flowing down a tube. For a given smoothness of tube, turbulence is encouraged by a high fluid velocity (v), large tube diameter (D) and high fluid density (ρ, rho); all these factors increase the fluid's momentum and thereby encourage any flow distortions to persist. Turbulence is discouraged by a high viscosity (η, eta) because this tends to damp out flow deviations. These factors can be combined as a dimensionless ratio called the *Reynolds' number* (Re):

$$\mathrm{Re} = (v.D.\rho)/\eta$$

The critical Reynolds' number at which turbulence sets in is around 2000 for steady flow down a rigid, straight uniform tube.

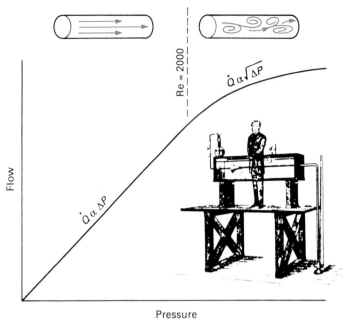

Figure 8.3 Pressure–flow relation for a Newtonian fluid in a rigid tube. Darcy's law, represented by the straight line through the origin, breaks down when turbulence develops. Inset shows Sir Osborne Reynolds' apparatus for studying the onset of turbulence; the flow-pattern (top) was visualized by injecting dye into the fluid

The critical value is smaller in blood vessels because blood flow is pulsatile and the vessels are neither straight nor uniform. Even so a critical Re is not normally reached in most vessels; for example, Re is only approximately 0.5 in arterioles. Turbulence does occur in the ventricles where it helps to mix the blood and produce a uniform arterial gas content. Turbulence also occurs in the human aorta during peak flow, and this sometimes creates an *'innocent' systolic ejection murmur* audible over the aortic area (Section 2.5). [Re reaches approximately 4600 in the root of the adult human aorta. Peak velocity is approximately 70 cm/s. The diameter is 2.5 cm. Blood density is $1.06\,\mathrm{g/cm^3}$. Blood viscosity is a 4 milliPascal s ($0.04\,\mathrm{g\,cm^{-1}\,s^{-1}}$).] Turbulence can also develop in leg arteries roughened by atheromatous plaques, and can cause a local *'bruit'* (murmur) audible through the stethoscope. Normal laminar blood flow is of course silent.

Single-file flow in capillaries

The diameter of most capillaries (5–6 µm) is less than the width of the human red cell (8 µm). Red cells are therefore compelled to proceed through capillaries in single file, and to deform into folded or parachute-like configurations even to enter the vessel, a fascinating and sometimes comic, cartoon-like spectacle when seen through the microscope. Since the cell spans the full width of the tube, parabolic flow is impossible and the bolus of plasma trapped between the cells is compelled to move along at uniform velocity, albeit with some internal eddying ('bolus flow' or 'plug flow'). Bolus flow eliminates some of the internal friction associated with lamina sliding against lamina. Friction between the cell and capillary wall is thought to be minimized by a thin film of plasma or by the endothelial glycocalyx, a cell surface coating of mucopolysaccharides. The glycocalyx is rich in negatively-charged sialic acid residue, and since the red cell surface is negatively charged too, electrostatic repulsion facilitates passage.

The efficiency of bolus flow depends critically on the deformability of the red cell, and this is impaired in many clinical conditions. The most dramatic of these is *sickle cell anaemia*, where the haemoglobin is abnormal. In hypoxic situations this causes the red cell to adopt a rigid sickle shape that reduces capillary flow, impairs tissue nutrition, and causes serious tissue damage (the 'sickling crisis'). Red cell flexibility is also impaired in *spherocytosis*, a condition in which many red cells are spherical rather than biconcave owing to a deficiency of spectrin, a fibrous 'skeleton' protein that coats the inner surface of normal red cell membranes. Spheres cannot fold easily and tend to burst (haemolyse) when forced through narrow channels, causing a 'haemolytic anaemia'. The haemolysis is particularly severe as spherocytes pass through special narrow channels inside the spleen, so splenectomy is often helpful in such cases.

The *polymorphonuclear leucocyte* is rounder and much stiffer than the red cell, and it moves less freely along the microvessels, often creating a little 'traffic jam' of red cells behind it. If the leucocyte adheres to the wall, as happens in small venules during inflammation, the resistance to flow can increase markedly. This is an important factor impairing microvascular flow during inflammation, and also in ischaemia of the myocardium and severe haemorrhagic hypotension.

8.3 Measurement of blood flow

In anaesthetized animals, flow or velocity can be measured directly in large vessels by an *electromagnetic velocity* meter (Section 6.5), or by a heated wire in the bloodstream (*hot-wire anemometry*), the wire cooling rate being proportional to fluid velocity. A third method is based on a brief intra-arterial injection of *radiolabelled microspheres* (typically of 15 μm diameter). The microspheres are washed into an organ in proportion to the flow it receives and lodge within its arterioles. The tissue can then be excised and its microsphere content determined by radioactive counting. The distribution of flow within the tissue can be assessed by dicing the tissue into small pieces and counting each separately.

In man, less direct methods are used, as follows.

Doppler ultrasound velocity meter

This non-invasive method, described in Section 6.3, is used to assess femoral artery blood flow in patients with ischaemic limb disease, and to assess placental blood flow in late pregnancy. A variant, the laser–Doppler flowmeter, uses a laser light beam rather than ultrasound and is useful for investigating superficial skin blood flow.

Measurement of blood flow using Fick's principle

The Fick principle, described in Section 6.1, can be used to measure blood flow in several other organs besides the lungs. To measure renal blood flow, para-aminohippuric acid (PAH) is injected intravenously and its rate of appearance in urine is measured. PAH is almost completely cleared from renal blood, so renal venous concentration is taken as zero, and the arteriovenous concentration difference is equated with the arterial concentration which is easily measured. Blood flow is then calculated as PAH excretion rate in urine (mg/min) divided by arterial concentration (mg/ml). The Fick principle has also been used to determine coronary and cerebral blood flow from the uptake of inhaled nitrous oxide gas from blood into these organs.

Venous occlusion plethysmography

This is used to measure blood flow in a limb, foot or digit. To measure forearm blood flow (Figure 8.4), an inflatable cuff is placed over

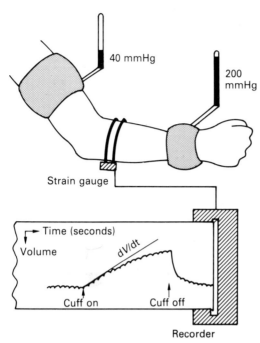

Figure 8.4 Venous occlusion plethysmography using a mercury-in-rubber strain gauge to record forearm circumference, from which volume can be calculated. Individual pulsations can be seen. The 'congesting cuff' (upper arm) occludes venous return and the wrist cuff eliminates hand blood flow from the measurement. The initial swelling rate (tangent to curve) measures forearm blood flow. Swelling rate tails off as venous back-pressure rises. After a few minutes (not shown here; see Figure 10.3) forearm blood volume stabilizes because venous pressure has exceeded cuff pressure and venous outflow resumes

the brachial vein and inflated quickly to 40 mmHg. This arrests the venous drainage but not the arterial inflow, so the forearm begins to swell with blood. The initial swelling rate equals arterial blood flow. The swelling rate is measured by a mercury-in-rubber strain gauge, which is a mercury-filled elastic tube wrapped around the limb. As limb circumference increases, the mercury column is stretched and narrowed, and its electrical resistance increases. This is measured with a Wheatstone bridge circuit and converted to change in forearm circumfer-

ence by a calibration factor. (In former years, swelling was measured by the displacement of air or water out of a rigid jacket around the limb, called a plethysmograph ('fullness record'). This is how the method's gargantuan name arose.) Another use of plethysmography, namely to study plasma ultrafiltration across the capillary wall, is shown later, in Figure 10.3.

Kety's tissue-clearance method

This measures microvascular blood flow in a small, local region of tissue. A rapidly diffusing solute is injected into the tissue as a local depot (Figure 8.5), from where it gradually diffuses across the capillary walls into the bloodstream and is washed away. If diffusion is fast enough, the concentration in the depot and incoming blood equilibrate during the blood's short residence in the capillary, and the rate of removal of solute is then directly proportional to capillary blood flow. This is called 'flow-limited exchange' and is explained more fully in Section 9.10. Fast-diffusing, lipid-soluble radioisotopes like xenon-133 and krypton-85 are suitable for this method, and their rate of removal is easily recorded by a gamma-counter over the depot. Kety pointed out in 1949 that, given the conditions outlined above, the isotope concentration declines exponentialy with time, so a plot of the logarithm of concentration (C_t) against time (t) is linear (see Figure 8.5). The slope of the log. plot (k) is called the removal rate constant and is given by the expression:

$$\log_e C_t = \log_e C_o - k.t = \log_e C_o - (\dot{Q}/V\lambda).t$$
$$(8.3)$$

where C_o is initial concentration, V is the solute's distribution volume and λ (lambda) is the solute partition coefficient between blood and tissue. Local blood flow per unit volume of tissue ($\dot{Q}/V$) is calculated from the slope (k). One problem in practice is that the tissue composition and blood flow may not be uniform, leading to complex multi-exponential clearance curves.

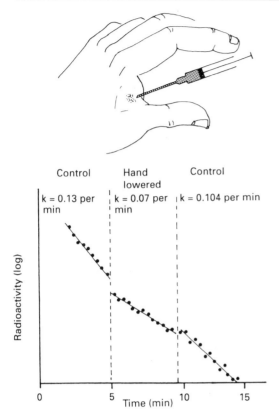

Figure 8.5 Tissue clearance method, using a cutaneous injection of xenon-133. With the hand at heart level the washout slope, k, was 13% per min (half-life 5.3 min; half-life is 0.693/k). The calculated blood flow was 9 ml min^{-1} 100 ml^{-1}. Lowering the hand 40 cm below heart level reduced blood flow to 5 ml min^{-1} 100 ml^{-1} due to local arteriolar constriction (see Chapter 12). (After Lassen, N. A., Henriksen, U. and Sejrsen, P. (1983) In *Handbook of Physiology, Cardiovascular System*, Vol. 3, Part 1, *Peripheral Circulation* (eds. J. T. Shepherd and F. M. Abboud), American Physiological Society, Bethesda, pp. 21–64)

8.4 Haemodynamics in arteries

Waveform of the arterial pressure pulse

Arterial pressure oscillates and the size of the oscillation, or 'pulse pressure', depends on the volume and speed of the ventricular ejection, the rate of runoff through the peripheral resistance vessels, and the distensibility of the artery wall (see Section 6.4). As ventricular ejection begins, input into the arterial system is much faster than runoff; arterial volume increases, even though 20–33% of the ejected blood flows away through the peripheral resistance during this phase. The arterial pressure rises steeply, forming the 'anacrotic limb' of the pulse (see Figure 8.6). Pressure reaches its maximum when the declining ejection rate transiently equals the runoff through the resistance vessels. Pressure then declines as ventricular systole weakens and runoff exceeds ejection rate. A notch on the descending limb *(dicrotic notch)* marks aortic valve closure, and as the valve cusps check the backflow they create a small secondary rise in pressure, the 'dicrotic wave'. As runoff continues, pressure gradually declines to the diastolic value.

Lesions of the aortic valve cause characteristic *abnormalities of the aortic waveform*. the aortic valve is narrowed by fibrosis (*aortic stenosis*), arterial pressure rises more sluggishly than normal during ejection and has an abnormal plateau (Figure 8.6, inset). In *aortic incompetence*, pressure decays abnormally quickly in diastole owing to reflux into ventricle. As a result, pulse pressure may be twice as big as normal, and may even cause relaxed limbs to jerk in time with the throbbing pulse.

Mean arterial pressure ($\bar{P}_a$)

Mean arterial pressure is not a simple arithmetic average of systolic and diastolic pressures, because the blood spends relatively longer near the diastolic level than near systolic level. The true, time-weighted average is nearer the diastolic value, and can be worked out by dividing the area under the pressure wave ($\int P . dt$) by time (see Figure 8.6). As a working approximation, however, a third of the pulse pressure is added to diastolic pressure:

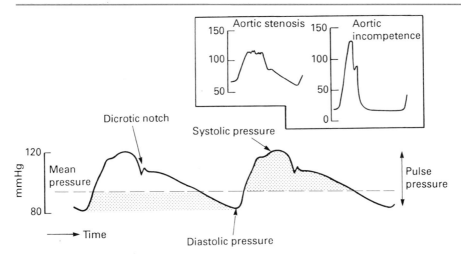

Figure 8.6 Pressure wave in human subclavian artery over two cycles recorded by an electronic pressure transducer. The mean pressure, averaged over time, is the pressure at which the area above the mean (grey area, $\int P . dt$) equals the area below the mean. Inset shows abnormal waveform in aortic valve stenosis (slow rise, prolonged plateau) and aortic incompetence (excessive pulse pressure, low diastolic pressure) (After Mills, C. J., Gale, I. T., Gault, J. H. *et al.* (1970) *Cardiovascular Research*, **4**, 405, omitting variable minor waves on the descending limb caused by reflections)

$$\bar{P}_a = P_{diast} + (P_{sys} - P_{diast})/3 \qquad (8.4)$$

This approximation is valid for the brachial artery waveform, where human pressure is normally measured. If, for example, brachial pressure is 110/80 mmHg, the pulse pressure is 30 mmHg and the mean pressure is 90 mmHg.

As explained earlier, Darcy's law can be written in a form which defines the two factors governing mean arterial pressure:

$$\bar{P}_a = CO \times TPR \qquad (8.5)$$

This will be referred to as the *'mean blood pressure equation'*. It is an important expression because it shows that mean arterial pressure is set by the size of the cardiac output and the total peripheral resistance.

Pulse pressure is the oscillation about the mean pressure. The size of this oscillation is set by arterial compliance, stroke volume, ejection rate and runoff as described in Section 6.4. Together, mean pressure and pulse pressure set the sytolic and diastolic pressures.

Measurement of arterial pressure

Direct methods

Arterial pressure was first measured by the vicar of Teddington, Stephen Hales, who in 1773 connected a vertical 9-foot (2.7 m) glass tube to the carotid artery of a horse via a goose trachea, and noted the height to which the blood rose in the tube. A century later the French medical physicist J. L. M. Poiseuille developed the smaller *mercury manometer*, which is still in use today. The principle behind manometry is that the vertical column of manometer fluid exerts a downward pressure which opposes the blood pressure, as in Figure 8.1. When the column reaches a stable height (h), the blood pressure must be equal to the pressure at the bottom of the column, namely ρgh (fluid density $\rho \times$ force of gravity g $\times h$). Since mercury is very dense ($\rho = 13.6 \, g/ml$), a column about 100 mm high suffices to balance blood pressure. Using his new mercury manometer, Poiseuille proved that there is little change in mean pressure along the arterial system, and therefore little resistance to flow along arteries.

The mercury manometer is a good way of measuring mean blood pressure but it cannot follow fast changes in pressure owing to the inertia of the mercury. To record the pressure waveform a fast-responding *electronic pressure transducer* is needed, and this was developed by the American scientists Lambert and Wood as a spin-off from aviation research during World War II. The transducer contains a metal diaphragm which deforms slightly when arterial pressure is applied to it via a catheter. The deformation of the diaphragm alters the resistance of a wire connected to it and the resistance is recorded. This produces a very fast response to pressure, but the transducer still has to be calibrated by a fluid column. For this reason, blood pressure is normally reported in mmHg or cmH$_2$O rather than standard international units (Pascals; see Appendix II for conversion factors).

Indirect measurement by sphygmomanometry

The mercury manometer is used in medical practice throughout the world to measure human blood pressure, by an indirect method called sphygmomanometry (Figure 8.7). A Riva-Rocci cuff, which is an inflatable rubber sac within a cotton sleeve, is wound around the upper arm, with the inflatable sac located medially over the brachial artery at heart level. The cuff is inflated initially to a pressure that obliterates the radial pulse. In a normal elderly subject this might be 180 mmHg, the applied pressure being measured by a mercury manometer. The applied pressure is transmitted through the tissues of the arm and occludes the artery. Auscultation of the brachial artery at the antecubital fossa (inner aspect of elbow) with a stethoscope therefore reveals no sound at this stage. Cuff pressure is then gradually lowered, and a sequence of sounds is heard.

1. When cuff pressure is just below systolic pressure, the artery opens briefly during each systole. The transient spurt of blood

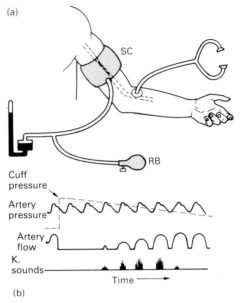

(a)

Cuff pressure

Artery pressure

Artery flow

K. sounds

Time

(b)

Figure 8.7 Measurement of human blood pressure. (a) Dashed line represents compressed brachial artery under the sphygmomanometer cuff (SC). Cuff pressure is controlled by the rubber bulb (RB) and measured by the mercury column. (b) Korotkoff sounds begin when cuff pressure is just below systolic pressure and diminish when cuff pressure is close to diastolic pressure

vibrates the artery wall downstream and creates a dull tapping noise called a Korotkoff sound. The pressure at which the Korotkoff sound first appears is conventionally accepted as systolic pressure, though it is actually about 10 mmHg less than the systolic pressure measured directly.

2. As cuff pressure is lowered further the Korotkoff sounds grow louder, because the intermittent spurts of blood grow stronger.

3. When cuff pressure is close to diastolic pressure, the artery remains patent for most of the cardiac cycle and the vibration of the vessel wall abruptly diminishes. This causes a sudden diminuendo of the Korotkoff sounds, and the cuff pressure at which this happens is accepted as the diastolic pressure (though it is about 8 mmHg higher than diastolic pressure

measured directly). A faint Korotkoff sound persists after the sudden diminuendo, and complete silence is often not attained until 8–10 mmHg below the true diastolic pressure.

In some hypertensive patients there is a silent period within the systolic–diastolic pressure range, which could lead to an erroneous under-estimation of systolic pressure if auscultation alone were used. It is therefore important, when first inflating the cuff, to palpate the radial artery and note the pressure at which the pulse disappears. This is a good measure of systolic pressure and avoids the possibility of missing hypertension.

A number of automated cuff-based systems for recording upper arm and finger blood pressure are also now available.

What is the 'normal' blood pressure?

That mythological polymath 'every school-boy' knows that 'normal' human blood pressure is 120/80 mmHg. For an adult male under certain conditions he would be right, but it is quite wrong to adopt 120/80 mmHg as the normal standard for a resting child, a pregnant woman in midterm or an elderly man. The lability of blood pressure is illustrated by the 24-h record shown in Figure 8.8, and some of the factors affecting blood pressure are as follows.

Age

Mean pressure increases progressively with age. In 3000 subjects studied in Wales, blood pressure is especially striking, and is of age, 125/80 mmHg (women) to 130/85 mmHg (men) at 30 years of age, and 180/90 mmHg at 70 years of age (see Figure 15.9, Chapter 15). The increase in pulse pressure is especially striking and is caused by reduced arterial compliance (see Figure 6.4). Reduced compliance is due to arteriosclerosis (hardening of the arteries by fibrosis and calcinosis), and is a virtually universal accompaniment to ageing. As a very rough rule, systolic pressure equals 100 mmHg plus age in years.

Sleep and exercise

Blood pressure can fall below 80/50 mmHg during sleep (see Figure 8.8). In exercise, mean blood pressure may either rise or fall, depending on the balance between increased

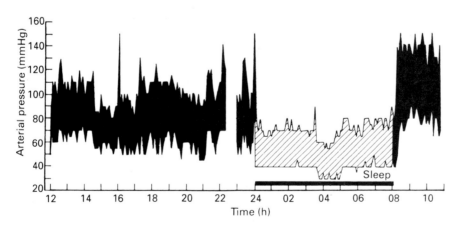

Figure 8.8 Arterial pressure in a normal subject recorded continuously for 24 h. Sleep (hatched period) lowered the pressure. A painful stimulus at 16.00 h and sexual intercourse at 24.00 h markedly raised pressure. (From Bevan, A. T., Honour A. J. and Stott, F. H. (1969) *Clinical Science*, **36**, 329, by permission)

cardiac output and reduced peripheral vascular resistance. In gentle dynamic exercise pressure can fall slightly, and even in heavy dynamic exercise, where cardiac output increases fourfold or more, the mean pressure increases by only 10–40 mmHg. In heavy static exercise such as weight-lifting, an 'exercise pressor reflex' can elevate pressure by approximately 60 mmHg (Section 15.3).

Gravity: direct effect

Pressure increases in arteries below heart level owing to the weight of the column of blood between the heart and artery. In a *foot* 115 cm below heart level, arterial pressure will increase by $115 \times 1.06/13.6$ cmHg (1.06 is the relative density of blood and 13.6 the relative density of mercury): this is 90 mmHg, so arterial pressure in the foot is increased to approximately 180 mmHg above atmospheric pressure. Conversely, pressure is reduced in the arteries above heart level and is only 60 mmHg or so in the human *brain* during standing. (Our problems are slight, though, compared with the giraffe's. To ensure cerebral perfusion, the giraffe has to generate an aortic pressure of approximately 200 mmHg.)

Gravity: indirect effect

Upon moving from lying to standing, arterial pressure changes at heart level due to changes in cardiac output and peripheral resistance. A transient fall in aortic pressure (which can produce a passing dizziness) is followed by a small but sustained reflex rise (Section 15.1).

Emotion and stress

Anger, apprehension, fear, stress and sexual excitement are all potent 'pressor' stimuli, i.e. they elevate blood pressure (see Figure 8.8). Even a telephone conversation raises pressure by around 10 mmHg compared with the relaxed state, while attending a meeting often raises it by 20 mmHg. Since a visit to the doctor is stressful for many patients, a solitary high pressure measurement is not in itself proof of the disease 'hypertension'; the measurement needs to be repeated with the patient relaxed. The pressor effect of stress is particularly harmful to patients with ischaemic heart disease, as the cautionary history of John Hunter in Section 7.10 illustrates.

Other factors

Arterial pressure fluctuates with *respiration*. In supine young adults, mean arterial pressure falls by a few mmHg with each inspiration, because of the reduction in left ventricular stroke volume. (In dogs, by contrast, pressure rises on inspiration because the inspiratory tachycardia (sinus arrhythmia) more than outweighs the fall in stroke volume.) The *Valsalva manoeuvre*, a forced expiration against a closed or narrowed glottis, causes a complex sequence of pressure changes which are described in Section 15.2. In *pregnancy*, blood pressure gradually falls and reaches a minimum at approximately 6 months, so in obstetrical practice a pressure of 130/90 mmHg would cause grave concern, even though it is merely close to the upper limit of normal for a non-pregnant woman. Even a *full bladder* can raise blood pressure. Many *pathological processes* also alter arterial pressure, such as dehydration, haemorrhage, shock, syncope (fainting), chronic hypertension, acute heart failure and valvular lesions like aortic incompetence. Some of these conditions are described in Chapter 16.

It will be clear from this brief survey that the yardstick used to assess a subject's blood pressure must be matched to age, sex, physiological and psychological condition.

Pulsatile flow in arteries

Flow along the aorta and major arteries is pulsatile and virtually ceases during diastole (Figure 8.9). This flow pattern arises from moment-to-moment changes in the pressure gradient along the arterial system. Pressure rises first in the proximal aorta, where the stroke volume is initially accommodated, so

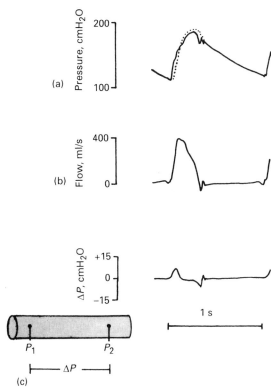

Figure 8.9 Pressure, flow and pressure gradient (ΔP over 5 cm) measured simultaneously in the ascending aorta of a normal human. The solid pressure line represents P_1, and P_2 has been reconstructed as the dotted line. Flow is virtually confined to the ejection phase and terminates with a brief backflow. Acceleration (not shown) has the same waveform as the pressure gradient trace. (After Snell, R. E., Clements, J. M., Patel, D. J., Fry, D. L. and Luchsinger, P. C. (1965) *Journal of Applied Physiology*, **20**, 691)

there is at first a pressure gradient from the proximal aorta to the peripheral arteries, which causes the blood already in the system to accelerate. The pressure pulse then spreads along the arterial tree (see later), taking an appreciable time to do so. Pressure in the human radial artery, for example, rises about 0.1 s later than in the aorta. Consequently, there comes a period when distal pressure is transiently higher than proximal pressure (Figure 8.9) and the pressure

gradient is reversed. The reversed pressure gradient does not instantly reverse the flow because the blood has acquired forward momentum, but it does steadily decelerate the flow. Thus, flow in the major arteries first accelerates and then decelerates over the initial third of the cardiac cycle. During the next two-thirds of the cycle, flow is virtually zero. The instantaneous flow is not governed by Darcy's law (which, as pointed out earlier, is a steady-state expression) but is governed by Newton's second law of motion, i.e. acceleration = force/mass.

The period of near zero flow gradually shortens as blood enters smaller arteries, and in the smallest arteries flow becomes continuous, albeit still pulsatile.

Transmission of the pressure wave

If arteries had rigid walls, pressure would rise virtually instantaneously throughout the arterial system, but they do not, and the pressure wave takes a finite time to pass along the arterial tree. The pressure pulse travels at around 4 m/s in young people and 10 m/s in the elderly. This is an order of magnitude faster than blood travels, mean blood velocity being approximately 0.2 m/s in the ascending aorta. One is reminded at this point of the White Queen's suggestion that Alice should practise believing at least six impossible things before breakfast. The difference between the pressure transmission velocity and blood velocity is, however, merely difficult to understand, not impossible (Figure 8.10). Since blood is essentially incompressible, the blood entering the proximal aorta during ejection has to create space for itself. This it does partly by distending the proximal aorta (which raises the pressure) and partly by pushing ahead the blood previously occupying the required space. As the displaced blood moves forward, it too must make space for itself, partly by distending the wall downstream (which raises the pressure there) and partly by displacing the blood ahead. This 'shunting' sequence repeats itself, very rapidly, along

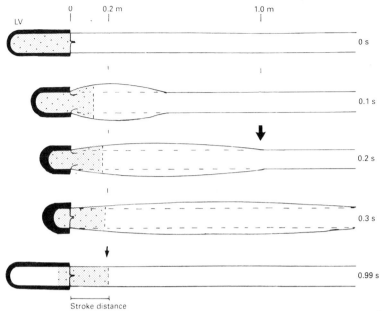

Figure 8.10 Sketch to illustrate transmission of the pressure pulse at 5 m/s along the arterial system. The left ventricle (LV) is shown ejecting 100 cm³ blood into an aorta of cross-section 5 cm²; the ejected blood travels only 20 cm per beat (small arrow, 1 s). This is the 'stroke distance'. The distension of the artery wall (the pulse) travels 1 metre in only 0.2 s (large arrow)

the arterial tree. The pulse is thus transmitted by a wave of wall distension (at 4–10 m/s) while the ejected blood itself advances only 20 cm (the 'stroke distance') in 1 s.

Since the wall deforms as it propagates the pulse, the transmission velocity is affected by wall stiffness: it increases as wall stiffness increases. Arterial stiffness is greater at high blood pressures and in elderly subjects, so pulse transmission is faster in elderly subjects. The measurement of transmission velocity, by timing the central and peripheral pulse, is a convenient way of assessing arterial distensibility in human subjects.

Change in the pressure waveform along the arterial tree

The shape of the pressure wave changes strikingly as it travels out to the periphery. The pulse pressure, far from damping out as one might imagine, actually grows taller and

steeper for some distance (Figure 8.11). This 'peaking' of the wave by around 50% is attributed partly to the tapering shape and increasing stiffness of the distal arterial tree and partly to the variation in transmission velocity with wall stiffness. The pulse pressure continues to increase as far as the third generation of arteries (e.g. femoral artery) but beyond this it becomes progressively damped out by the viscous properties of the blood and artery wall (see Figure 1.6). As the oscillations in pressure and flow dwindle the blood reaches the resistance vessels (arterioles).

8.5 Vascular resistance

Resistance to flow in tubes: Poiseuille's law

The resistance to laminar flow arises exclusively from the internal friction between

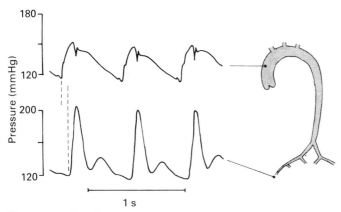

Figure 8.11 Simultaneous records of the pressure-wave in the canine ascending aorta and femoral artery. The dashed lines show the time required to propagate the pulse, namely 86 ms foot-to-foot. (From Noble M. I. M. (1979) *The Cardiac Cycle*, Blackwell, Oxford, by permission)

adjacent laminae of fluid and has nothing to do with friction between tube and fluid – which is zero because of the zero-slip condition (see Figure 8.2). Nevertheless, resistance is greatly affected by tube geometry because the radius of the tube affects the rate of shear (sliding) of the laminae. If the same flow is forced through a narrow tube and a wide tube, the velocities are greater in the narrower tube (since mean velocity equals flow/cross-sectional area), so the shear rates are higher in the narrower tube; and high shear rates produce more internal friction.

The properties which determine resistance were elucidated in 1840 by the Parisian physician, Jean Leonard Marie Poiseuille, in an extraordinarily meticulous study of water flowing through glass capillary tubes. Poiseuille established that the resistance (R) to the steady laminar flow of a Newtonian fluid such as water (or plasma) along a straight cylindrical tube is proportional to tube length (L) and fluid viscosity (η); and is inversely proportional to tube radius raised to the fourth power (r^4):

$$R = 8\eta \, . \, L/\pi r^4 \qquad (8.6)$$

Combining this definition of resistance with Darcy's law (equation 8.1a) we get an expression for flow through a tube, called *Poiseuille's law*:

$$\dot{Q} = (P_1 - P_2) \, . \, \frac{\pi \, . \, r^4}{8\eta L} \qquad (8.7)$$

Poiseuille's law describes flow along a single tube. If several tubes are arranged in *series*, the overall resistance is the sum of the individual resistances. However, if the tubes are connected in *parallel* (e.g. capillaries), the same driving pressure will obviously produce more flow, because the conducting capacities of the tubes summate. If there are N tubes of equal conductance K, the net conductance is NK. Resistance is the reciprocal of conductance, so the net resistance is $1/NK$.

Armed with Poiseuille's law, we can now consider the total systemic resistance which, as explained in Section 1.6, is sited chiefly in the arterioles and tiniest arteries.

Tube geometry: importance of arteriolar radius

Resistance is equisitively sensitive to vessel radius due to the fourth power term in Poiseuille's law. A fall in radius from approximately 1 cm in the human aorta to

0.01 cm in an arteriole will in itself increase resistance a hundred million times, and this is essentially why arterioles are the main site of resistance. Of course, the radius of a capillary is even smaller (approximately 0.000 3 cm), so why does the capillary network not offer an even greater resistance than the arteriolar network? The pressure drop per unit length of vessel (gradient dP/dx, a measure of the vessel's intrinsic resistance) is in fact five times greater in capillaries than arterioles but the pressure drop across the whole capillary bed, approximately 30 mmHg, is smaller than that across the arteriolar bed (40–50 mmHg) because of (1) the huge number of capillaries in parallel arrangement, (2) the shortness of capillaries (approximately 0.5 mm), and (3) the occurrence of bolus flow rather than laminar flow in capillaries.

The radius of an arteriole is actively controlled by the tension of smooth muscle in its wall. Contraction narrows the lumen (vasoconstriction) and relaxation produces vasodilatation. Owing to the fourth-power effect on resistance, active changes in radius constitute an extremely powerful mechanism for regulating both the *local blood flow* to a tissue and the central *arterial pressure* (equation 8.5). A mere 16% reduction in arteriolar radius will in theory halve the blood flow to an organ, if viscosity is unchanged (see later).

Wall tension, vasoconstriction and vasodilatation

Laplace's law in outline   Blood vessels are distensible, so the width of a given vessel depends on blood pressure (which tends to distend it), surrounding pressure (which tends to compress it) and the tension in the wall (which counterbalances the pressure drop across the wall). The key point to note here is that the amount of tension in the wall needed to counteract a given pressure drop across the wall *depends on the radius of the vessel*: the bigger the vessel, the greater the wall tension needed to offset a given transmural pressure difference. This general principle is commonly known as *Laplace's law*. It applies to both spheres (e.g. heart, see Section 7.6) and tubes (below).

Wall force and stress in a thick-walled tube   The classical analysis of the tension or force in the wall of a homogeneous tube is delightfully simple, as follows. The circumferential force per unit length of wall (F/L) is often called the wall *'tension'* (T; Figure 8.12). This resists the internal distending force caused by the internal pressure (P_i) pressing on the internal surface. This *internal distending force* is the pressure times area acted on in one direction. For a tube of internal radius r_i and unit length, the area in one direction is $2r_i$ (Figure 8.12), so the internal distending force is $P_i \times 2r_i$. We must not forget, however, that the outer surface (radius r_o) is at the same time being compressed by the outside pressure P_o, so there is also an *external compressive force*, of size $P_o \times 2r_o$. At mechanical equilibrium the wall tension on each side of the tube ($2T$) must be equal and opposite to the net transmural distending force $P_i 2r_i - P_o 2r_o$. Since the '2's cancel out, we reach Love's classical equation for mechanical equilibrium in a tube:

$$T = F/L = P_i r_i - P_o r_o \qquad \cdot (8.8)$$

A related common term is wall *stress* (S). Stress is force per unit surface area in a solid (same units as pressure in a fluid). For a tube of wall thickness w and unit length, $S = T/w$.

Wall force in a thin-walled tube   When a tube has a very thin wall relative to its radius – as for example in a capillary – r_i and r_o are nearly equal. Love's equation (8.8) then simplifies to $T = \Delta P r$. This is *Laplace's law for a thin tube*, and as noted above it states that for a given transmural pressure drop ΔP, the smaller the radius, the smaller the tension in the wall. Since a capillary has a very small radius, the tension in its wall is relatively low, despite the substantial blood pressure inside it.

Tension in wall of arterial vessels   In an artery or arteriole, the wall has a significant

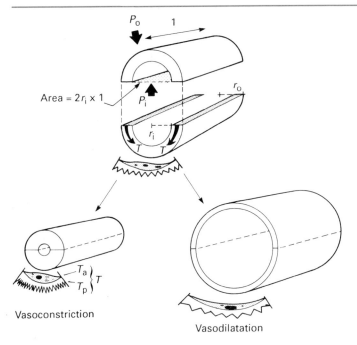

Figure 8.12 Wall mechanics in a blood vessel. The internal pressure (P_i) acting over area $2r_i$ tends to push the two halves of the cylinder apart. This is opposed by the external pressure (P_o) and by the tension in the wall on each side of the cylinder (T). The tension is the sum of the force exerted by active smooth muscle (T_a) and the force exerted by passive elastic elements (T_p) represented here as springs. T_a and T_p change in opposite directions during vasoconstriction and vasodilatation to produce mechanical stability. (After Azuma, T. and Oka, S. (1971) *American Journal of Physiology*, **221**, 1301–1308)

thickness relative to internal radius, so Laplace's law for a thin tube is then at best an approximation. Love's equation (8.8) tells us the absolute force in the vessel wall, but in physiology and medicine we are not so much interested in absolute wall forces as in the *extra* force (tension) in the fibres and contractile cells of the wall needed to counterbalance the blood pressure – 'extra' meaning over and above the forces when internal and external pressures are equal (see Appendix II, 'Laplace in a tube' for detail). Taking into account the fact that the artery wall is a composite material containing much water as well as stress-bearing fibres and cells, it has been suggested that the extra tensile stress in the fibrous elements and cells, T_{extra}, upon raising blood pressure (P_i) above outside pressure (P_o) is given approximately by

$$T_{\text{extra}} = (P_i - P_o)r \qquad (8.9)$$

where r is approximately the mean radius, $(r_i + r_o/2)$ (M. Colding-Jørgensen, P. Sejrsen and M. J. Mulvany, personal communication). This can be considered another form of Laplace's law. It says that the *tension in the wall fibres increases with radius at a given blood pressure, or with blood pressure at a given radius.*

Mechanics of vasoconstriction and vasodilatation The total fibre tension T_{extra} is the sum of two components, namely *active tension* in the vascular smooth muscle cells and *passive tension* in the collagen and elastin of the wall. When the cells begin to *contract*, the immediate effect is to raise wall tension, so there is mechanical disequilibrium (expression 8.9) and the radius begins to fall. As

Laplace's law shows, a reduced radius will only reach a stable value if the *net* wall tension is reduced, assuming that blood pressure remains the same. The fall in net wall tension is achieved by 'unloading' the passive fibres, i.e. their tension falls as the vessel radius is decreased by the contracting cells (Figure 8.12). Without this, vasoconstriction would be a highly unstable process. Conversely, *vasodilatation* is achieved by relaxation of the smooth muscle cells. This reduces the active tension, producing mechanical disequilibrium. The internal distending pressure then pushes the wall out to a bigger radius, until a point is reached where the rising passive tension in the stretched collagen and elastin grows big enough to re-establish mechanical equilibrium (Figure 8.12).

Viscosity of blood

The word viscosity stems from 'viscum', the Latin for mistletoe, because mistletoe berries contain a thick glutinous fluid. Viscosity was defined by Isaac Newton as 'defectus lubricitatis' or lack of slipperiness, meaning that it is a measure of the internal friction within a moving fluid, analogous to friction between two moving solid surfaces.

Viscosity is defined formally as the ratio of shear stress to shear rate. *Shear stress* is the shearing or sliding force applied per unit area of contact between two laminae (N/m^2), and it depends on the axial pressure gradient. *Shear rate* is the change in velocity per unit distance radially (see Figure 8.2), so its units are $(m/s)/m$, i.e. s^{-1}. The viscosity of water is 0.001 Newton-s/m^2 at 20°C, which is usually expressed as 1 milliPascal-second or 1 centiPoise. The viscosity of a fluid relative to water is easily and accurately measured with a simple capillary viscometer. The time taken for the test fluid to flow between two marks in a glass capillary tube is simply divided by the time taken by water under the same pressure head. With a simple fluid like water or plasma, the viscosity is unaffected by the tube radius or shear rate,

and such a fluid is called Newtonian. Whole blood by contrast has anomalous, non-Newtonian properties (see later).

Viscosity of plasma

The viscosity of water decreases as temperature rises, and at body temperature (37°C) it is only 69% of its viscosity at room temperature (20°C). In plasma, the presence of voluminous protein molecules (albumin and globulins) raises the viscosity by 70% so the viscosity of plasma is 1.2 mPa s at 37°C. In *myeloma* a cancer of globulin-secreting cells, the globulin concentration and viscosity rise to pathological levels. Moreover, the globulins are themselves abnormal and some can cause red cells to agglutinate (attach to each other) under cool conditions. The viscosity can then increase so dramatically in cold fingers that perfusion is badly impaired and necrosis (severe damage and tissue death) of the fingertips ensues.

Importance of haematocrit

The addition of red cells to plasma greatly increases the amount of internal friction during flow, so blood viscosity is dominated by haematocrit (Figure 8.13). Haematocrit is the red cell volume expressed as a fraction or percentage of the blood volume. At a haematocrit of 47% the relative viscosity of human blood is approximately 4, as measured in a wide-bore viscometer at high shear rates (the significance of these conditions will be explained shortly). At this haematocrit, there are frequent collisions between the red cells during flow, and were it not for the great flexibility of the red cell the viscosity would be even higher. If the cells are hardened by glutaraldehyde, the relative viscosity rises to 100. Achieving the optimal haematocrit for oxygen delivery is a delicate balancing act: on the one hand a high haematocrit increases the oxygen-carrying capacity of the blood but on the other it also raises viscosity, which either reduces the flow or increases arterial pressure and cardiac work. Each species has an optimal haematocrit in this respect. In the camel, for

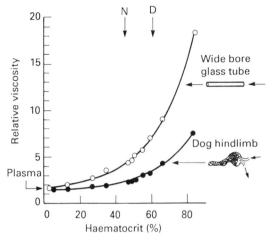

Figure 8.13 Effect of haematocrit on the viscosity of blood relative to water. Open circles: viscosity measured in a high-velocity glass viscometer. Closed circles: smaller effective viscosity in the vasculature of an isolated dog hindlimb, due to the Fåhraeus–Lindqvist effect – see text. N, normal haematocrit; D, haematocrit at which cells are packed so tightly that they begin to deform even at rest. (After the classic experiment of Whittaker, S. R. F. and Winton, F. R. (1933) *Journal of Physiology*, **78**, 339–369)

example, the red cells are less flexible than human cells, and the camel's haematocrit is only 27%.

Abnormalities of haematocrit can have serious haemodynamic effects. *Polycythaemia*, a raised haematocrit, develops either as a physiological adaptation to chronic hypoxia (e.g. in high altitude climbers and residents) or as a pathological condition called polycythaemia rubra vera, in which an overproduction of red cells by the bone marrow raises the haematocrit as high as 70%. At haematocrits above 63% the red cells are so closely packed that they are deformed even at rest, doubling the viscosity and raising the resistance to flow. As a result, polycythaemia rubra vera causes hypertension and a sluggish blood flow, which in turn predisposes to cerebral thrombosis and coronary thrombosis (strokes and heart attacks). Conversely, *anaemia* reduces viscosity and resistance. In order to maintain blood pressure, cardiac output has to

increase, and if this situation is prolonged a form of cardiac failure called high-output failure can develop. These examples illustrate the importance of the homeostasis of viscosity for normal cardiovascular functioning.

Non-Newtonian viscosity of blood. I – Effect of tube radius

In 1933 Whittaker and Winton made the remarkable observation that the effective viscosity of blood in the peripheral circulation is only half that of the same blood measured in a wide-bore viscometer (see Figure 8.13). Just before this, in 1931, Fåhraeus and Lindqvist made a related finding – the apparent viscosity of blood in a viscometer depends on the radius of the tube through which the blood is driven (Figure 8.14a), which is not the case for plasma or water. In tubes of diameter greater than 1 mm (small arteries) the viscosity of blood is independent of bore, but below 1 mm diameter the apparent viscosity decreases. In tubes of diameter 30–40 μm, which is the size of many arterioles, the relative viscosity is only approximately 2.5, and in capillary-size tubes (approximately 6 μm), blood viscosity reaches a minimum value almost as low as that of plasma. This constitutes a remarkable and important device for minimizing the pressure needed to perfuse the microcirculation, and explains the low viscosity of blood *in vivo* shown in Figure 8.13. The *Fåhraeus–Lindqvist effect*, as it is known, arises from several factors. In capillaries, the single-file pattern of flow lowers the viscosity. In arterioles, the viscosity is reduced by the peripheral plasma stream produced by axial flow (see Figure 8.2). Since shear rates are highest peripherally, a reduction in friction at that location has a particularly marked effect on the overall viscosity. This effect declines in wider tubes because the thickness of the marginal layer becomes insignificant relative to tube radius.

Fåhraeus described another curious consequence of axial flow; the concentration of red

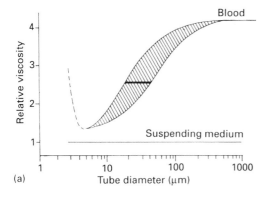

(a)

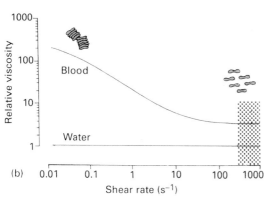

(b)

Figure 8.14 The anomalous viscous properties of blood flowing through glass tubing. (a) Fåhraeus–Lindqvist effect: viscosity decreases as tube diameter is reduced. Hatched area indicates spread of data. The effective viscosity of blood in the intact circulation is approximately 2.5 (black bar), implying that the functional diameter of the resistance vessels is approximately 30 μm (arterioles). At diameters smaller than a blood capillary, viscosity rises again (dashed line). (b) Effect of shear rate on viscosity. Dotted region shows typical shear rates *in vivo*. Sketches show red cell aggregation into rouleaux at low shear rates and disaggregation at high rates. ((a) After Gaetghens, P. (1981) In The *Rheology of Blood, Blood Vessels and Associated Tissues* (eds D. R. Gross and N. H. C. Wang), Sijthoff and Noordhoff, Amsterdam; (b) from Chien, S., Usami, S. and Skalak, R. (1984), see Further Reading)

cells in blood flowing along a narrow tube (the dynamic or tube haematocrit) is lower than the central haematocrit in the feeding

and draining vessel. In a tube of radius 15 μm, for example, fed from a central reservoir of haematocrit 40%, the dynamic haematocrit is only approximately 24%. This is a little hard to digest at first acquaintance. The explanation lies in the difference between axial and marginal stream velocities (see Figure 8.2). Let us consider, as a simple example, arterial blood of haematocrit 50% feeding an arteriole in which the cells have twice the velocity of plasma owing to their more axial location. If the haematocrit in the parent artery and vein is to remain at 50% (which it must, since the circulation is in a steady state) equal volumes of plasma and red cells must pass through the arteriole in a given time. Since the cell velocity is twice the plasma velocity in our example, equal volume flows are only possible if the concentration of red cells in the arteriole is half that in the parent blood. This is achieved by the red cells speeding away from the plasma at the tube entrance, thinning out rather like traffic entering a fast road from a congested slip road.

Non-Newtonian viscosity. II – Effect of shear rate

The viscosity of blood varies not only with tube diameter but with velocity too, or more accurately with shear rate (see Figure 8.14b). Shear rate, it will be recalled, is the change in fluid velocity per unit distance normal to the direction of flow. At very low flows and shear rates, viscosity can become very high, whereas at physiological flows and shear rates (around 1000 per s) viscosity is relatively low. Reduction in viscosity with increasing shear rate is attributed to deformation and lining-up of the deformed cells with the flow lines, and to a tank-tread motion of the red cell membrane around its interior. At low flows in horizontal tubes, partial sedimentation of the cells within the tube contributes to the rise in viscosity. Low flow also allows the red cells to adhere to each other to form 'rouleaux', which resemble stacks of coins. It is thought that such changes probably occur in veins *in vivo* if blood flow is sluggish.

8.6 Pressure–flow curves for entire vascular beds

The conditions under which Poiseuille's law is strictly valid include a steady flow (cf. pulsatile flow *in vivo*) of a Newtonian fluid (cf. blood) along a long straight vessel (cf. branched, curved and tapering vasculature) with rigid walls (cf. distensible blood vessels). So one certainly has to be cautious in applying Poiseuille's law to the circulation! In the lungs and in perfused hindlimbs with little vascular muscle tone, the pressure–flow relation is relatively linear at physiological pressure: but there is a positive pressure intercept at zero flow, and a curved relation at low pressures (see curve labelled 'blood' in Figure 8.15). The curvature indicates that resistance decreases as pressure rises. This is caused by (1) the elasticity of the arterioles,

which permits radius to increase and therefore resistance to decrease as pressure rises, and (2) alterations in blood viscosity with shear rate. The latter seems to be the main factor, because perfusing a dog's hindlimb with saline produces a more linear pressure–flow relation, extrapolating virtually through the origin (Figure 8.15).

In circulations with good arteriolar tone, a curious and physiologically-important pressure–flow relation exists, called an *autoregulation curve*. Flow increases with pressure up to a certain point, but the slope of the relation then flattens and thereafter flow changes relatively little with pressure, until pressure exceeds about 180 mmHg. A nearly constant flow in the face of a rising pressure indicates that resistance is *rising* in proportion to the pressure. This phenomenon, called autoregulation, is caused by active vasoconstriction and is described further in Section 12.3. Autoregulation occurs in most organs *in vivo* except the lung.

8.7 Haemodynamics in veins

Venous distension curve

Peripheral venules and veins are thin-walled, voluminous vessels and they contain roughly two-thirds of the circulating blood. They act as a variable reservoir of blood for the thoracic compartment and thereby influence the cardiac filling pressure.

The volume of blood in a peripheral vein depends on the venous blood pressure and on active wall tension, as illustrated in Figure 8.16. The effect of pressure on venous volume is particularly steep between zero pressure and 10 mmHg because the thin-walled vein deforms easily. At a transmural pressure of 1 mmHg, the vein is almost collapsed and has a narrow elliptical profile. As pressure rises towards 10 mmHg, the elliptical profile becomes progressively rounder, enabling the vein to accommodate large volume change with just a few mmHg change in pressure. The maximum distensibility, which occurs at approximately

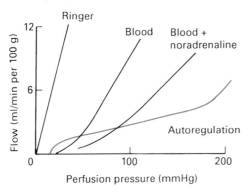

Figure 8.15 Pressure–flow curves for dog skeletal muscle. When the arterioles are in good physiological condition, autoregulation is present. When this is abolished, steeper curvilinear relations are seen: the curvature is caused by changes in resistance with pressure. Noradrenaline causes vasoconstriction and increases resistance. Perfusion with mammalian Ringer's solution (a physiological salt solution) produces a steeper line due to its low viscosity, and the line is almost straight because the anomalous viscous effect of blood is removed. (From Pappenheimer, J. R. and Maes, J. P. (1942) *American Journal of Physiology*, **137**, 187–199; and Stainsby, W. N. and Renkin, E. M. (1961) *American Journal of Physiology*, **201**, 117–122, by permission)

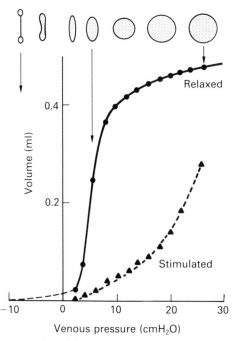

Relaxed

Stimulated

Figure 8.16 Venous pressure–volume curve, in relaxed state (filled circles) and at maximum contraction (triangles). The change in cross-section of the vein with pressure is shown schematically above. (Canine saphenous vein, from Vanhoutte, P. M. and Leusen, I. (1969) *Pfluger's Archiv*, **306**, 341–353, by permission)

4 mmHg, is estimated to be approximately 100 ml/mmHg for the human venous system – over 50 times greater than the compliance of the arterial system. Below zero transmural pressure, the vein collapses into a dumb-bell shape and any flow is confined to the marginal channels. Above 10–15 mmHg the profile is fully circular and since the stretched collagen in the wall is relatively inextensible the volume is less sensitive to pressures over 15 mmHg.

The other factor influencing venous volume is active tension in the smooth muscle of the venous tunica media. In the gastrointestinal, hepatic, renal and cutaneous circulations, the vein wall is innervated by sympathetic vasomotor nerves. Sympathetically-excited venoconstriction reduces the capacitance of these peripheral veins (see Figure 8.16, lower curve)

and displaces blood into the thoracic compartment. This provides an important mechanism by which the nervous system can regulate the filling pressure of the heart.

Peripheral and central venous pressures

Blood enters venules at heart level at a pressure of approximately 12–20 mmHg, and by the time it reaches named veins like the femoral vein, pressure has fallen to approximately 8–10 mmHg. The subsequent venous resistance is very small (except in collapsed vessels) so the 8–10 mmHg pressure head suffices to drive the cardiac output from the periphery into the central veins and right ventricle, where the diastolic pressure is 0–6 mmHg.

In intensive care units, central venous pressure (CVP) is often monitored directly via a catheter advanced into the subclavian vein or superior vena cava. In the routine clinical examination of the cardiovascular system, however, the CVP is assessed indirectly by inspection of the neck veins (see Figure 8.17). The external jugular vein runs over the sternomastoid muscle and the internal jugular vein runs deep to it. With the subject in a semi-supine position the lower part of the external jugular vein is normally distended while the upper part is collapsed (an effect of gravity). From the venous pressure–volume curve, we know that transmural pressure is zero at the point of collapse of a vein. CVP is therefore equal to the pressure exerted by the vertical column of blood between this point and the right atrium. If, for example, the point of collapse (zero pressure) is 7 cm vertical distance above the right atrial midpoint, CVP is 7 cm of blood (7.4 cmH$_2$O). The position of the atrium cannot of course be observed directly but from anatomical studies we know that the right atrial midpoint is approximately 5 cm lower than the manubriosternal angle, which is readily located. Thus by measuring the vertical distance between the point of collapse and

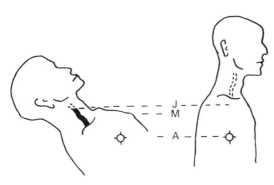

Figure 8.17 Estimation of central venous pressure (CVP) in a semi-supine human subject. CVP is the pressure at the point where the venae cavae enter the right atrium. This is equal to the vertical distance between point of collapse of the jugular vein (J) and right atrium (A). (The atria serve as a standard reference level when measuring circulatory pressures.) Since point A cannot be seen, the height of J above the manubriosternal angle (M) is measured instead; M–A is approximately 5 cm. CVP = (J–M) + 5 (cmH$_2$O). In the upright position the jugular vein is normally collapsed

the manubriosternal angle, and adding 5 cm, CVP can be estimated. Although the accuracy is only of the order ±2 cm, this is sufficient to detect the grossly elevated CVP which characterizes right ventricular failure (see Chapter 16). The normal subject has to be semi-supine because in the upright position the point of collapse is hidden below the clavicle: in right ventricular failure by contrast the CVP may be so high that the venous pulse is visible in the neck even when the patient is upright.

Effect of posture and altered gravity

The adoption of a standing position (orthostasis) increases the pressure in any blood vessel below heart level and reduces it in any vessel above heart level, owing to the drag of gravity on the vertical column of fluid between the heart and the vessel. This is particularly important in veins because their volume is particularly sensitive to transmural pressure.

Veins below heart level

Upon tilting a human subject upright, a transitory closure of the venous valves in the limbs prevents any significant backflow of blood away from the heart. Pressure in the dependent veins then rises steadily over approximately 30–60 s because blood continues to flow into the veins from the arterial system, and as it does so it opens the venous valves and re-establishes an uninterrupted column of blood between the heart and the feet. The weight of this fluid column raises venous pressure in the feet tenfold, from approximately 10 mmHg supine to nearly 100 mmHg upright (see Figures 8.18 and 8.21). There is no counterbalancing rise in extramural pressure (unless the subject is immersed in water), so the veins distend: this is plainly visible in one's own hand on lowering it below heart level. In a human adult, about 500 ml of extra blood accumulate over approximately 45 s in the distended veins of the lower limbs. This is usually called venous 'pooling', but the phrase is misleading in that a pool is static whereas the venous blood is of course flowing continuously. Most of the additional blood comes ultimately from the intrathoracic compartment, so the CVP falls, impairing stroke volume by the Frank–Starling mechanism and provoking a transitory arterial hypotension and, sometimes, dizziness (postural hypotension; Section 15.1). A handcount among medical students indicates that nearly all healthy individuals occasionally experience this orthostatic dizziness, especially when warm and venodilated.

Caveat: flow in a siphon or 'How gravity does not work'

Gravity acts equally on venous and arterial fluid columns; consequently, the pressure difference between the arteries and veins at any vertical level is not directly altered by orthostasis (see Figure 10.5), and nor therefore is blood flow. The assumption by some students that venous flow decreases in the dependent leg 'because blood has to go uphill against gravity' is utterly spurious,

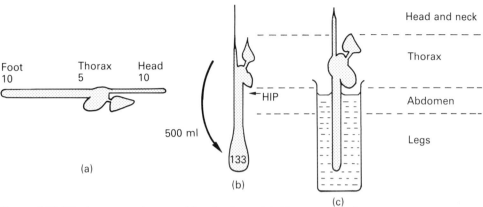

Figure 8.18 Displacement of venous blood volume (pink) on moving from supine position (a) to standing (b). The thoracic compartment includes the central veins, heart and pulmonary blood; the lungs are shown disproportionately small here. Numbers are typical pressures in cmH_2O. The hydrostatic indifferent point (HIP) is the point where pressure is unaltered by tilting. (c) shows how immersion in water increases central volume and CVP. (After Gauer, O. H. and Thron, H. L. (1963) *Handbook of Physiology, Circulation*, Vol. 3 (eds. W. F. Hamilton and P. Dow, American Physiological Society, Bethesda, pp. 2409–2440)

for it ignores the fact that gravity has an equal effect on the arterial column. The circulation through the limb or brain in fact resembles flow through a U-tube siphon, and flow through a rigid siphon is the same whether it is vertical, horizontal or upside down (Figure 8.19). Indeed, if blood vessels were completely rigid, gravity would have no overall effect on the circulation. Limb blood flow does in fact decline with dependency as can be seen in Figure 8.5, but this is not because 'blood has to go uphill'; it is because (1) the orthostatically-induced fall in cardiac output elicits a reflex increase in vasoconstrictor nerve activity to limb arterioles, and (2) there is also a local arteriolar constriction in response to the rise in local transmural pressure.

Veins above heart level

In vessels above heart level, the effect of gravity is to reduce blood pressure. When the transmural pressure falls to zero or less, the unsupported superficial veins collapse (Figures 8.16 and 8.18). Deeper veins are better supported and do not collapse completely. Veins within the rigid cranial cavity are a special case and do not collapse because

gravity reduces the pressure of the cerebrospinal fluid around them too, so the transmural pressure hardly changes.

When gravity alters

Air pilots experience altered g forces during aerobatic manoeuvres. A pilot pulling out of a steep dive can experience +3g to +4g along the body axis, and venous pooling in the lower body is so severe that the stroke volume falls rapidly and the pilot experiences a 'blackout' due to cerebral hypoperfusion. To prevent this, an anti-gravity suit is worn; bags inflate automatically around the legs to raise extramural pressure and minimize venous distension during turns. Conversely, in an inverted loop-the-loop manoeuvre a high negative g force is experienced, i.e. gravity is directed towards the head. This distends the retinal vessels and causes a 'redout' of vision. In space travel, the circulation is subjected to zero gravity for long periods but as this is not dissimilar to a supine posture or to floating in water, it presents no special problem for the cardiovascular system until the return to positive gravity.

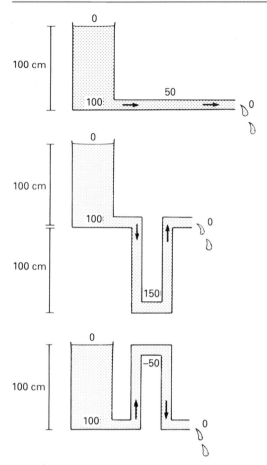

Figure 8.19 The siphon effect in a rigid U-tube. The feed-tank produces a pressure head of $100\,cmH_2O$ to drive the flow. Flow passes through either a straight tube or a U-tube of equal resistance. The net pressure difference driving flow is the same in each case, so the flow is identical in all three situations (siphon principle). Numbers refer to pressure in cmH_2O at various points

Oscillations in venous pressure and flow

Pressure is pulsatile in veins close to the right atrium, such as the jugular veins. The pulse pressure is a few mmHg, just sufficient to move the overlying skin and render itself visible but too small to be palpable, unlike the arterial pulse. The waveform of the venous pulse was described fully in Section 2.3. Figure 8.20 relates the pressure waves to the oscillations in venous flow. Blood flow in central veins displays two spurts per cycle. Peak flow occurs during the x descent of the pressure wave and is caused by atrial relaxation. This inflow may be boosted by ventricular systole because the ballistic effect of firing out a mass of blood propels the ventricle downwards (like the recoil of a gun: Newton's law of action and reaction), stretching the atria and helping to suck blood into them. The second flow-spurt, during the y descent, is due to the tricuspid valve opening in diastole. This second spurt is boosted by the elastic recoil of the ventricular walls when end-systolic volume is low (e.g. exercise). Thus flow through the

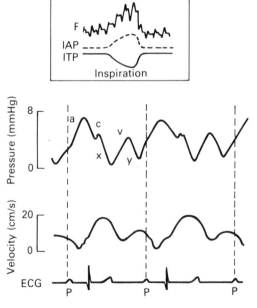

Figure 8.20 Pressure and flow in human superior vena cava over two cycles. Inset shows effect of breathing on venous return. F, flow in thoracic inferior vena cava; IAP, intra-abdominal pressure; ITP, intra-thoracic pressure. (After Brecher, G. A. (1956) *Venous Return*, Grune and Stratton, New York and Wexler, L., Bergel, D. L., Gabe, T. *et al.* (1968) *Circulation Research*, **23**, 349–359)

great veins, while primarily driven by the upstream pressure of about 8 mmHg (pressure from behind or *'vis a tergo'*), is aided by two transient reductions in downstream pressure due to the motion of the heart (suction from in front or *'vis a fronte'*).

Venous flow can also be assisted by two non-cardiac factors: the skeletal muscle pump and the effect of breathing, as described next.

Skeletal muscle pump

When a skeletal muscle contracts it compresses the veins within it, expelling their blood into the central veins. Venous valves prevent retrograde flow and ensure that the emptied segments refill from the periphery during muscle relaxation (Figure 8.21). Rhythmic exercise thus has a pumping effect, with several beneficial consequences. (1) The pump redistributes venous blood from the periphery into the central veins, and this prevents CVP from falling during exercise (cf. Figure 7.10). The muscle pump may even increase CVP slightly and move the ventricle up the Starling curve. (2) Like any pump, the muscle pump lowers pressure in the feed line: distal venous pressure falls because as the muscle relaxes blood drains rapidly from the distal veins into the empty muscle veins.

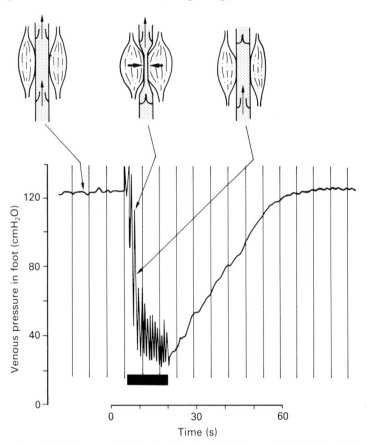

Figure 8.21 Pressure in the dorsal vein of the human foot during quiet standing, interrupted by rhythmic contraction of the calf muscles for a short period (black bar). Insets illustrate how the muscle pump operates. The subject, a physiologist, evidently has competent venous valves (as is of course to be expected of a physiologist!). (Unpublished data of Levick, J. R. and Michel, C. C.)

At the same time, closure of the proximal valves interrupts the vertical column of blood between limb and heart. This reduces venous pressure in the foot and calf from around 90–100 mmHg in immobile orthostasis to 20–40 mmHg during walking, running, cycling, etc. As a result, the arteriovenous pressure difference driving blood flow through the calf muscle increases by 50–60%. (3) The muscle pump reduces capillary filtration pressure in the legs too since capillary pressure is close to venous pressure, and this reduces the tendency of a dependent limb to swell during exercise.

If the venous valves become *incompetent*, the muscle pump becomes ineffective. Since the vertical blood column can no longer be effectively broken up, the veins are subjected to a chronically-raised pressure load which leads to permanent distension (*varicose veins*). In addition the distal tissues swell due to the unrelieved, high capillary filtration pressure and this can provoke trophic skin changes and ulceration, usually just above the ankle (*venous ulcer*).

Respiratory pump

Flow in the vena cava increases during inspiration (see Figure 8.20, inset). This is because the fall in intrathoracic pressure expands the intrathoracic veins, and at the same time the diaphragm compresses the abdominal contents, raising the abdominal venous pressure and enhancing venous flow from abdomen to thorax. Conversely, vena caval flow slows during expiration, especially during forced expiration or a Valsalva manoeuvre (Chapter 15). Coughing can elevate intrathoracic pressure to 400 mmHg, and *paroxysmal coughing* can impede venous inflow to such a degree that fainting results.

The respiration-related oscillations in venous return evoke oscillations in stroke volume and blood pressure. Right ventricle stroke volume rises during inspiration owing to increased right ventricular filling. Left ventricular stroke volume on the other hand falls in inspiration because the stretched

pulmonary vessels have a greater capacitance and this reduces the left side filling pressure. The situation reverses during expiration, so the output of the two ventricles is equal when averaged over the respiratory cycle. Because left ventricular output falls on inspiration and rises on expiration it is common to find that systemic blood pressure has a similar respiration-related cycle.

8.8 Summary

Blood flow is laminar in arteries and veins, turbulent in the ventricles and bolus pattern (single file) in capillaries. Except for turbulent flow, flow (Q) is linearly proportional to the pressure drop across a tube ($P_1 - P_2$) and inversely proportional to resistance (R); $Q = (P_1 - P_2)/R$.

In man, *tissue blood flow* can be determined via the Fick principle (e.g. renal blood flow using PAH), venous occlusion plethysmography (limbs), Doppler ultrasound (accessible major arteries and veins), laser Doppler (skin) and radio-isotope clearance (skin, muscle).

Arterial pressure can be measured by sphygmomanometry. The pulsatile wave has a characteristic dicrotic notch, caused by aortic valve closure. Mean brachial artery pressure is approximately diastolic pressure + one-third of the pulse pressure; the latter is systolic pressure minus diastolic pressure. Mean pressure is determined by cardiac output × total peripheral resistance, and varies with age, exercise, emotional stress, sleep, posture and many other factors. The pressure wave is transmitted rapidly along the arterial tree and the propagation rate depends on arterial wall stiffness.

Vascular resistance. Since pressure drops from ~ 80 mmHg to ~ 35 mmHg between the small arteries and the start of capillaries, it follows that the arterioles and terminal arteries are the chief site of resistance. Resistance is determined by the factors in Poiseuille's equation, namely $8\eta L/\pi r^4$, where η is blood viscosity, L is length and r is lumen radius. The *radius* of resistance vessels is controlled by the tension of smooth muscle in the media. This provides a powerful (r^4) way of regulating both local blood flow and arterial blood pressure. Vessel radius is related to wall tension and local pressure by Laplace's law. The *viscosity* of blood depends mainly on the haematocrit (raised in polycythaemia, reduced in anaemia), but also varies with tube radius (η decreases in microvessels, facilitating microvascular flow; the Fåhraeus–Lindqvist effect) and velocity (η rises at very low shear rates).

Venous pressure at heart level is $10\,mmHg$ or less. Small changes in venous pressure have large effects on venous blood volume due to the collapsible nature of veins. Venous smooth muscle tone actively regulates peripheral venous blood volume in many tissues (e.g. skin, splanchnic circulation). Peripheral veins thus serve as variable blood 'reservoirs'. Distension of leg veins by gravity in the upright posture is responsible for a fall in CVP and stroke volume. This is partly offset by the muscle pump during movement.

Further reading

Reviews and chapters

Blomqvist, C. G. and Stone, H. L. (1983) Cardiovascular adjustments to gravitational stress. In *Handbook of Physiology, Cardiovascular System*, Vol. 3, Part 1, *Peripheral Circulation* (eds J. T. Shepherd and F. M. Abboud), American Physiological Society, Bethesda, pp. 1025–1063

Caro, C. G., Pedley, T. J., Schroter, R. C. and Seed, W. A. (1978) *The Mechanics of the Circulation*, Oxford University Press, Oxford

Chien, S. (1992) Blood cell deformability and interactions: from molecules to micromechanics and microcirculation (Zweifach Lecture). *Microvascular Research*, **44**, 243–254

Chien, S., Usami, S. and Skalak, R. (1984) Blood flow in small tubes. In *Handbook of Physiology, Cardiovascular System*, Vol. 4, *Microcirculation* (eds E. M. Renkin and C. C. Michel), American Physiological Society, Bethesda, pp. 217–250

Goldsmith, H. L., Cokelet, G. R. and Gaehtgens, P. (1989) Robin Fåhraeus: evolution of his concepts in cardiovascular physiology. *American Journal of Physiology*, **257**, H1005–H1015

McDonald, D. A. (1974) *Blood Flow in Arteries*, Edward Arnold, London

Noble, M. I. M. (1979) *The Cardiac Cycle*, Blackwell, Oxford

Pappenheimer, J. R. (1984) Contributions to microvascular research of Jean Leonard Marie Poiseuille. In *Handbook of Physiology, Cardiovascular System*, Vol. 4, *The Microcirculation* (eds E. M. Renkin and C. C. Michel), American Physiological Society, Bethesda, pp. 1–10

Pickering, T. G. (1990) Physiological aspects of non-invasive ambulatory blood-pressure monitoring. *News in Physiological Sciences*, **5**, 176–179

Zweifach, B. W. and Lipowsky, H. H. (1984) Pressure-flow relations in blood and lymph microcirculations. In *Handbook of Physiology, Cardiovascular System*, Vol. 4, *Microcirculation* (eds E. M. Renkin and C. C. Michel), American Physiological Society, Bethesda, pp. 251–307

Research papers

Reinke, W., Gaehtgens, P. and Johnson, P. C. (1987) Blood viscosity in small tubes : effect of shear rate, aggregation, and sedimentation. *American Journal of Physiology*, **253**, H540–H547

Sutton, D. W. and Schmid-Schönbein, G. W. (1989) Hemodynamics at low flow in resting vasodilated rat skeletal muscle. *American Journal of Physiology*, **257**, H1419–1427

Toska, K. and Eriksen, M. (1993) Respiration-synchronous fluctuations in stroke volume, heart rate and arterial pressure in humans. *Journal of Physiology*, **472**, 501–512

Chapter 9

Solute transport between blood and tissue

The heart and vasculature exist for one fundamental purpose: the delivery of metabolic substrate to the cells of the organism. This delivery takes place across the thin walls of capillaries, which thus subserve the ultimate function of the cardiovascular system. The capillary wall is also the site of fluid exchange between plasma and interstitial fluid, which governs the volume of each compartment (Chapter 10). In addition, endothelial cells of capillaries and larger vessels have many active functions dependent on cellular metabolism, some of which are covered here and some in Chapter 12.

9.1 Microvessel heterogeneity and density

Types of microvessel

The smallest arteries branch into first-order arterioles with muscular walls innervated by sympathetic nerves. These branch further to give rise to terminal arterioles, whose walls contain smooth muscle but few vasomotor nerves, control being dominated at this level by local metabolites. The terminal arteriole gives rise to a cluster or module of capillaries (Figure 9.1) and the smooth muscle tone in the terminal arteriole determines whether the capillary module is well perfused with blood ('open' capillaries) or not ('closed' capillaries). A few tissues, such as mesentery, have a ring of smooth muscle at the capillary entrance, the 'precapillary sphincter', governing capillary perfusion, but most tissues lack these. Another specialized structure is the arteriovenous anastomosis, a broad muscular vessel bypassing the capillary network in the skin of the extremities (fingers, nose, ear); it is involved in temperature regulation (see Chapter 13). The capillaries themselves are only 5–8 μm in diameter ('capillary' means hair-like), and were first

proved to exist by Malpighi, a pioneer of microscopy who observed capillaries in a frog lung in 1661. The venous ends of capillaries unite to form pericytic venules (postcapillary venules) whose walls contain pericytes but no smooth muscle. These too are exchange vessels. Smooth muscle reappears in the walls of venules of diameter 30–50 μm.

Heterogeneity of length and blood flow

The non-uniformity within a microcirculation is striking. Capillaries vary in length (typically 500–1000 μm), in blood flow and in dynamic haematocrit even within the same tissue at the same time. Blood flow waxes and wanes every 15 s or so in some capillary modules and can stop briefly due to spontaneous rhythmic contractions in the terminal arterioles (*vasomotion*). This influences both solute exchange and fluid exchange (see Chapter 10). In well-perfused capillaries, the blood velocity is typically 300–1000 μm/ s and the transit time is 0.5–2 s; this is the time available for plasma to unload oxygen, glucose, etc., and load up with carbon dioxide, etc. Mean transit time can fall to approximately 0.25 s in exercise.

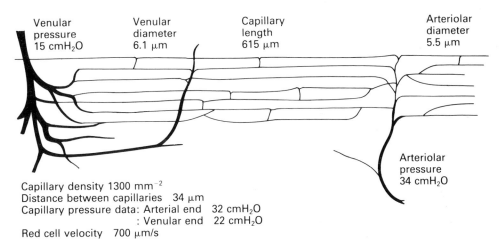

Venular pressure 15 cmH$_2$O
Venular diameter 6.1 μm
Capillary length 615 μm
Arteriolar diameter 5.5 μm

Arteriolar pressure 34 cmH$_2$O

Capillary density 1300 mm^{-2}
Distance between capillaries 34 μm
Capillary pressure data: Arterial end 32 cmH$_2$O
: Venular end 22 cmH$_2$O
Red cell velocity 700 μm/s

Figure 9.1 Capillary bed in relaxed cremaster muscle of a rat, with a terminal arteriole feeding a module of 14 capillaries. Numbers are means of observations. (From Smaje, L. H., Zweifach, B. W. and Intaglietta, M. (1970) *Microvascular Research*, **2**, 96–110, by permission)

Capillary density and its functional importance

Skeletal muscle contains one or more capillaries per muscle fibre (300–1000 capillaries per mm^2 of muscle). The number of capillaries packed into a tissue is functionally important because it determines (1) the total area of capillary wall available for exchange between blood and tissue (e.g. 100 cm^2/g in muscle), and (2) the intercapillary spacing and therefore the maximum blood-to-cell distance, which has a large effect on diffusion time (see Table 1.1). In keeping with this, endurance exercise training results in new capillary formation, and capillary/fibre ratios as high as 6–8 have been found in the gastrocnemius of long-distance runners. In the myocardium and brain, where oxygen consumption is high and sustained, the capillary density is even greater than in skeletal muscle, providing around 500 cm^2 surface per gram tissue. In the lung, capillary area is extremely high (3500 cm^2/g).

9.2 Structure of exchange vessels

The term 'exchange vessel' actually embraces both sides of the anatomical capillary bed because some oxygen diffuses through the walls of terminal arterioles and some fluid crosses the walls of pericytic venules. True anatomical capillaries are of three ultrastructural types: continuous, fenestrated and discontinuous (in order of increasing permeability to water).

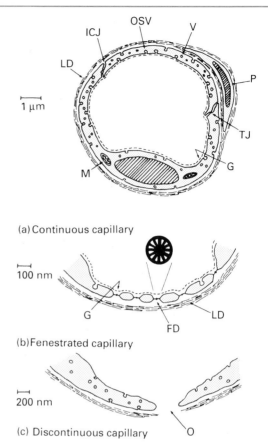

(a) Continuous capillary

(b) Fenestrated capillary

(c) Discontinuous capillary

Figure 9.2 Sketches of capillary wall in transverse section, based on electron micrographs. FD, fenestral diaphragm; inset shows diaphragm *en face*; G, glycocalyx; ICJ, intercellular junction; LD, lamina densa of basal lamina; M, mitochondrion; O, open intercellular gap; OSV, open surface vesicle; P, pericyte; TJ, tight part of junction; V, vesicle. Scale only approximate

Continuous capillary

Continuous capillaries are found in muscle, skin, lung, fat, connective tissue and the nervous system. The circumference is formed by 1–3 flattened endothelial cells resting on a basement membrane (Figure 9.2). Because the wall is only 1 cell thick, diffusion distance is very small (approximately 0.5 μm). Pericytes, or 'Rouget cells', partly envelop the capillary and there is some evidence that pre-

and postcapillary pericytes can contract, although the significance of this is unclear. The endothelial cell contains mitochondria, endoplasmic reticulum, a Golgi apparatus and filaments of the contractile proteins actin and myosin. The latter form distinct stress fibres in spleen endothelium, and splenic capillaries appear to be actively contractile. Most capillaries are thought to be non-contractile under physiological conditions, but contraction of venular endothelial cells can occur in acute inflammation (Section 10.11).

Certain endothelial features are particularly important for solute transfer, namely the intercellular junction, vesicle system and surface coat (glycocalyx). Their structure is as follows.

Intercellular junctions

These are parallel-sided clefts occupying 0.1–0.3% of the capillary surface. They are almost certainly the transcapillary route taken by most fluid and by metabolites like glucose. In cross-section the cleft is 15–20 nm wide for most of its length, and this is much wider than the diameter of a glucose molecule (0.9 nm) or even albumin (7.1 nm). At one to three points along the cleft, the adjacent cell membranes come into very close proximity and form 'tight junctions', but these junctions do not provide a continuous seal around the cell perimeter. Freeze-fracture electron microscopy, which displays the junctional membrane *en face*,

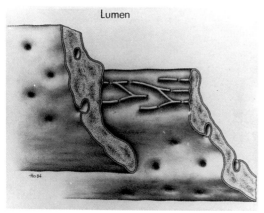

Figure 9.3 Three-dimensional reconstruction of tight junction between two endothelial cells, based on serial thin sections. The cleft is typically 500–1000 nm long, from lumen to outside, and 15–20 nm wide. Small lipophobic solutes and water can circumvent the junctional strands. They might also pass through discrete interruptions in them. (From Bundgaard (1984) *Journal of Ultrastructural Research*, **88**, 1–17, by permission)

reveals the tight junctions as lines of membrane particles (junctional strands, Figure 9.3). The junctional strands run round the cell perimeter but are interrupted by two kinds of break. (1) Short gaps of 5–11 nm occur occasionally between individual particles. (2) The junctional strands sometimes come to an abrupt end leaving a tortuous but open route through the intercellular cleft. The overlap of other strands prevents this tortuous bypass from being seen in a single transverse section, but serial transverse sections confirm its existence. In pericytic venules, which are actually more permeable than capillaries, the overlap of the junctional strands is less marked. Conversely, in brain capillaries, which have a very low permeability to fluid, the strands are numerous and complex and extend without interruption around the perimeter to form a true seal (zonula occludens), as in tight epithelia.

Endothelial vesicles and vesicular transport

About a quarter of the cytoplasmic volume is occupied by vesicles of diameter 60 nm, which are thought to be involved in transporting macromolecules into the cell (endocytosis) and, more controversially, across it (transcytosis). Some vesicles open directly onto the cell surface by a stalk 20 nm wide while others look as though they are floating free in the cytoplasm. This led to the idea that vesicles might ferry plasma proteins across the cell, loading up at the surface, detaching and diffusing across the cell to release their load at the abluminal side. Ultrathin serial sections, however, reveal that free-floating vesicles are mostly an illusion; 99% of seemingly 'free' vesicles are connected, out of the plane of section, to one or other surface via surface vesicles as in Figure 9.4(a). The vesicular system is thus a racemose invagination of the plasmalemma resembling a bunch of grapes. Nevertheless, these structures might still play a role in macromolecular transport by a process involving transient fusion and exchange of contents between the luminal and abluminal

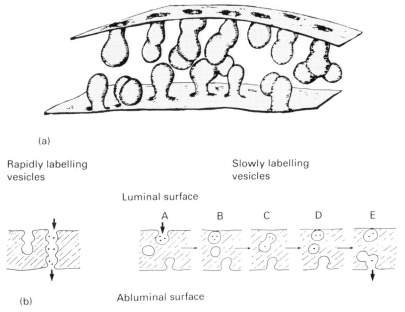

Figure 9.4 Diagrams of the endothelial vesicle system. (a) Reconstruction of serial sections. Vesicles are a racemose invagination of the surface plasmalemma, with hardly any truly free-floating vesicles. (b) Frames A–E show how a slow transcytosis of protein molecules (black dots) might occur from the plasma to interstitium by fusion and mixing of contents (frame C) between luminal-linked and abluminal-linked vesicles. A few abluminal vesicles label unusually rapidly, perhaps because they are part of a multivesicular transendothelial channel (left). ((a) From Frokjaer-Jensen, J. (1983) *Progress in Applied Microcirculation*, **1**, 17–34, by permission; (b) from Clough, G. and Michel, C. C. (1981) *Journal of Physiology*, **315**, 127–142, by permission)

systems, as in Figure 9.4(b). Very rarely, two or three vesicles are seen to be fused to create a continuous channel across the endothelial cell, the 'multivesicular channel', and these too may contribute to plasma protein passage (Figure 9.4b, left).

Glycocalyx

The endothelial surface is coated with a thin layer of negatively-charged material called the glycocalyx, as revealed by cationic (positive charged) probes (Figure 9.5). The glycocalyx covers the intercellular cleft and fenestrae, and lines the surface vesicles too. It consists of a meshwork of fibrous molecules with protein cores and sugar-based side chains, namely sialoglycoproteins such as podocalyxin, and gly-cosaminoglycans such as heparan sulphate. There is growing evidence that this meshwork acts as a macromolecular sieve (Section 9.8).

Basal lamina

The basal lamina (often called basement membrane) is 50–100 nm thick and consists of a dense region (lamina densa) separated from the cell by a lighter region (lamina rara). The lamina densa consists of a network of type IV collagen molecules and negatively-charged heparan sulphate proteoglycan. It is attached to the cell by a cross-shaped glycoprotein called laminin. The basal lamina endows the capillary with sufficient strength to withstand blood pressure. The tension in the capillary wall is low, owing to the small radius of curvature (see Laplace's

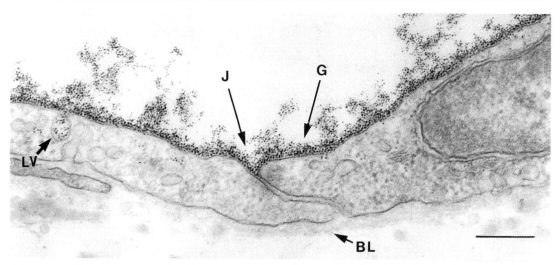

Figure 9.5 Electron micrograph of frog mesenteric capillary perfused with a solution of cationized ferritin (diameter 11 nm). Lumen at the top. The cationic molecules (black dots) bind to and delineate the glycocalyx (G). On the left, some ferritin molecules are seen labelling a vesicle (LV). The intercellular junction in the centre (J) appears impermeable to them. The cationized ferritin was found to reduce hydraulic conductance (see 'the protein effect', Section 9.8), whereas native ferritin, which does not bind to the glycocalyx, does not affect conductance. BL, basal lamina. Bar = 0.2 μm. (From Turner, M. R., Clough, G. and Michel, C. C. (1983) *Microvascular Research*, **25**, 205–222, by permission)

law, Section 8.5). The stress, however, can be very high, comparable with the mean stress in an artery wall, because stress is tension divided by wall thickness, and the latter is very thin. In Goodpasture's syndrome, weakening of the capillary basal lamina by autoantibodies directed against type IV collagen results in bleeding into the alveolar and glomerular spaces.

The basal lamina retards but does not prevent the passage of protein molecules. In renal glomerular capillaries a double lamina densa holds back very large macromolecules such as ferritin, and a high negative charge density helps hold back negatively charged proteins.

Fenestrated capillary

Fenestrated capillaries are an order of magnitude more permeable to water and small hydrophilic solutes than most continuous capillaries. They occur in tissues specializing in fluid exchange (renal glomerulus and

tubules, exocrine glands, intestinal mucosa, ciliary body, choroid plexus, synovial lining of joints) and also in endocrine glands. The endothelium is perforated by small circular windows, the fenestrae (diameter 50–60 nm), which allow plasma within 0.1 μm of the extravascular space. Fenestrae are the major route by which water and metabolites cross fenestrated capillaries. The fenestrae are mostly not open holes but are bridged by an extremely thin membrane, the fenestral diaphragm (thickness 4–5 nm) which is sandwiched between the glycocalyx and basement membrane. Viewed *en face* the diaphragm resembles a cartwheel, being perforated by about 14 wedge-shaped apertures of arc-length 5.5 nm (see Figure 9.2b). In renal glomerular capillaries, however, diaphragms are totally absent.

Discontinuous capillary

Discontinuous or sinusoidal capillaries possess some intercellular gaps over 100 nm wide and a discontinuity in the underlying basal lamina. As a result, these capillaries are permeable even to plasma proteins. They occur wherever red cells need to migrate between blood and tissue, i.e. bone marrow, spleen and liver.

9.3 Transport processes: diffusion, reflection, convection

The passage of water and solutes across the capillary wall is a passive process requiring no energy expenditure by the endothelium. *Fluid movement* across the wall is a process of hydraulic flow down pressure gradients set up by the heart. (Water molecules also diffuse extremely rapidly across the wall but this diffusion is bidirectional and no net transport results.) *Metabolite exchange* is mainly a process of passive diffusion down concentration gradients set up by tissue metabolism. To a minor extent, metabolites are also swept along in the transcapillary stream of fluid ('convective transport'), but the stream is relatively slow and this form of solute transport can often be neglected (see footnote to Table 9.2). Diffusion of small solutes across the capillary wall is very rapid, as shown by the timed sequences of photographs in Figure 9.6. *Macromolecules* diffuse more slowly than metabolites like glucose, so convective transport across the capillary wall is relatively more important in their transport.

To understand capillary exchange, we must therefore consider the nature of diffusion and convection across a porous membrane and equip ourselves with a basic kit of transport expressions.

Free diffusion and Fick's law

Diffusion was studied by Adolf Fick, Professor of Physiology at Wurzburg, and Fick's first law of diffusion (1855) describes the rate of diffusion, i.e. the mass of solute transferred by diffusion per unit time (J_S) – Figure 9.7(a). Fick's law can be summarized thus:

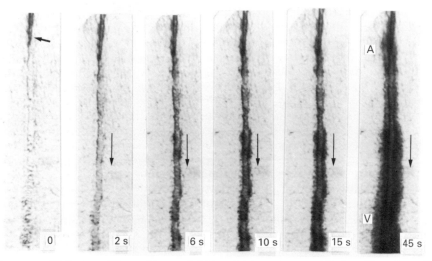

Figure 9.6 Diffusion of Evans blue, a lipid-insoluble molecule of Stokes–Einstein radius 1.3 nm, out of a frog mesenteric capillary. Tip of the perfusing micropipette just visible (thick arrow); thin arrows show direction of flow. Permeability can be determined from change in optical density with time. By 15–45 s an arteriovenous gradient of permeability is clearly visible (A–V); venous capillaries and pericytic venules are normally more permeable than arterial capillaries, probably due to their less extensive junctional strands. (From Levick, J. R. (1972) Doctoral thesis, Oxford)

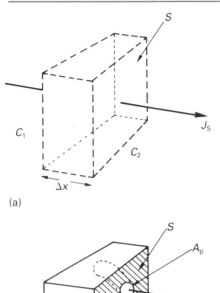

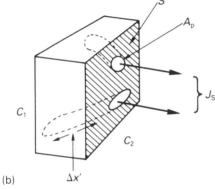

Figure 9.7 (a) Free diffusion in bulk solution. The solute traverses an unimpeded layer of fluid of thickness Δx and surface area S, driven by concentration difference $C_1 - C_2$. J_S is the diffusion rate (moles/s). (b) Membrane reduces J_S by confining solute to pores of total area A_p. The pathlength through the pore, $\Delta x'$, can exceed the membrane thickness Δx

$$J_S = -DS\frac{\Delta C}{\Delta x} \qquad (9.1)$$

Diffusion rate depends on the concentration difference driving diffusion (ΔC) and the distance across which diffusion is occurring (Δx), the ratio $\Delta C/\Delta x$ being the concentration gradient. Diffusional transport also depends on surface area (S), and the diffusion coefficient (D), which represents the intrinsic velocity of the solute. The negative sign indicates that solute flux occurs down the concentration gradient. The diffusion coefficient (D) depends on temperature, solvent viscosity and solute size. Small molecules diffuse faster than big ones, and for most solutes D is inversely proportional to the cube root of the molecular weight. The diffusion coefficient is often used to calculate the effective *radius* of a molecule, idealized as a sphere (the Stokes–Einstein radius or diffusion radius; see Table 9.1 and Appendix II).

Effect of a membrane on diffusion, and meaning of 'permeability'

Diffusion through a large volume of solvent is called free diffusion. When a solute diffuses across a membrane, however, several factors slow the diffusional process.

Available area If the solute is confined to solvent-filled pores penetrating the membrane, the area available for diffusion is reduced from the total surface (S) to the pore area (A_p) (Figure 9.7b). Moreover, for a molecule of radius 'a', the centre of the molecule can get no closer to the pore rim than distance 'a', so only a fraction of the pore space is available to the molecule. If the pore is a cylinder of radius r, the available fraction is $(r - a)^2/r^2$ (Figure 9.8). This geometrical effect is called *steric exclusion*. Owing to steric exclusion, the concentration of solute in pore water is less than the concentration in bulk solution and the ratio of the two concentrations at equilibrium is called the equilibrium partition coefficient ϕ (phi). For a neutral cylindrical pore, ϕ equals the fractional available space, $(r - a)^2/r^2$. Thus steric exclusion reduces the pore area available for diffusion to $A_p \times \phi$.

Pathlength If the pores run obliquely through the membrane, as endothelial junctions mostly do, the diffusion distance ($\Delta x'$) is greater than the membrane thickness (Δx), as illustrated in Figure 9.7(b).

Intrapore diffusion Whenever a solute molecule moves through water it experiences frictional resistance, called hydrodynamic drag; this is what governs the

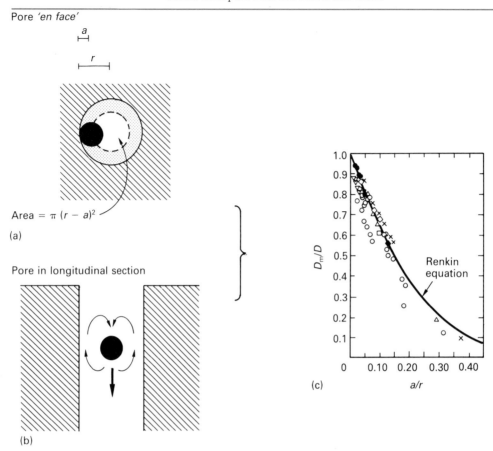

Pore 'en face'

Area = $\pi (r - a)^2$

(a)

Pore in longitudinal section

(b)

(c)

Figure 9.8 A spherical molecule of radius 'a' diffusing through a water-filled cylindrical pore of radius r. (a) End-on or 'bird's eye' view of pore, showing steric exclusion of the molecule centre from an annulus of fluid (pink). (b) Longitudinal section through the pore. Arrows indicate how solute movement necessitates solvent flow, giving rise to enhanced hydrodynamic drag within the narrow confines of the pore. (c) Plot of reduced diffusion across a membrane (D_m) relative to the free diffusion coefficient (D) as the ratio of molecular size to pore size increases (a/r). The membranes were mica sheets containing pores of known, uniform radius produced by bombardment with uranium fission fragments. The 'Renkin equation' is $D_m/D = $ steric exclusion $\times$ hydrodynamic drag (restricted diffusion) $= (1 - a/r)^2 \times (1 - 2.1\,a/r + 2.09(a/r)^3 - 0.95(a/r)^5)$. (From Beck, R. B. and Schultz, J. S. (1972) *Biochimica Biophysica Acta*, **255**, 273–303, by permission)

diffusion coefficient. The hydrodynamic drag on a solute inside a pore rises progressively as the solute radius approaches pore radius in size, because the water slips less easily past the solute molecule in the confined space of a pore (Figure 9.8b). As a result, the solute's diffusion coefficient within the pore (D') is smaller than its free diffusion coefficient in bulk solution (D) and this is called '*restricted diffusion*'. The restriction to diffusion increases rapidly when solute size/pore size exceeds one-tenth; for example, the restricted diffusion coefficient is half the free value when solute radius is 15% of pore radius (Figure 9.8c).

Because of the above effects, Fick's law is modified by the presence of a membrane and becomes:

$$J_S = -D' \frac{A_p}{\Delta x'} \phi \, \Delta C \qquad (9.2)$$

This expression tells us the factors responsible for a membrane's 'permeability'. The permeability of a membrane (P) is, by definition, the rate of diffusion of solute across unit area of membrane per unit concentration difference, or in symbols: $P = J_S/S\Delta C$. Rearranging this to get J_S,

$$J_S = -PS\Delta C \qquad (9.3)$$

Comparing equation (9.3) with equation (9.2), we see that permeability P is governed by the restricted diffusion coefficient (D'), the pore length ($\Delta x'$) and the fractional pore area available to the solute ($A_p \, \phi/S$). Measurements of capillary permeability can therefore provide valuable insights into the porosity of the wall.

Reflection and reflection coefficients

Two additional parameters are needed to characterize exchange across capillaries besides permeability, namely the 'reflection coefficient' and 'hydraulic conductance'. The reflection coefficient (σ; sigma), is an index of the membrane's molecular selectivity, as illustrated in Figure 9.9. It is defined as the osmotic pressure that a given difference in solute concentration exerts across the test membrane divided by the full osmotic pressure that the same concentration difference exerts across a perfect semi-permeable membrane; thus σ equals $\pi_{\text{effective}}/\pi_{\text{ideal}}$. If the solute passes through the membrane as freely as water, it exerts no osmotic pressure and $\sigma = 0$. If the solute is totally reflected by the pores, it exerts its full osmotic potential and $\sigma = 1$. For most hydrophilic molecules at the capillary wall, reflection is partial and σ is between 0 and 1. The size of σ is related to the partition coefficient ϕ:

$$\sigma = (1 - \phi)^2 \qquad (9.4)$$

and as explained earlier ϕ (and therefore σ) depends on the ratio of solute radius to pore radius a/r. Reflection coefficients are thus a useful guide to pore size.

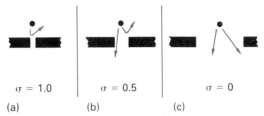

$\sigma = 1.0$ (a) $\sigma = 0.5$ (b) $\sigma = 0$ (c)

Figure 9.9 The osmotic reflection coefficient (σ) depends on the molecular selectivity of a membrane (see text)

Convection and hydraulic conductance (L_p)

The rate of fluid movement across a membrane depends on the pressure gradients and on the *hydraulic conductance* of the membrane. The latter is defined as the filtration rate (J_V) produced by unit pressure difference acting across unit area of membrane, and is usually symbolized by L_p or K. Hydraulic conductance, like the other properties considered above, depends on the porosity of the membrane.

Solute transport by *convection* (wash along or 'solvent drag') depends not only on the filtration rate but also on the reflection coefficient. This is because only the fraction of solute that is not reflected, namely $(1 - \sigma)$, can be washed into a pore. This is important for macromolecule transport (Sections 9.7 and 10.4).

9.4 Measurement of permeability

Because of its physiological importance, capillary permeability has been intensively investigated. To measure capillary permeability, three sets of measurement are required (see equation 9.3): (1) the rate of solute transfer, (2) the membrane area, and (3) the concentration difference across the wall.

Solute diffusion rate across the capillary wall can be measured by direct optical methods in individual capillaries perfused with dyes or fluorescent markers (see Figure 9.6). In whole organs the transfer of rapidly diffusing solutes (e.g. glucose) across the entire microvascular bed can be determined by the Fick principle (Section 6.1), i.e. transfer rate = blood flow × arteriovenous concentration difference. With slowly-exchanging solutes like albumin, arteriovenous differences are slight. Instead, net transfer by all processes (diffusion, convection and vesicles) is given by pre-nodal lymph flow × concentration in lymph.

The anatomical area of the capillary walls (S) can be measured in tissue sections, but the value *in vivo* is often less certain because perfusion of some capillaries is intermittent.

Mean concentration difference across the capillary wall (ΔC) is particularly difficult to measure because the average plasma concentration is not simply the arithmetic average of venous and arterial concentrations. Concentration falls non-linearly along a capillary, declining most steeply at the inlet where the transmural concentration gradient and efflux is highest (Figure 9.10). One method that takes account of this is the *multiple-tracer dilution technique*. This techni-

que has also revealed some important consequences of curvilinear concentration profiles along a capillary (e.g. how blood flow affects exchange) so the method is presented next.

Multiple-tracer dilution technique

A solution containing a diffusible test solute and a non-exchanging reference solute (usually radiolabelled albumin) is injected rapidly into the organ's main artery. A series of venous blood samples is collected over the next few seconds and analysed. The concentration of test solute in the venous effluent is found to fall below that of the reference solute because some test solute has diffused out of the capillaries (Figure 9.11). The reference concentration indicates what the test solute concentration would have been if no exchange had taken place. From this the fraction of the test solute that is extracted during its passage through the capillary bed (extraction, E) is calculated for each sample. The extraction must be measured at several, increasing blood flows ($\dot{Q}$) in order to check that exchange is not being limited by

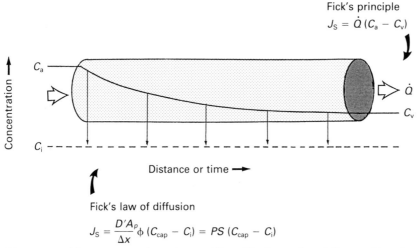

Fick's principle

$$J_S = \dot{Q}\,(C_a - C_v)$$

Fick's law of diffusion

$$J_S = \frac{D'A_p}{\Delta x}\phi\,(C_{cap} - C_i) = PS\,(C_{cap} - C_i)$$

Figure 9.10 The concentration of a rapidly diffusing solute falls non-linearly along a capillary from arterial level (C_a) to venous level (C_v). Thin arrows indicate size and direction of diffusional flux. $\dot{Q}$ is blood flow. If interstitial concentration (C_i) is constant (or zero) and permeability is uniform, the concentration profile is exponential, and the mean plasma concentration C_{cap} equals $C_i + \{(C_a - C_v)/\ln((C_a - C_i)/(C_v - C_i))\}$ For other symbols, see text equation (9.2)

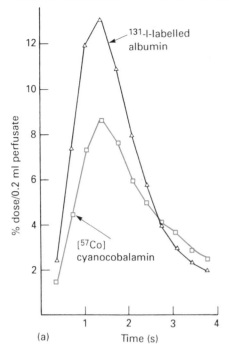

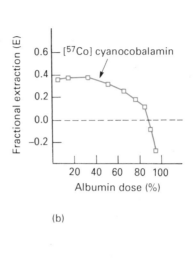

(b)

(a)   Time (s)

Figure 9.11 Multiple-tracer dilution method in the cat salivary gland. (a) Concentration of test solute, radiolabelled vitamin B_{12} (cyanocobalamin, radius 0.84 nm) and reference solute, radioiodinated serum albumin (radius 3.6 nm), in successive samples of venous effluent. The marker content is expressed as a percentage of the mass injected intra-arterially in a brief bolus. The lines cross at 3 s because B_{12} that has reached the interstitium begins to diffuse back into the plasma as plasma concentration falls below interstitial concentration. (b) Extraction of B_{12}, calculated as (arterial concentration − venous concentration)/arterial concentration, for successive venous samples. Extraction falls as interstitial concentration rises and becomes negative (i.e. reverses) when the concentration gradient reverses. (From Mann, G. E., Smaje, L. H. and Yudilevich, D. L. (1979) *Journal of Physiology*, **297**, 335–354, by permission)

delivery rate, rather than by capillary permeability; the former situation causes permeability to be underestimated (Section 9.10). The permeability–surface area product (PS) for the whole capillary bed can then be calculated from the extraction and plasma flow ($\dot{Q}$) using the Renkin–Crone expression:

$$E = 1 - \exp(-PS/\dot{Q}) \qquad (9.5)$$

which is based on an exponential concentration profile along the capillary. The Renkin–Crone expression is an important one and will be returned to in Section 9.10, for it tells us how blood flow affects solute exchange. (For those who like to understand the origin of an expression, equation (9.5) is the result

of substituting the expression for mean intracapillary concentration in the legend of Figure 9.10 into the definition of permeability (equation 9.3) with C_i set to zero.)

9.5 Permeation of lipid-soluble molecules

The lipid-solubility of a molecule dramatically influences its permeation through the capillary wall. Capillary permeability to the lipid-soluble molecule oxygen, for example, is many thousand times greater than permeability to lipid-insoluble glucose. The second main factor affecting permeation is the solute's molecular size; capillary permeability to glucose (M_w 180) is nearly 1000 times greater than to albumin (M_w 69000; Table 9.1). Solutes thus fall into three main classes: lipid-soluble molecules, small lipid-insoluble molecules and large lipid-insoluble molecules (macromolecules).

Taking the lipophilic molecules first, capillary permeability increases in proportion to the solute's oil:water partition coefficient, indicating that these molecules traverse the capillary wall by dissolving in the lipid cell membrane. Virtually the entire capillary surface is available for diffusion and this explains the high permeability. The oil:water partition coefficient is approximately 5 for *oxygen* and 1.6 for *carbon dioxide*, so capillaries are extremely permeable to respiratory gases: indeed, the permeability to oxygen is so high that some gas exchange even occurs in arterioles, and the haemoglobin saturation can fall to approximately 80% before the blood even enters the true capillaries. *Anaaesthetic agents* and the flow-tracer *xenon* also fall into this class of solute.

9.6 Permeation of small lipid-insoluble molecules: small pore concept

Hydrophilic solutes like electrolytes, glucose, lactate, amino acids, vitamin B_{12}, insulin and many drugs cannot easily penetrate the endothelial cell membrane but they can cross the capillary wall via paracellular water-filled channels. This is why the permeability of capillaries to water and small lipid-insoluble molecules is two to three orders of magnitude higher than the permeability of cells to these molecules. The permeability of a protein-retaining dialysis membrane on the other hand is an order of magnitude higher than capillary permeability. This comparison, supported by calculations of the pore area needed to explain permeability values, led Pappenheimer, Renkin and Borrero to propose, in 1951, that the capillary wall is penetrated by small aqueous channels occupying a tiny fraction of the capillary surface (less than 0.1% in dog hindlimb capillaries)–the small pore theory.

Table 9.1 Capillary permeability to various solutes

Solute	M_w	$D(cm^2/s, \times 10^5)$	a(nm)	Membrane	Permeability (cm/s, $\times 10^6$)
Oxygen	32	2.11	0.16	continuous capillary	~100 000
Urea	60	1.90	0.26	continuous capillary	26–28
Glucose	180	0.91	0.36	continuous capillary	9–13
Sucrose	342	0.72	0.47	continuous capillary	6–9
				cerebral capillary	0.1
				fenestrated capillary	> 270
Albumin	69 000	0.085	3.55	continuous capillary	0.03–0.01
				fenestrated capillary	0.04

M_w, molecular weight in Daltons. D, free diffusion coefficient in water at 37°C. a, Stokes–Einstein diffusion radius. Continuous capillaries of cat leg, dog heart and human forearm, fenestrated capillaries of cat salivary gland (After Renkin, E. M. (1977) *Circulation Research*, **41**, 735–743; Clough, G. E. and Smaje, L. H. (1984) *Journal of Physiology*, **354**, 445–455; Landis, E. M. and Pappenheimer, J. R. (1963) *Handbook of Physiology, Cardiovascular System, Circulation*, Vol. II (eds W. F. Hamilton and P. Dow), American Physiological Society, Bethesda, pp. 961–1034)

Restricted diffusion and equivalent pore size

It was the discovery of restricted diffusion across the capillary wall, by Pappenheimer and his co-workers in 1951, that firmly established the 'small pore theory' of capillary permeability. The permeability of hindlimb capillaries to hydrophilic solutes declines as molecular size increases, and falls off more steeply than the free diffusion coefficient (Figure 9.12). This happens in artificial porous membranes too when solute diameter becomes a significant fraction of the channel width, and is caused by steric exclusion and restricted diffusion (see Figure 9.8). Restricted diffusion in the capillary wall indicates that narrow aqueous channels must perforate the wall, and the degree of restriction enables the equiva-

lent radius of the channels to be calculated (see legend to Figure 9.8 for details). It emerges that the channels in the walls of cardiac, skeletal muscle and intestinal capillaries restrict diffusion to the same degree as cylindrical pores of radius 4–5 nm. It must be emphasized that nobody believes that the small pores are actually cylindrical tubes, only that some of their properties can be equated with those of tubes. The true nature of small pores is considered in Section 9.8.

Another way of estimating the size of the small pores is to measure the reflection coefficient. The capillary reflection coefficient for plasma albumin (radius 3.55 nm) is typically 0.8–0.9, from which an equivalent pore radius of 4.6–5.3 nm is easily calculated (see equation 9.4).

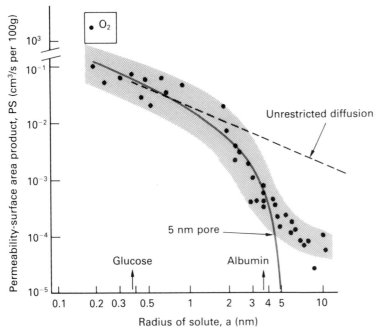

Figure 9.12 Effect of molecular size (Stokes–Einstein diffusion radius) on permeability in continuous capillaries. Points refer to lipophobic solutes except for oxygen. Dashed line of slope −1 shows effect of fall in free diffusion coefficient with molecular size. Red line shows decline in permeability in cylindrical pores of radius 5 nm (see Figure 9.8). Small solutes conform to line for 5 nm-radius pores but the permeability to solutes larger than albumin indicates the existence of a few larger pores too. Data from mammalian skeletal muscle and skin except for oxygen (lung). Solutes range from urea to immunoglobulins. (After Renkin, E. M. and Curry, F. E. (1978) In *Membrane Transport in Biology*, Vol. IV (eds G. Giebisch, D. C. Tosteson and H. H. Ussing), Springer-Verlag, Berlin, pp. 1–45)

Differences in permeability due to differences in pore density

The permeability of capillaries to small lipophobic solutes varies greatly between tissues. The permeability of frog mesenteric capillaries and salivary gland capillaries is over 10 times larger than the permeability of muscle capillaries. The hydraulic conductance of the wall varies similarly, in linear proportion to solute permeability. If pore radius (r) were different in the various capillaries, hydraulic conductance would increase disproportionately more than permeability, owing to the r^4 effect in Poiseuille's hydraulic law. Since this is *not* the case, channel width must be the same in capillaries with a high or low permeability. The physiological variation in permeability between organs with continuous or fenestrated capillaries is not due to differences in pore size but is due to differences in the total area of the wall occupied by pores and/or the pore length.

By dividing the hydraulic conductance (proportional to r^4 in a tube) by the solute permeability (proportional to r^2), an equivalent tube radius can again be calculated. The radius works out, however, to be 9 nm, which is incompatible with the estimates of 4–5.3 nm based on restricted diffusion and reflection. This discrepancy indicates that the channels are not in reality cylindrical tubes. Even if the channels are assumed to be parallel-sided slits, like the endothelial clefts, a similar discrepancy still occurs. A solution to this classical puzzle is offered by the relatively new fibre-matrix theory, which is described in Section 9.8.

9.7 Permeation of large lipid-insoluble molecules: large pore concept

The permeability of most capillaries to plasma protein is less than a millionth of the permeability to oxygen. The permeability can be assessed either by recording the extravascular accumulation of radiolabelled albumin after an intravascular injection or by collecting the prenodal lymph, which transports escaped plasma protein out of the tissue. Plasma protein is found in lymph at 20–70% of the plasma concentration, demonstrating that normal capillary beds have a finite low permeability to macromolecules. This should not be thought of as some lamentable 'leak'. On the contrary, it is a functional necessity, both for interstitial defence by immunoglobulins and for the transfer of protein-bound substances like iron, copper, vitamin A, lipids, thyroxine, testosterone and oestradiol.

The permeability versus *molecular size plot again*

Permeability declines steeply as solute radius approaches 3.5 nm (albumin) because solute width is approaching the width of the small pores. Beyond this point, however, the slope of the permeability plot flattens, and the permeability to larger macromolecules declines only slightly more than one would expect from the decline in free diffusion coefficient (see Figure 9.12). The persistence of a finite permeability to macromolecules that are too large to penetrate the small pore system led Grotte, in 1956, to propose the coexistence of a tiny population of large pores of radius 20–30 nm. Measurements of the reflection coefficient have confirmed this: the 'admitted fraction' $(1 - \sigma)$ decreases rapidly with solute radius between 1 nm and 3.5 nm but does not fall to zero even for molecules as large as fibrinogen (Stokes–Einstein radius 10 nm).

Transport through the large pore system

Calculations suggest that there is about one large pore per 12 000 small pores. The large pore system therefore contributes little to the transport of small solutes or fluid. In the discontinuous capillaries of liver, however, the large:small pore ratio is higher, approximately 1:100. Conversely, renal glomerular capillaries and cerebral capillaries may lack a large pore system entirely.

Large pores, like small pores, are a functional concept and their actual physical nature is controversial (Section 9.8). This makes it difficult to be dogmatic about how macromolecular transport occurs. The processes that might be involved are diffusion, convection and vesicular transport. A rise in filtration rate increases the rate of transport of macromolecules across the capillary wall many-fold, and this shows that convective transport (solvent drag) through hydraulically continuous large pores dominates protein transport at moderate to high filtration rates. Diffusion or vesicular transport might be more important at low filtration rates.

Effects of macromolecular size and charge

Large proteins like fibrinogen undergo more reflection by the capillary wall than do smaller proteins like albumin, so the larger plasma proteins are less abundant in interstitial fluid. This process is called 'molecular sieving' and is considered further in Section 10.4.

The permeation of a macromolecule is affected by its charge, as well as size. Many capillaries, such as glomerular vessels, are less permeable to net negatively-charged macromolecules like albumin than to neutral or positively-charged ones of similar size. This is due to repulsion of the molecule by the fixed negative charges of the glycocalyx and basement membrane. The charge effect is most marked for the smaller macromolecules which are known to pass partly through the small pores, so the charge effect probably arises mainly in the small pores.

9.8 In search of pores

Anatomical location of the small pores

The small pore system is a set of channels of equivalent radius 4.0–5.5 nm occupying less than 0.1% of the capillary surface in continuous capillaries. The intercellular cleft is generally regarded as the region where the small pores are located because: (1) intercellular clefts occupy only 0.1–0.3% of the surface, and (2) small lipid-insoluble molecules like ferrocyanide, lanthanum ions and microperoxidase can penetrate the cleft, as shown in Figure 9.13. The tight junctions are an obstacle to passage through the cleft, despite the fact that the opposing membranes do not actually fuse at the junction. These obstacles can be circumvented, however, by a tortuous, open pathway around the ends of the junctional strands and/or via the inter-particle gaps (see Figure 9.3). The differences in permeability between organs appear to be due principally to differences in the fraction of the cleft's surface area that is functionally 'open' (i.e. not sealed by tight junctions). In muscle capillaries, for example, only approximately 10% of the intercellular cleft needs to be open to account for the wall's permeability; in the more permeable capillaries of frog mesentery it is about 50% and in the relatively impermeable cerebral capillaries less than 0.1%. The fenestra, when present, is a second site for small pores, as indicated by the fact that capillary permeability increases in proportion to the number of fenestrae per capillary.

Fibre matrix theory

The location of the small pores is reasonably certain, but their physical nature remains controversial because the dimensions of the clefts and fenestrae do not correspond adequately with those deduced for small pores: the cleft is too wide (15 nm) and the fenestral diaphragm too thin. In 1980, Michel and Curry proposed the 'fibre matrix theory' to resolve such difficulties (Figure 9.14). The glycocalyx is a matrix of fibrous molecules covering the entrance to the intercellular clefts and fenestrae, and they suggested that this matrix may be dense enough to function like small pores, i.e. the spaces between the molecular chains may be narrow enough to restrict solute diffusion, increase hydraulic resistance and reflect macromolecules. The uniformity of the glycocalyx would explain

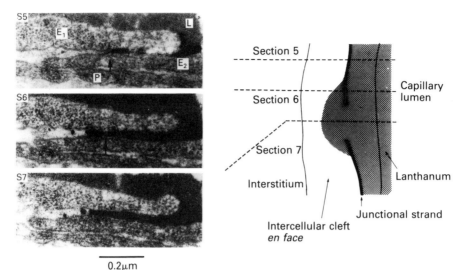

0.2μm

Figure 9.13 Three consecutive sections through a continuous capillary perfused with a solution of lanthanum ions (black) for 10 s prior to fixation. The intercellular cleft is shown *en face* in the sketch. The tight junction (arrow) blocks passage (Section 5) but is circumvented by an open pathway at the end of the junctional strand (Section 7). An intermediate section (6) gives the false impression that the tight junction itself is permeable. L, lumen; E, endothelium; P, pericyte. (After Adamson, R. H. and Michel, C. C. (1993), see Further Reading)

why the albumin reflection coefficient is about the same (0.8–0.9) in both highly permeable capillaries and less permeable ones. Also, while cylindrical and slit-pore models predict unreasonable values for small-pore radius from hydraulic data (the 'puzzle' mentioned in Section 9.5), the fibre matrix equations produce no such inconsistency. This is because Poiseuille's law does not apply to irregular porosities with discontinuous walls; such channels offer less hydraulic resistance for a given reflection coefficient.

An observation which highlights the importance of the glycocalyx is *'the protein effect'*. When albumin is washed out of a capillary, P and L_p increase and σ decreases. This indicates that albumin normally helps maintain the narrowness of the notional small pores, and albumin is known to bind to glycocalyx via its cationic arginine groups. Moreover cationized ferritin, which as Figure 9.5 shows likewise binds to the glycocalyx, has the same permeability-reducing effect. The protein effect is thought to be due to the

adherent protein molecules changing the density and spacing of the matrix (Figure 9.14). An exciting aspect of this hypothesis is that it opens up the possibility of modifying capillary permeability therapeutically by changing the density and pattern of the fibre matrix.

A further plasma protein, orosomucoid, also appears to bind to the capillary wall and enhances its selectivity against negatively-charged solutes.

Large pores

In discontinuous capillaries there are open intercellular gaps which are undoubtedly the large pores (see Figure 9.2). In healthy continuous and fenestrated capillaries the nature of the large pore is still controversial, there being three main candidates (see Figure 9.18). (1) The occasional *intercellular cleft* might open wider than normal and loosen its fibre matrix. Gaps of 50–500 nm have indeed been seen occasionally in venules but they are so rare that the investigator is never

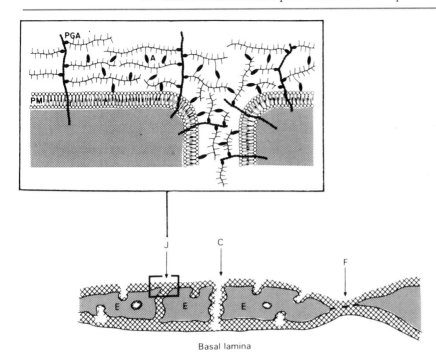

Figure 9.14 Fibre matrix model of capillary permeability. Glycocalyx covers the endothelium (E) and fenestra (F) and intercellular junction (J). It also lines the vesicles. The multivesicular transcellular channel (C) is shown as a clear route, representing the large pore system; these are very few in number. (Inset) Putative details of matrix structure. Proteoglycan fibres (PGA) bind albumin (A) via its positively-charged arginine groups. Molecular sieving is governed by the mesh size while the number of channels (J, F, C) influences total hydraulic and diffusional permeability. PM, plasmalemma membrane. (From Michel, C. C. (1980) *Journal of Physiology*, **309**, 341–355 and Curry, F. E. (1986) *Circulation Research*, **59**, 367–380, by permission)

sure whether they are normal or artefact. (2) The rare *transendothelial channels* formed by fused vesicles (see Figures 9.4 and 9.18) are about the right size to serve as large pores, being 15–35 nm in radius. (3) Some form of transport by the invaginated *vesicular system* is conceivable. Macromolecules like gold-labelled albumin and ferritin (radius 5.5 nm) undoubtedly enter the luminal vesicles (see Figure 9.5) and some minutes later appear in abluminal vesicles. The mechanism might be a transient fusion of luminal and abluminal systems with an exchange of contents, but how much this contributes to net protein transport is not clear. Protein transport is certainly not an active process for it is not abolished by metabolic poisons or tissue cooling. Moreover, the increase in net protein

transport when filtration pressure is increased implies that there exists a hydraulically conductive 'large pore', i.e. a continuous channel. At normal low filtration rates, however, the observed protein flux is greater than expected for conductive channels alone, so it may turn out that both conductive channels and some form of vesicular transport are important at normal capillary pressures.

9.9 Carrier-mediated transport across cerebral capillaries

Although cerebral capillaries are highly permeable to oxygen and carbon dioxide they are exceptionally impermeable to small lipophobic molecules like K^+, L-glucose, sucrose, mannitol, polar dyes, catecholamines and plasma proteins. This gives rise to the concept of a *'blood-brain barrier'* whose function is to protect the delicate neuronal circuits from interference by plasma solutes. The barrier is created by the dense complex junctional strands which form a continuous seal around the endothelial cell perimeter (zonula occludens), and by the scantiness of the vesicular system. These structural specializations are probably induced by the surrounding astrocytes whose 'feet' cover over 80% of the abluminal surface of the cerebral capillary.

The brain's chief energy source is glucose in its natural dextro-rotatory form (D-glucose, dextrose). D-glucose, unlike its stereo-isomer L-glucose, rapidly crosses the blood-brain barrier by *facilitated diffusion*. It binds reversibly to a specific carrier protein in the endothelial cell membrane, very like the glucose carrier in red cell membranes, and this renders the capillary wall selectively permeable to D-glucose. The movement of the glucose is nevertheless a passive diffusion down the concentration gradient set up by neuronal activity, and is not an active transport. Because receptor sites are involved, glucose transport displays the characteristic phenomena of *saturation* at high concentrations, *stereospecificity* (D-glucose is transported but L-glucose is not) and *competitive inhibition* by analogues like deoxyglucose and galactose. Carriers also exist for the metabolic acids lactate and pyruvate and for adenosine. There are three distinct carriers for amino acids: one for large neutral amino acids like phenylalanine, one for anionic amino acids like glutamate and one for cationic amino acids like arginine. There is evidence also for facilitated diffusion of adenosine across the coronary endothelium.

Cerebral endothelium also seems capable of active ionic transport. If brain interstitial K^+ concentration rises due to neuronal electrical activity, K^+ is pumped out across the abluminal membrane of the endothelial cell, where a Na^+–K^+ ATPase is located (rather as in a tight epithelium). This stabilizes the level of K^+ in brain interstitium and probably explains why cerebral endothelium has five to six times as many mitochondria as muscle endothelium.

9.10 Effect of blood flow on exchange rate

To illustrate how blood flow influences solute exchange, let us consider a simple and rather artificial situation in which the pericapillary concentration is held constant. This is in fact the situation during the first few seconds of an indicator diffusion experiment (see Figure 9.11), since the pericapillary concentration of test solute is zero at the early times. Under these conditions the limiting factor for solute exchange can be either the rate at which plasma delivers solute (flow-limited exchange) or the rate at which the wall allows solute across (diffusion-limited exchange).

Flow-limited exchange

The permeability of a capillary to lipophilic solutes (e.g. oxygen) and very small lipophobic solutes is so high that the solute equilibrates with the pericapillary fluid within the plasma transit time. Consequently, exchange involves only the initial segment of the capillary (see Figure 9.15, curve F). If flow is increased, an equilibrium may still be reached before the end of the capillary, albeit a little further downstream, and the arteriovenous concentration difference is unaltered (curve F'). From the Fick principle (Section 6.1), we know that solute transfer is directly proportional to blood flow if the arteriovenous difference is constant, and this is how lipid-soluble molecules like antipyrine behave (Figure 9.15b). A rise in blood flow is thus an important way of increasing the transfer of lipid-soluble substances. A classic example of this is O_2 *uptake in the lung*, where pericapillary (i.e. alveolar), P_{O_2} is held virtually constant by ventilation, and where blood P_{O_2} equilibrates with alveolar P_{O_2} before the end of the capillary is reached.

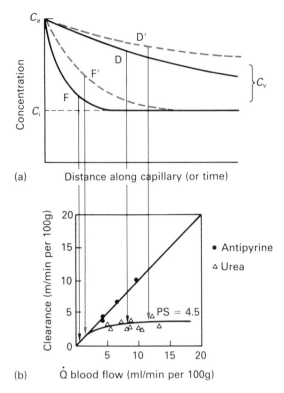

Figure 9.15 (a) Plasma concentration of a diffusible solute along a capillary. If plasma equilibrates with interstitium (C_i) before the end of the capillary, exchange is flow limited (curve F). Raising blood flow causes more of the downstream capillary wall to participate in exchange (curve F′) and increases the transfer rate. If plasma fails to equilibrate with interstitium, exchange is limited by the diffusion barrier (curve D). Raising blood flow now limits the time for diffusion so extraction falls and venous concentration rises (curve D′): this offets the effect of blood flow, and solute transfer barely increases. (b) Effect of blood flow on rate of solute clearance (solute transfer rate from plasma to interstitium per unit arterial concentration) in skeletal muscle. The lipid-soluble solute antipyrine undergoes flow-limited exchange; so too does urea at low flows. At flows $>10\,\mathrm{ml/min^{-1}}\,100\,\mathrm{g^{-1}}$, urea undergoes diffusion-limited exchange and the plateau equals PS for urea. ((a) After Michel, C. C. (1972) In *Cardiovascular Fluid Dynamics* (ed. D. Bergel), Academic Press, London; (b) From Renkin, E. M. (1967) In *International Symposium on Coronary Circulation* (1966) (eds G. Marchetti and B. Taccardi), Karger, Basel, pp. 18–30, by permission)

Consequently, raising blood flow (cardiac output) increases oxygen uptake rate proportionately. Permeability cannot be measured when exchange is flow-limited, because the fraction of capillary wall involved in exchange is unknown. Instead, the solute transfer rate is a measure of blood flow (see Figure 9.15b, antipyrine line; Figure 8.5, xenon; and Figure 6.1, oxygen).

Diffusion-limited exchange

Bigger lipophobic molecules like inulin and cyanocobalamin (vitamin B_{12}) cross the capillary wall too slowly to equilibrate with pericapillary fluid during the normal transit time (Figure 9.15a, curve D). The same is true for smaller molecules like glucose if the blood transit time is shortened sufficiently by raising the blood velocity. The exchange rate is then limited not by flow but by the diffusional resistance of the capillary wall. Diffusion-limited exchange is relatively insensitive to blood flow because raising the blood flow reduces the time spent in the capillary; extraction falls and venous concentration rises (curve D′). By applying the Fick principle, we find that the effect of the rise in blood flow is largely offset by the fall in $C_a - C_v$, and solute exchange increases relatively little. This is illustrated by the urea curve in Figure 9.15b.

The above examples show that a crucial factor in solute transfer is the ratio of the diffusing capacity of the wall (*PS*) to the blood flow ($\dot{Q}$). If the diffusing capacity is high relative to flow, exchange is flow-limited; conversely if flow is high relative to diffusing capacity the exchange is diffusion-limited. The concepts of flow-limited exchange and diffusion-limited exchange are actually extremes of a continuous spectrum, and the whole spectrum is described by the Renkin–Crone expression (equation 9.5). The latter tells us how extraction varies with the $PS/\dot{Q}$ ratio. As a rough rule exchange can be regarded as flow-limited if $PS/\dot{Q}$ is 5 or more and diffusion-limited if it is less than 1. For glucose in a skeletal muscle capillary $PS/\dot{Q}$ can vary between about 5 at rest (low blood flow; flow-limited exchange) and 1 during exercise (high blood flow; diffusion-limited exchange).

The 'mixed regime' As noted above, the concepts of flow-limited exchange and diffusion-limited exchange are simply extremes of a continuous spectrum. Inbetween, there exists a mixed regime, where end-capillary solute concentration has not equilibrated with the tissue, but is nevertheless well below the arterial value. Here, increasing blood flow produces a significant rise in end-capillary concentration (the effect of shortened residence time in the capillary). The resulting increased mean capillary concentration drives a modest increase in transfer rate (Fick's law of diffusion), but not by as much as the flow increase (e.g. less than two-fold for a doubling of flow).

Oxygen transport to muscle O_2 transport in the *lung* is a good example of flow-limited exchange, as pointed out under 'flow-limitation'. In *skeletal muscle*, O_2 transfer across the capillary wall itself is again flow-limited (because the wall is extremely permeable to respiratory gases); but capillary wall resistance is only a tiny part of the diffusional resistance of the total path from blood to muscle mitochondrion. The resistance of the whole transport pathway is substantial because of the distance involved (up to 25 μm, cf. 0.3 μm in lung); the importance of distance Δx is shown in equation (9.1). As a result, O_2 transfer from blood to muscle fibre is in the mixed regime referred to above. Venous P_{O_2} (40 mmHg at rest, about 15 mmHg in maximal exercise) is well below arterial P_{O_2} (100 mmHg) but does not reach equilibrium with mitochondrial P_{O_2} (<5 mmHg in exercise). There is a large drop in P_{O_2} from capillary to a point just within the muscle fibre sarcoplasm (a distance of several μm), but within the muscle fibre the P_{O_2} is relatively uniform. This is due to the presence of myoglobin, which is present in red muscle at concentrations up to 7 g/kg. Myoglobin greatly speeds up the rate of diffusion of O_2 at low P_{O_2}'s, because oxygen

can 'hop' from one unoccupied binding site to the next (*facilitated diffusion*).

9.11 Physiological regulation of exchange rate

In a steady state, the rate of transfer of oxygen and nutrients across the capillary wall must keep pace with the rate of consumption by the tissue. In exercising muscle, for example, oxygen consumption can increase 20–40 fold, and this requires a corresponding increase in transcapillary transfer rate. This is achieved by three mechanisms: capillary recruitment, an increased concentration gradient across the wall and increased blood flow. In the case of O_2 there is also increased diffusion velocity through muscle myoglobin as intracellular P_{O_2} falls.

Capillary recruitment

In skeletal muscle, each capillary supplies a surrounding envelope of muscle, called a Krogh cylinder (Figure 9.16). The radius of the Krogh cylinder depends on capillary density. A low capillary density or, equivalently, perfusion of only a fraction of the existing capillaries produces a broad Krogh cylinder and a poor oxygen tension at its periphery. In resting skeletal muscle, half to three-quarters of the capillaries are either not perfused or perfused only sluggishly at any moment, owing to vasomotion in the terminal arterioles (Section 9.1). During exercise the metabolic dilatation of terminal arterioles increases the number of well-perfused capillaries, and this not only increases the *surface area* for exchange but also reduces the *diffusion distance*, i.e. radius of the Krogh cylinder (Figure 9.16). Diffusion distance is especially important for gas exchange, because the main diffusional resistance in the overall blood-to-tissue pathway is not at the capillary wall but in the tissues, due purely and simply to the greater length of the extravascular pathway (> 10 μm). The main fall in oxygen concentration is thus not from

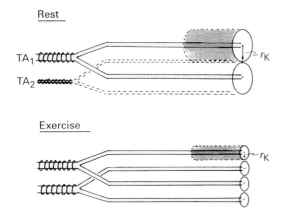

Rest

TA$_1$

TA$_2$

r_K

Exercise

r_K

Figure 9.16 Diagram illustrating the Krogh cylinder concept and capillary recruitment in exercising skeletal muscle. At rest, contraction of terminal arteriole 2 (TA$_2$) stops the perfusion of one capillary module (dashed lines) so the Krogh cylinder radius is large (r_K). Metabolic vasodilatation during exercise dilates terminal arteriole 2, increasing the perfused capillary area and reducing the maximum diffusion distance r_K. Strictly, the Krogh 'cylinder' is really a hexagonal column

plasma to pericapillary space but from pericapillary space to cell interior. The intracellular P_{O_2} is only approximately 20 mmHg in resting muscle, despite a blood P_{O_2} of 100 mmHg (arterial) to 40 mmHg (venous).

Tissue concentration gradient

An increased cellular metabolic rate lowers the intracellular concentration of glucose, oxygen, etc., and this increases the concentration difference between plasma and the cell. In combination with the shortened cell-to-capillary distance, this raises the concentration gradient ($\Delta C/\Delta x$) driving solute from the plasma to the cell. For glucose, for example, the mean concentration difference across the capillary wall increases from approximately 0.3 mM in resting muscle to approximately 3 mM during heavy exercise (Table 9.2).

Table 9.2 Transport of glucose from blood to 100 g skeletal muscle *in vivo*

	Rest	Heavy exercise	Fractional change (exercise/rest)
Glucose consumption rate (J_s) †	1.4 μmol/min	60 μmol/min	43 ×
Arterial concentration (C_a)	5 mM	5 mM	–
Venous concentration (C_v)	4.44 mM	4 mM	0.9 ×
Extraction (E)	11.2%	20%	1.8 ×
Blood flow	2.5 ml/min	60 ml/min	24 ×
Perfused capillary density	250/mm^2	1000/mm^2	} 4 ×
Diffusion capacity (PS)	5 cm^3/min	20 cm^3/min	
Mean concentration difference across capillary wall (ΔC)*	0.3 mM	3 mM	10 ×
Mean pericapillary concentration (C_i)	4.7 mM	2 mM	0.4 ×
Krogh cylinder radius	36 μm	18 μm	0.5 ×

*ΔC is calculated as J_s/PS – see equation (9.3).
† Diffusion, and not fluid filtration, is the dominant transcapillary transport process for glucose and other small solutes. This is clear from a simple calculation based on the consumption by resting skeletal muscle (1.4 μmol/min^{-1} 100 g^{-1}). Net transcapillary fluid flow is 0.005 ml/min^{-1} 100 g^{-1} and since plasma contains 5 μmol glucose per ml, the maximum convective transport of glucose is 0.025 μmol/min. This is a mere 2% of the total glucose transfer. The major process driving a metabolite across the capillary wall is thus diffusion.
(After Crone, C. and Levitt, D. G. (1984) In *Handbook of Physiology, Cardiovascular System*, Vol. IV, *Microcirculation* (eds E. M. Renkin and C. C. Michel), American Physiological Society, Bethesda, pp. 431)

Blood flow

Blood flow usually increases in proportion to an organ's metabolic rate (Figure 9.17), and if exchange is flow-limited (e.g. oxygen transfer), the flux into the pericapillary space increases in proportion to blood flow for a given pericapillary concentration. Metabolites such as glucose and urea are flow-limited at resting blood flows but become diffusion-limited at the high flows that occur in exercise. Once the exchange process has become diffusion-limited, further rises in blood flow have only a small benefit.

The various factors that increase glucose delivery to exercising muscle fibres are brought together in Table 9.2 and Figure 9.17.

9.12 Active functions of endothelium

In addition to its passive functions as a porous membrane, endothelium has many active metabolic functions. (1) It secretes *structural components*: the glycocalyx and basal lamina. (2) The endothelial cell produces several *vasoactive substances*, for example, prostacyclin (PGI_2), a vasodilator and anti-platelet aggregating factor. Arterial endothelium secretes endothelium-derived relaxing factors and endothelin (see Chapter 12). An endothelial surface enzyme converts circulating angiotensin I into the vasoactive form angiotensin II, and degrades the circulating vasoactive substances bradykinin and serotonin. (3) There is evidence that *carbonic anhydrase*, an enzyme catalysing the conversion of plasma HCO_3^- to carbon dioxide, occurs as another surface enzyme in lung microvessels. (4) Another cluster of activity concerns the *clotting system*, endothelium being a producer of thromboxane and von Willebrand factor (factor VIII-related substance). Von Willebrand's disease is a genetically-determined failure of endothelial cells to synthesize this haemostatic factor, resulting in a prolonged bleeding time. (5) Endothelium is also involved in the *defence*

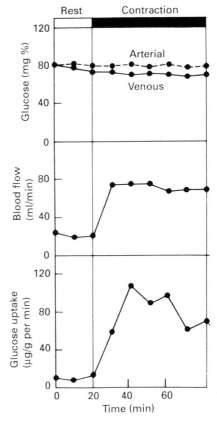

Figure 9.17 Glucose transfer rate from plasma to dog skeletal muscle (lower panel) calculated by the Fick principle from the data in the upper panels. Uptake rate = blood flow × arteriovenous concentration difference. Increased exchange in moderate exercise is achieved partly by increased blood flow and partly by increased extraction, i.e. widening of the arteriovenous difference. (After Chapler, C. K. and Stainsby, W. N. (1968) *American Journal of Physiology*, **215**, 995–1004)

against pathogens. Venular endothelium interacts with polymorphs and lymphocytes during inflammation as the first step in white cell emigration. Production of adhesive molecules by the endothelium is an important step in this process, as described in the next chapter. The endothelial cell also undergoes a contractile process in inflammation, mediated via a rise in intracellular Ca^{2+} concentration, which leads to gap formation (Section 10.11).

9.13 Summary

A dense network of fine, thin-walled capillaries subserves nutrient and water exchange between tissue and blood. Oxygen, glucose, etc., cross the capillary wall by diffusion down metabolism-dependent concentration gradients. Water, by contrast, flows down a pressure gradient. The three types of capillary, namely continuous, fenestrated and discontinuous capillaries, form a hierarchy of increasing permeability to water and small lipophobic solutes. Solutes fall into three classes as regards permeation:

1. Lipid-soluble molecules, like the respiratory gases and anaesthetics, diffuse directly through the endothelial cell membrane, so the capillary is extremely permeable to them.
2. Small, lipid-insoluble molecules, like glucose and amino acids, diffuse through aqueous pathways in the endothelial intercellular clefts and fenestrations. Since this 'small pore system' occupies only a small percentage of the capillary surface area, permeation is much slower than for lipid-soluble molecules. Also, the narrowness of the pores (functional radius 4–5 nm) slows the transfer of the larger solutes, owing to partial steric exclusion and restricted diffusion. Pore size may be determined by the mesh size in a network of fibrous molecules, the glycocalyx, that covers the intercellular junctions and fenestrae. Blood-brain barrier capillaries have exceptionally tight intercellular junctions, and permeation of glucose and amino acids into the brain is by facilitated diffusion across the endothelial cell membrane, mediated by specific intramembrane transport proteins.
3. Even very large, lipid-insoluble molecules such as plasma proteins of radius >5 nm cross the capillary wall slowly, implying the existence of a limited 'large pore system'. Large pore identity remains controversial; such transfer could be the result of vesicular transport.

The rate of passive transfer of solutes can be increased hugely (e.g. in exercising muscle) by a combination of (a) increased concentration gradients due to increased tissue metabolic rate, (b) recruitment of previously underperfused capillaries as the feeding arterioles undergo metabolic vasodilatation (reducing the radius of the Krogh cylinder), and (c) increased capillary blood flow. The effect of blood flow depends on whether solute exchange is flow-limited or diffusion-limited. If the ratio of permeability to flow is high (flow-limited exchange, e.g. oxygen), then raising flow increases the exchange rate. If the ratio is low (diffusion-limited case, e.g. large lipophobic solutes), raising flow has little effect on exchange.

Endothelium has many active metabolic functions too. These include secretion of structural components (glycocalyx, basal lamina), secretion of vasoactive substances (prostanoids, endothelium-derived relaxing factors), enzymatic conversion of circulating vasoactive hormones and autacoids (e.g. angiotensin, bradykinin, 5HT) and the secretion of certain clotting factors (thromboxane, von Willebrand factor).

Although the active functions of endothelial cells are very exciting, and important in regulation of arteriolar tone, we must not lose sight of the fact that the single most important function of the endothelium is to determine the permeability of the capillary wall. The transfer of material across the capillary wall is summarized in Figure 9.18, but the concepts of John Pappenheimer and Gene Renkin, originators of pore theory, and Charles Michel and Roy Curry, developers of fibre matrix theory, might also be summarized less prosaically as follows:

The Pappenheimer pore's so small
You cannot make it out at all,
Though many sanguine doctors hope
To see one through the microscope –
Rectangular or round in shape
With many nanometres gape.
Some say the pore contains a fluff
Of glyco-proteinaceous stuff,
Whose fibres subdivide the space

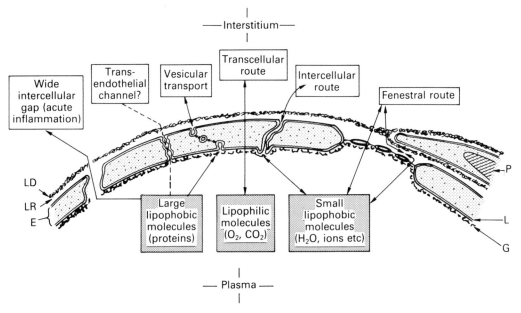

Figure 9.18 Main transport pathways across the capillary wall. Flux of small proteins through the small pore system is not shown. While water passes mainly through the small pore system as shown, some also passes directly through the cell membrane and some through the large pore system. E, endothelium; G, glycocalyx; L, lipid plasma membrane; LR, LD, lamina rara and lamina densa of basement membrane; P, pericyte. (From Levick, J. R. (1983) In *Studies in Joint Disease*, 2nd edn (eds A. Maroudas and E. J. Holborow), Pitman, London, pp. 153–240, by permission)

Constructing there a random lace
'Til albumin, a protein, lands
And tidies up those tangled strands,
Through which there flows dilute sal-ine.
All this has never yet been seen,
But Scientists, who ought to know,
Assure us that it must be so.
Oh let us never, never doubt
What nobody is sure about.

(With apologies to Hilaire Belloc)

Further reading

Reviews and chapters

Bradbury, M. W. B. (1993) The blood-brain barrier. *Experimental Physiology*, **78**, 453–472

Crone, C. (1984) The function of capillaries. In *Recent Advances in Physiology 10* (ed. P. F. Baker), Churchill Livingstone, London, pp. 125–162

Curry, F. E. (1994) Regulation of water and solute exchange in microvessel endothelium: studies in single perfused capillaries. *Microcirculation*, **1**, 11–26

Honig, C. R., Gayeshi, T. E. J. and Groebe, K. (1991) Myoglobin and oxygen transfer. In *The Lung: Scientific Foundations* (eds R. G. Crystal and J. B. West), Raven Press, New York, pp. 1489–1496

Hudlicka, O., Egginton, S. and Brown, M. D. (1988) Capillary diffusion distances – their importance for cardiac and skeletal muscle performance. *News in Physiological Science*, **3**, 134–138

Michel, C. C. (1988) Capillary permeability and how it may change. *Journal of Physiology*, **404**, 1–29

Renkin, E. M. (1985) Capillary transport of macromolecules: pores and other endothelial pathways. *Journal of Applied Physiology*, **58**, 315–325

Rippe, B. and Haraldsson, B. (1987) How are macromolecules transported across the capillary wall? *News in Physiological Science*, **2**, 135–138

Ryan, U. S., Ryan, J. W. and Crutchly, D. J. (1985) The pulmonary endothelial surface. *Federal Proceedings*, **44**, 2603–2609

Vane, J. R., Gryglewski, R. J. and Botting, R. M. (1987) The endothelial cell as a metabolic and endocrine organ. *Trends in Pharmacological Science*, **8**, 491–496

Wissig, S. L. and Charonis, A. S. (1984) Capillary ultrastructure. In *Edema* (eds N. C. Staub and A. E. Taylor), Raven Press, New York, pp. 117–142

Wittenberg, B. A. and Wittenberg, J. B. (1989) Transport

of oxygen in muscle. *Annual Reviews of Physiology*, **51**, 857–878

Research papers

Adamson, R. H. and Michel, C. C. (1993) Pathways through the intercellular clefts of frog mesenteric capillaries. *Journal of Physiology*, **466**, 303–327.

He, P. and Curry, F. E. (1993) Albumin modulation of capillary permeability: role of endothelial cell $[Ca^{2+}]_i$. *American Journal of Physiology*, **265**, H74–H82

Wagner, R. C. and Chen, S. C. (1991) Transcapillary transport of solute by the endothelial vesicular system: evidence from thin serial section analysis. *Microvascular Research*, **42**, 139–150

Chapter 10
Circulation of fluid between plasma, interstitium and lymph

Impelled by the pressure within the capillaries, fluid filters slowly across the capillary wall, passes through the interstitial space and returns to the bloodstream via the lymphatic system. The entire plasma volume (except the protein) circulates in this fashion in under a day, so the maintenance of a normal plasma and interstitial volume depends on capillary and lymphatic function. Pathological processes affecting these vessels can give rise to inflammatory swelling and lymphoedema, respectively, while abnormalities of the filtration forces can cause other forms of oedema (excess fluid in the tissue).

10.1 Starling principle of fluid exchange

Fluid movement across the capillary wall is a passive process driven by the pressures acting on either side of the wall. Capillary blood pressure drives filtration into the tissue, as pointed out by Carl Ludwig in 1850; and the osmotic 'suction' pressure of the plasma proteins promotes absorption from the tissue, as Ernest Starling stated in 1896 (Figure 10.1). A very simple experiment led Starling to the view that the capillary wall is a semipermeable membrane across which plasma proteins exert an osmotic pressure. He injected saline into the tissue spaces of a dog's hindlimb and found that the saline was absorbed into the bloodstream, as revealed by haemodilution. Starling also showed that the osmotic pressure of the plasma 'colloids' (i.e. proteins) was large enough to counteract capillary pressure and produce absorption. Following Starling's usage, the osmotic pressure of plasma protein is still called the 'colloid osmotic pressure' (or oncotic pressure). Starling recognized that it is colloid osmotic pressure that retains water within the circulation, and this discovery led to the use of colloid solutions as plasma volume expanders for wounded soldiers in World War I, and subsequently to the development of modern therapeutic colloids like urea-linked gelatin (Haemaccel) – a striking example of the practical benefit that can accrue from 'pure' research.

The modern form of the 'Starling principle' is as follows. The net rate and direction of fluid movement across any given segment of capillary wall (J_V) depends on the net filtration pressure, which is the hydraulic pressure drop minus the colloid osmotic pressure drop across the wall (Figure 10.1). The drop in hydraulic pressure is capillary pressure (P_c) minus interstitial pressure immediately outside the wall (P_i); and the osmotic pressure difference is plasma colloid osmotic pressure (π_p) minus the colloid osmotic pressure of interstitial fluid immediately outside the wall (π_i). In other words:

Filtration rate $\propto$

$$\{(\text{Hydraulic drive}) - (\text{Osmotic suction})\}$$

or in symbols

$$J_V \propto \{(P_c - P_i) - (\pi_p - \pi_i)\}$$

The proportionality factor depends on the surface area of wall (S) and the wall's hydraulic conductance (L_p; Section 9.3). Writing in the proportionality factors, we get:

$$J_V = L_p.S.\{(P_c - P_i) - (\pi_p - \pi_i)\} \qquad (10.1)$$

This is not quite complete, however, because the capillary wall is not a perfect semipermeable membrane; it is slightly permeable to plasma proteins. As explained in Section 9.3, osmotic pressure is not fully exerted across a leaky membrane, and the ratio of the osmotic pressure actually exerted ($\Delta\pi_{\text{effective}}$) to the

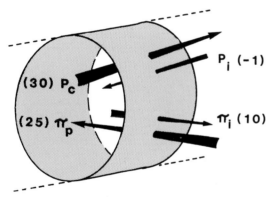

Figure 10.1 The Starling principle. The four pressures governing fluid exchange are capillary pressure (P_c), pericapillary interstitial pressure (P_i), plasma protein osmotic pressure (π_p) and pericapillary interstitial protein osmotic pressure (π_i). Typical values given in mmHg above atmospheric; -1 mmHg is $760 - 1 = 759$ mmHg so the P_i arrow points into the capillary. Intravascular values from warm human skin at heart level. (From Levick, J. R. and Michel, C. C. (1978) *Journal of Physiology*, **274**, 97–109). Interstitial values from human subcutaneous tissue (Aukland, K. (1987) *Advances in Microcirculation*, **13**, 110–123)

full osmotic pressure exerted by the same concentration difference across a perfect membrane ($\Delta\pi_{\text{ideal}}$) is called the reflection coefficient (σ);

$$\sigma = \Delta\pi_{\text{effective}}/\Delta\pi_{\text{ideal}} \qquad (10.2)$$

For plasma proteins, σ is typically 0.75–0.95, meaning that only 75–95% of the potential osmotic pressure difference across the wall is exerted in reality. It must be stressed that this is not due to the presence of protein in the interstitium, but is a reduction of the osmotic pressure exerted by the protein concentration difference, whatever that difference. Thus the osmotic pressures in the filtration equation are reduced by factor σ, and the correct expression for fluid movement is:

$$J_V = L_p S\{(P_c - P_i) - \sigma(\pi_p - \pi_i)\} \qquad (10.3)$$

This is called the *Starling equation* and is central to understanding clinical oedema (see later). The Starling equation applies to each consecutive small segment of the capillary wall, where P_c, etc., can be regarded as uniform. Over the whole length of the vessel the capillary pressure changes and the effects of this are considered later (Section 10.6).

Proof of the Starling principle in single capillaries

The cannulation of individual capillaries was pioneered by an American medical student, Eugene Landis, in 1926, and the method has proved a powerful tool for investigating transcapillary flow. Figure 10.2 shows a modern form of Landis' method. A single capillary is cannulated and perfused with red cells suspended in an albumin solution of known colloid osmotic pressure (COP). The vessel is then blocked downstream by a glass rod. If ultrafiltration occurs out of the blocked segment, red cells creep towards the block as the lost fluid is replaced from the pipette. Conversely, if absorption of interstitial fluid occurs, the red cells are pushed back towards the pipette. Transcapillary flow is calculated from the cell velocity and pressure is measured through the micropipette. Key observations are as follows. (1) The initial filtration rate is linearly proportional

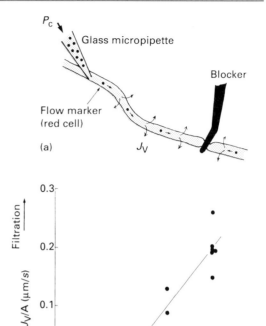

(a)

(b)

Figure 10.2 (a) Modified Landis red cell method for measuring fluid exchange in a single capillary of frog mesentery. Filtration rate is red cell velocity × cross-section of filtering segment (πr^2). Measurements are made at several capillary pressures. (b) Initial filtration rate per unit wall area (J_V/A) as a function of capillary pressure. Intercept at zero filtration equals effective osmotic pressure ($\sigma\pi$, $15\,\text{cmH}_2\text{O}$) exerted *in vivo* by the albumin solution, whose COP *in vitro* (π) was $22\,\text{cmH}_2\text{O}$. The slope equals hydraulic conductance (L_p). (From Michel, C. C. (1980) *Journal of Physiology*, **309**, 341–355, by permission)

to capillary pressure and the steepness of the relation represents wall conductance (L_p). L_p can be actively regulated. It is doubled by atrial natriuretic peptide, for example, and is greatly increased by agents that raise intracellular Ca^{2+} (Section 10.11). (2) Filtration rate is zero when capillary pressure is close to the perfusate's COP, and lowering the pressure beyond this point produces a transient absorption of interstitial fluid. This unequivocally proves Starling's hypothesis, namely, that the capillary wall acts like an osmometer membrane. (3) The capillary pressure that produces zero filtration is equal, on average, to 82% of the perfusate's COP. Since the interstitial pressures are probably negligible in the mesentery, the reflection coefficient for albumin is about 0.82 in these vessels.

Fluid exchange in whole organs

Changes in the weight or volume of a tissue are often used to assess filtration rate in whole organs, including human limbs, as in Figure 10.3. If capillary pressure is raised by congesting the venous outflow, filtration rate increases linearly with pressure. Conversely, if plasma COP is raised, the filtration rate decreases, in accordance with the Starling equation. The slope relating initial tissue swelling rate to capillary pressure is called the capillary filtration coefficient or capacity. It represents the sum of the hydraulic permeabilities of all the exchange vessels within the tissue, i.e. the sum of their surface area $\times$ conductance values, $\Sigma(L_p S)$. The capillary filtration capacity in 100 ml of human forearm is 0.003–0.005 ml min^{-1} per mmHg rise in venous pressure. In cat intestine, where the mucosal capillaries are fenestrated, it is 20 times higher.

The Starling principle relates primarily to a short segment of capillary wall over a brief period of time, since each pressure term is then invariant. For the whole capillary bed, however, capillary pressure changes with distance along the capillary, and can also vary with time, so we must consider this pressure in a little more detail.

10.2 Capillary pressure and its control

Pressure in the exchange vessels is the most variable of the four Starling pressures, and is

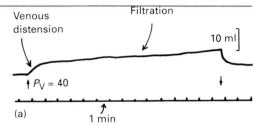

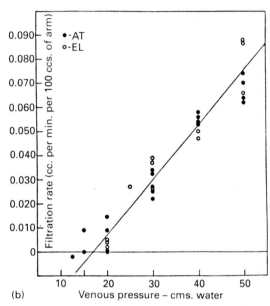

Figure 10.3 Capillary filtration in the human forearm. (a) Forearm volume measured by plethysmography (see Section 8.3). First arrow marks inflation of a venous congesting cuff around upper arm to 40 cmH$_2$O, and second arrow deflation. Blood volume changes account for the initial step. (b) Filtration rate (swelling rate after > 2 min) at a series of venous pressures. The slope, 0.003 ml min^{-1} mmHg^{-1} venous pressure per 100 ml forearm, depends on the aggregate capillary filtration coefficient. (From the classic work of Krogh, A., Landis, E. M. and Turner, A. H. (1932) *Journal of Clinical Investigation*, **11**, 63–95)

the only one under nervous control. It is influenced by distance along the capillary, arterial and venous pressures, vascular resistance and gravity.

Axial distance

Pressure falls by about 1.5 mmHg per 100 µm

along the mammalian capillary owing to the vessel's hydraulic resistance (see Figure 10.11). In human skin at heart level, for example, pressure falls from 32–36 mmHg at the arterial end of the capillary loop to 12–25 mmHg at the venous end, the exact values depending on skin temperature.

The average pressure is lower in portal circulations (hepatic sinusoids approximately 6–7 mmHg, renal tubular capillaries approximately 14 mmHg), in the pulmonary circulation (approximately 10 mmHg) and in fluid-absorbing tissues (e.g. gut mucosal capillaries, 14 mmHg).

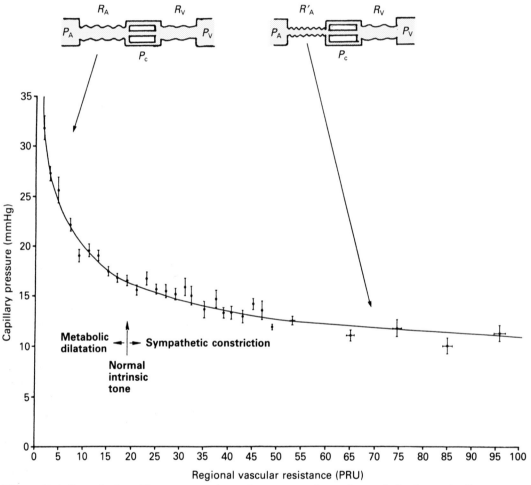

Figure 10.4 Control of capillary pressure by resistance vessel tone in cat skeletal muscle. Pressure was measured towards the venous end of the capillary bed at a fixed venous pressure of 7 mmHg (P_V) and arterial pressure 100 mmHg (P_A). The peripheral resistance unit (PRU) reflects mainly precapillary resistance. Inset shows how precapillary resistance (R_A) affects capillary pressure (P_c).

{Blood flow from artery to midcapillary equals $(P_A − P_c)/R_A$. Flow from midcapillary to vein equals $(P_c − P_V)/R_V$. Since the two flows are virtually equal, $P_A − P_c/R_A = (P_c − P_V)/R_V$. This gives the Pappenheimer–Soto Rivera equation defining capillary pressure: $P_c = (P_A + P_V R_A/R_V)/(1 + R_A/R_V)$.}

(Data from Maspers, M., Björnberg J. and Mellander, S. (1990) *Acta Physiologica Scandinavica*, **140**, 73–83 by permission)

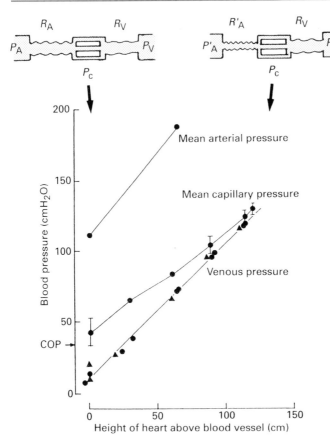

Figure 10.5 Pressure in nailfold skin capillaries of the human foot measured by direct micropuncture with the foot at various distances below heart level. Popliteal artery pressure and dorsal foot vein pressure increase with distance below heart level in the expected fashion, but capillary pressure increases relatively less. Top inset illustrates the vasoconstrictor response that buffers the capillary pressure rise. (From Levick, J. R. and Michel, C. C. (1978) *Journal of Physiology*, **274**, 97–109, by permission)

Pre- to postcapillary resistance ratio

Capillary pressure must be inbetween arterial pressure and venous pressure but the precise value, whether closer to venous or arterial pressure, depends on the resistance of the precapillary vessels (R_A) and postcapillary vessels (R_V). If precapillary resistance is high, the capillary is well shielded from arterial pressure; the precapillary pressure drop is great and capillary pressure is close to venular pressure (Figure 10.4). If postcapillary resistance is relatively high and precapillary resistance relatively low, the situation is somewhat like a hosepipe whose outlet is squeezed – the pressure rises until it nearly equals supply pressure, namely arterial pressure. Mean capillary pressure depends on the balance between these two effects, i.e. on the ratio of pre- to postcapil-

lary resistance (R_A/R_V). The exact relation is derived in the legend of Figure 10.4.

The value of R_A/R_V is typically 4 or more in systemic organs, so capillary pressure is more sensitive to venous pressure than to arterial pressure. This is why venous congestion affects filtration rate so markedly in Figure 10.3.

The pre- to postcapillary resistance ratio is actively controlled by central mechanisms (sympathetic vasoconstrictor nerves and circulating hormones) and by local mechanisms (myogenic response and tissue metabolites), as shown in Figure 10.4. An example of central regulation is provided by skin vasodilatation following a rise in core temperature; reduced sympathetic vasoconstrictor activity lowers R_A/R_V to about 2, which raises mean capillary pressure to over 25 mmHg (in excess of plasma COP) and enhances filtration. This is why fingers swell and rings feel tighter in hot weather. An example of local regulation is seen in the human foot during standing, as described next.

Importance of gravity

Both arterial and venous pressures increase linearly with vertical distance below heart level, reaching 180 mmHg and 90 mmHg, respectively in the feet of a standing man of average height (Figure 10.5). Capillary pressure inevitably increases too, but does so by a smaller amount than either the arterial or venous pressure, because local vasoconstriction raises R_A/R_V to 20–30 and shifts the capillary pressure very close to the lower, venous limit of its range. The local vasoconstriction is called the 'veni-arteriolar response'. Its mechanism may be partly myogenic, though it also seems to require the local presence of sympathetic nerve terminals. Despite the protective effect of the veni-arteriolar response, capillary pressure reaches approximately 95 mmHg in the motionless dependent foot and exceeds plasma COP throughout most of the lower body in the upright position.

10.3 Colloid osmotic pressure of plasma

How does osmotic flow occur?

The process of osmosis across a semipermeable membrane is illustrated in Figure 10.6. In a solution under atmospheric pressure, the pressure exerted on an imaginary plane within the liquid arises partly from bombardment by solvent particles and partly from bombardment by solute particles. Since these effects together add up to atmospheric pressure, it follows that the pressure exerted by the solvent is less than atmospheric pressure. (The situation is rather like that in a gas mixture where each gas has a partial pressure, which is less than the total pressure.) The solute thus lowers the energy level of the solvent. Since the solute cannot enter the pore of a semipermeable membrane, the pore contains pure solvent. If there is pure solvent on the opposite side of the membrane at atmospheric pressure, a pressure gradient exists between the pore exit (solution side, solvent at less than atmospheric pressure) and pore entry (solvent side, solvent at atmospheric pressure), and this drives solvent through the pore. The intrapore pressure gradient can be cancelled out by raising the solution's hydrostatic pressure or by lowering pressure on the solvent side. Flow then ceases, and the hydrostatic pressure required to produce this equilibrium is called 'osmotic pressure'. It should be noted that, contrary to a common belief that water moves through the membrane by diffusion during osmosis, it actually *flows* hydraulically along an intrapore pressure gradient. Experiments confirm that osmotic flow obeys a hydraulic law, *not* Fick's law of diffusion.

Total osmotic pressure of plasma versus *colloid osmotic pressure*

Osmotic pressure is a 'colligative' property, like freezing point depression, which means that it depends on the number of particles in solution but not on their chemical identity. The osmotic pressure (π) of an 'ideal' dilute solution is described by van't Hoff's law, namely $\pi = RTC$, where R is the gas constant, T the absolute temperature and C the molar concentration of particles: RT is 25.4 atmospheres per mole/litre at 37°C. Since plasma contains about 0.3 moles of particles per litre, mostly as sodium, chloride and bicarbonate ions, the van't Hoff osmotic pressure is enormous (7.6 atmospheres or 5800 mmHg). However, this *potential* osmotic pressure is simply not exerted across the capillary wall because (1) the high permeability of the small pore system to electrolytes (except in the brain) quickly establishes an electrolyte equilibrium between plasma and interstitium, and (2) the average reflection coefficient of the capillary wall to electrolytes is only approximately 0.1. Thus it is only the plasma proteins ('colloids'), at a

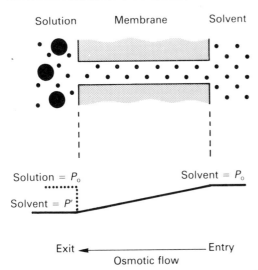

Figure 10.6 Osmotic flow between a solution (left) and solvent (right) exposed to equal pressure, P_o (atmospheric pressure). Owing to the presence of solute, the 'partial pressure' P' of solvent within the solution (i.e. its energy level) is less than P_o. This sets up a hydraulic pressure gradient within the pore which produces an osmotic flow of solvent into the solution. (After Mauro, A. (1981) In *Water Transport Across Epithelia* (eds Ussing, H. H., Bindslev, N., Lassen, L. A. and Sten-Knudsen, D.), Munksgaard, Copenhagen, pp. 107–110)

concentration of merely 0.001 moles/litre, that exert a sustained osmotic pressure across the capillary wall.

Non-ideal nature of plasma colloid osmotic pressure (COP)

Plasma COP is 21–29 mmHg in man, corresponding to 65–80 g protein/litre. In mammals like dog, rabbit and rat, the COP is only about 20 mmHg, and in amphibia it is even lower, 9 mmHg. Albumin comprises only half of the plasma protein by weight but is responsible for two-thirds to three-quarters of the plasma COP because its molecular weight (69 000) is half that of gamma globulins (150 000) and hence its molar concentration is higher. Plasma COP thus depends on the albumin:globulin ratio as well as total protein concentration. Albumin

exerts a negative feedback on the rate of albumin synthesis by the liver, which accounts for the stable level of the plasma COP in a given species.

Protein COP is 'non-ideal', i.e. it considerably exceeds the COP predicted from van't Hoff's ideal law (Figure 10.7). The excess COP is due partly to the space taken up by the voluminous protein molecules (0.7 ml/g), which increases their effective concentration, and partly to their charge. The albumin molecule carries a net negative charge of -17 at pH 7.4 and this attracts an excess of Na^+ ions into the albumin solution (the *Gibbs–Donnan effect*). These ions are confined

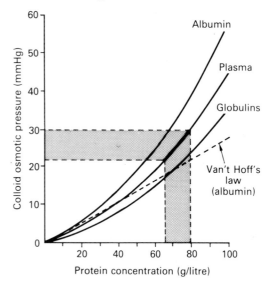

Figure 10.7 Osmotic pressure of human plasma proteins in isotonic saline (pH 7.4, 37°C). Shaded region shows the normal range for human plasma. Dashed line is the van't Hoff law prediction for albumin. The actual COP deviates from this, and is given, in mmHg, by polynomial equations:

albumin $\pi = 0.28C + 1.8.10^{-3}C^2 + 1.2.10^{-5}C^3$
plasma $\pi = 0.21C + 1.6.10^{-3}C^2 + 0.9.10^{-5}C^3$
globulins $\pi = 0.16C + 1.5.10^{-3}C^2 + 0.6.10^{-5}C^3$

where concentration C is g/l. (From Scatchard, G. *et al.*, summarized by Landis, E. M. and Pappenheimer, J. R. (1963) In *Handbook of Physiology 2, Circulation III* (eds W. F. Hamilton and P. Dow), American Physiological Society, Washington, pp. 961–1034) electrostatically to the albumin side of the membrane, so they are osmotically effective and account for roughly a third of albumin's COP.

10.4 Colloid osmotic pressure of interstitial fluid

Over half the plasma protein in the body is actually in the interstitial compartment (16% body weight) rather than in the smaller plasma compartment (4% body weight). The whole-body average interstitial concentration is estimated to be 20–30 g/litre. To assess the protein levels in individual tissues, interstitial fluid can be collected by inserting a nylon wick into the tissue and allowing the fluid to equilibrate with it. Alternatively, since interstitial fluid and prenodal lymph probably have a similar composition, a prenodal lymph duct can be cannulated for fluid collection. Human leg lymph contains 15–20 g/litre of plasma protein, intestinal lymph 30–40 g/litre and lung lymph 40–50 g/litre. These protein levels represent between 23% (leg) and 70% (lung) of the plasma concentration. Interstitial COP is therefore *far from negligible*, and substantially reduces the absorptive force into plasma ($\pi_p - \pi_i$: Table 10.1).

Effect of fluid filtration on interstitial protein concentration

There is a continuous escape of plasma proteins from blood to interstitium (Section 9.7), yet the concentration of plasma proteins in interstitial fluid is always less than in plasma. This is because there is a simultaneous input of water from the capillaries. In the steady state the interstitial protein concentration (C_i) depends on the rate of protein arrival relative to the rate of water arrival. If protein mass m enters the interstitium in time t (flux J_s) and if water volume V enters the interstitium at the same time (flow J_v), then:

$$C_i = \frac{m/t}{V/t} = \frac{J_s}{J_v} \tag{10.4}$$

The idea that concentration can be set by the ratio of two fluxes is illustrated in Figure 10.8(a).

Because of the above process, there is an important inverse relation between interstitial protein concentration and capillary filtration rate, as illustrated in Figure 10.8(b). If water filtration were to cease altogether, interstitial concentration would gradually rise to plasma level due to diffusion. When capillary pressure and filtration rate are increased, interstitial protein concentration falls because the water flow increases more than the protein flux. Protein flux increase too, due to increased convective transport, but this is not as marked

Table 10.1 Starling pressures in human subcutaneous tissue (mmHg)

	Normal subjects	Congestive cardiac failure
Chest		
Plasma COP	26.8	23.3
Interstitial fluid COP	15.6	10.5
Interstitial fluid pressure	−1.5	−1.4
Ankle		
Plasma COP (arterial)	26.8	23.3
Interstitial fluid COP	10.7	3.4 } mild
Interstitial fluid pressure	0.1	0.4 } oedema

COP = colloid osmotic pressure. Interstitial fluid from a soaked wick. Interstitial pressure by wick-in-needle method. (From Noddeland, H., Omvik, P., Lund-Johansen, P. *et al.* (1984) *Clinical Physiology*, **4**, 283–297)

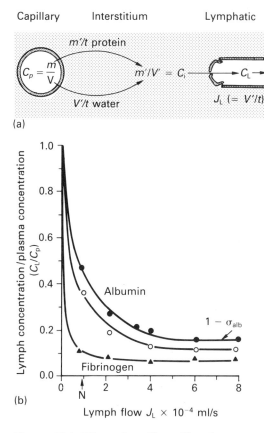

(a)

(b)

Figure 10.8 Effect of capillary filtration rate on interstitial protein concentration and COP. (a) Mass of protein transferred by all processes into the interstitium in a given time (m'/t or J_s) is diluted by the volume of capillary filtrate over the same period (V'/t or J_v) to form interstitial fluid (concentration C_i). This drains away as lymph ($C_L = C_i$). (b) Effect of net filtration rate (equal to lymph flow, J_L) on lymph/plasma concentration ratio (C_L/C_p) in dog paw. Filtration rate was varied by venous congestion. N is normal value. Curves are for albumin (●, radius 3.55 nm), γ-globulin (○, radius 5.6 nm) and fibrinogen (▲, radius 10 nm). At high flows C_L/C_p falls to a limit, namely $1 - \sigma$. (From Renkin, E. M. *et al.* (1977), plotted by Curry, F. E. (1984) *Handbook of Physiology, Cardiovascular System*, Vol. IV, Part II *Microcirculation* (eds E. M. Renkin and C. C. Michel), American Physiological Society, Bethesda, pp. 309–374, by permission)

as the rise in water flow, owing to the reflection of protein by the small pore system.

There is a limit to the decline in interstitial protein concentration, which is set by the average reflection coefficient of the capillary wall to plasma proteins. At high filtration rates protein transport by diffusion or vesicles is relatively negligible and macromolecular sieving is maximal, so the ratio of interstitial concentration to plasma concentration (C_i/C_p) equals the non-reflected fraction of solute $(1 - \sigma)$.* If for example, the reflection coefficient is 0.9 (90%), then 10% of the solute is not reflected and the minimal value of C_i/C_p is 0.1. This approach is often used to assess σ.

We see, then, that interstitial COP is not only a *determinant* of filtration rate (equation 10.3), but also a *function* of filtration rate (equation 10.4). This has important physiological consequences, as explained in Sections 10.6 and 10.10.

10.5 Interstitial pressure and nature of interstitial space

The biopolymer network

To understand the fourth Starling term, interstitial fluid pressure, we must recognize that the interstitial space is not simply a pool of liquid, but has a complex biochemical structure (Figure 10.9). The space is intersected by periodic collagen fibrils of diameter 20–50 nm (collagen types I and III) and microfibrils of diameter approximately 10 nm (collagen type VI), and the interfibrillar spaces are themselves subdivided by a class of fibrous molecule called glycosaminoglycan (GAG). These are long-chain polymers of amino sugars, and the chief types are hyaluronate, keratan sulphate,

*This is easily proved. If transport is predominantly convective, protein transport rate (J_s) equals filtration rate (J_v) × plasma concentration (C_p) × non-reflected fraction $(1 - \sigma)$. Substituting $J_vC_p(1 - \sigma)$ for J_s in equation (10.4), we get $C_i/C_p = 1 - \sigma$.

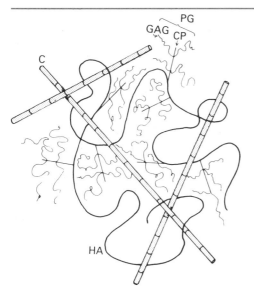

Figure 10.9 Organization of interstitial matrix. Components include collagen fibrils (C, large rods), hyaluronate molecules (HA, long un-branched heavy line) and proteoglycans (PG), composed of a protein core (CP, thin straight lines) and sulphated glycosaminoglycan side chains (GAG, thin curly lines). Microfibrils and glycoproteins not shown. Interstitial fluid is located in the inter-molecular spaces. (From Granger, H. J. (1981) In *Tissue Fluid Pressure and Composition* (ed. A. R. Hargens), Williams and Wilkins, Baltimore, pp. 43–96, by permission)

dermatan sulphate, heparan sulphate and chondroitin sulphate. The sulphated GAGs are up to 40 nm long, whilst hyaluronate is several micrometres along. The sulphated GAGs are covalently bound at one end to a linear protein core, itself up to 400 nm long, to create a brush-shaped molecule called a proteoglycan. The molecular weight of a proteoglycan can be up to 2.5 million in cartilage. The proteoglycans are immobilized by attachment to the long strands of hyaluronate (M_w 1–6 million) and by entanglement within the scaffolding of collagen fibrils. The whole system forms a three-dimensional network of molecular fibres. The sulphate and carboxyl groups of the GAGs represent fixed negative charges and this has an important effect on interstitial pressure (see later).

Near-immobilization of water

Interstitial fluid occupies the minute spaces within the network of fibrous molecules. The average effective radius of these spaces ranges from a mere 3 nm (cartilage) to 30 nm (Wharton's jelly). The resistance to flow through such tiny spaces is very high and as a result interstitium behaves much like a gel; Wharton's jelly in the umbilical cord is a classic example. Cells are not so much 'bathed' in interstitial fluid (a traditional but misleading metaphor) as 'set' in a gel. The gel is functionally important in (1) preventing a flow of interstitial water down the body under the drag of gravity, (2) impeding bacterial spread, and (3) influencing the interstitial pressure–volume relation (Section 10.7).

Meaning of 'interstitial fluid pressure'

The term 'interstitial fluid pressure' is not quite as straightforward as it sounds because the free energy level of the liquid depends not just on mechanical pressure but also on the influence of the interstitial GAGs, and both these effects are rolled into one in the Starling term 'interstitial pressure' (P_i). Wharton's jelly (umbilical cord) nicely illustrates the influence of the GAGs: if a slice of the jelly is brought into contact with saline at atmospheric pressure it imbibes the saline and swells. The swelling tendency is due to the osmotic pressure of the trapped GAGs, which in turn is caused mainly by their fixed negative charges via the Gibbs-Donnan effect (Section 10.3). If a subatmospheric pressureis applied to the fluid in contact with the gel, imbibition can be halted, and the pressure which produces an equilibrium is called the 'gel swelling pressure'.

With the help of this background information, we can understand what physiologists traditionally call the 'interstitial fluid pressure'. If we imagine a GAG-free fluid phase, such as plasma ultrafiltrate, brought into contact with the interstitium, the pressure which must be applied to the free fluid to prevent it either flowing into the interstitium or drawing fluid out of it equals the Starling term 'interstitial fluid pressure'. In other words, it is the pressure at which a free fluid phase has the same potential energy as the fluid within the interstitial matrix.

Measurements of interstitial fluid pressure

Because fluid mobility is so low in the interstitium, the fluid is exceedingly slow to equilibrate with saline in an inserted hypodermic needle, making pressure measurement difficult. Guyton overcame this problem in 1960 by creating an artificial pool of free fluid, which was allowed to equilibrate with the surrounding interstitium for several weeks (Figure 10.10). The artificial pool was formed by surgically implanting a hollow perforated capsule under the skin, and leaving it to fill with fluid. After several weeks, a hypodermic needle was inserted through one of the perforations to measure the pressure of the intracapsular fluid, which was assumed to be in equilibrium with the surrounding interstitial fluid. Intracapsular pressure was found to be subatmospheric (around -5 mmHg), and this discovery

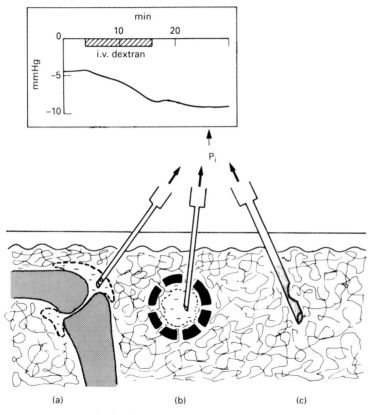

Figure 10.10 Methods for measuring interstitial fluid pressure. (a) Where a pool of free interstitial fluid exists naturally, as in a joint cavity, pressure can be measured via a hypodermic needle. (b) Guyton's capsule, a chronic method (see text). (c) Wick-in-needle, an acute method developed by Fadnes, Reed and Auckland; saline between the nylon filaments in the tip equilibrates with interstitial fluid via the side hole. The multiple channels within the nylon wick facilitate pressure transmission. Inset illustrates how pressure in the giant interstitial cavity of a knee grows more subatmospheric when capillary absorption is induced by a high plasma COP (i.v. dextran infusion over hatched period) (From Levick, J. R. (1983) In *Studies in Joint Disease* 2, (eds A. Maroudas and E. J. Holborow), Pitman, London, pp. 153–240)

evoked a lively controversy since interstitial pressure was formerly regarded as slightly positive. Guyton pointed out, however, that subatmospheric pressure could explain why untethered skin hugs concave surfaces such as the anatomical snuffbox (base of first metacarpal) and ankles.

Later, more rapid techniques such as the wick-in-needle method (see Figure 10.10 legend for details) have confirmed that the equilibrium pressure is indeed slightly sub-atmospheric in many tissues and in inter-stitial spaces like the joint space and epidural space (-1 to -3 mmHg). This accords with what we now know about the imbibition pressure exerted by the interstitial matrix. The maintenance of the subatmospheric pressure in the face of a continual input of fresh capillary ultrafiltrate is probably due to suction of fluid from the tissues by lymphatic vessels (see later). Pressure is above atmo-spheric, however, in encapsulated organs like the kidney ($+1$ to $+10$ mmHg), in certain muscles, myocardium, bone marrow and flexed joints.

10.6 Imbalance of Starling pressures: filtration and absorption

There is still much to be learned about the 'fine tuning' of the Starling forces *in vivo*. The size of the component terms and their balance varies greatly between tissues: con-trast for example, the dependent foot where capillary pressure is far higher than plasma COP and the lung where pressure is much lower than plasma COP. Yet both these tissues filter fluid and produce lymph.

The filtration fraction

Virtually all tissues form lymph, including the lung, so there is normally a net filtration of fluid out of the microcirculation. The fraction of plasma filtered per transit (the filtration fraction) is actually very small in most tissues, around 0.2–0.3%, but since 4000 litres or so of plasma pass through an adult

subject's microcirculation each day, a large volume of fresh interstitial fluid is generated over the course of a day, perhaps as much as 8 litres. Lymphatic drainage ensures that the interstitial volume remains normal despite this. In certain tissues, such as the renal glomerulus, salivary gland and dependent foot the filtration fraction is around a hundred times higher, being 20% in glomer-ular capillaries.

Critical capillary pressure for zero filtration

Figure 10.11 shows typical Starling pressures along a capillary in mammalian muscle, mesentery or warm skin at heart level. Plasma colloid osmotic pressure does not change significantly because the filtration fraction is small, but capillary pressure falls progressively with distance. We can work out the critical capillary pressure at which filtration would cease (the nul-flux or iso-gravimetric pressure) from the Starling prin-ciple: it is $\sigma(\pi_p - \pi_i) + P_i$. For the values in Figure 10.11(a) (and taking $\sigma = 0.9$), the nul-flux pressure works out to be 12.5 mmHg. Pressure does not actually fall as low as 12.5 mmHg until the larger venules are reached, however, and is well above this in well-perfused capillaries. Well-perfused ca-pillaries are thus commonly in a state of filtration over virtually their whole length.

The transience of fluid absorption

The flow of lymph is quite low and this leads physiologists to believe that some of the capillary filtrate is reabsorbed directly into the bloodstream. When and where this absorption takes place, however, is not well understood. Textbooks have traditionally depicted fluid filtration out of the arterial half of the capillary and reabsorption into the venous half, because P_c is less than π_p in the downstream segment (the Landis model of exchange). But as shown in Figure 10.11(a), this view is untenable for well-perfused capillaries when modern measurements of interstitial COP and interstitial pressure are taken into account. *Vasoconstriction*, how-ever, can reduce the capillary pressure

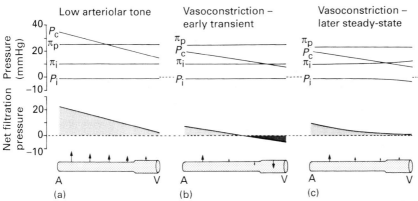

Figure 10.11 Change in pressures and fluid exchange with axial distance; symbols as in text. The shaded net filtration pressure equals $(P_c - P_i) - \sigma(\pi_p - \pi_i)$, and σ is taken to be 0.9. Bottom sketches represent the exchange vessels from arterial end of capillary (A) to pericytic venules (V) and arrows indicate direction of fluid exchange. Values are typical of skin, muscle and mammalian mesentery. (a) Well-perfused capillary. (b) Immediate effect of precapillary vasoconstriction, before interstitial forces have had time to change. (c) Later, during vasoconstriction. The transient absorption period has caused π_i to rise and P_i to fall, re-establishing a steady state in which there is again filtration throughout the vessel

sufficiently for the Landis filtration–absorption model to develop transiently, as illustrated in Figure 10.11(b). The downstream absorption cannot be maintained as a permanent state, however, because the absorption process raises the interstitial protein concentration and π_i, and lowers P_i, and these changes gradually abolish the net absorptive force (Figure 10.11(c)); the absorption fades away with time.

Both theory and experiment indicate that reabsorption cannot be sustained by capillaries with a finite permeability to plasma protein, except under very special conditions (see later). The reason is that the normal low value of pericapillary protein concentration is entirely dependent on filtration being present, as illustrated in Figure 10.8. If filtration ceases, protein accumulates outside the wall and progressively reduces the COP difference upon which absorption depends, until finally absorption ceases. An experiment proving that sustained absorption is not in general possible, no matter how much P_c is reduced, is illustrated in Figure 10.12.

It is probable therefore that reabsorption occurs transiently in most tissues during periods of arteriolar vasoconstriction, and occurs chiefly at the venous end of the microcirculation. Fortunately, from the point of view of fluid balance, the absorption rate across the venular walls is enhanced by their greater hydraulical conductance, which is another facet of the arteriovenous gradient of permeability illustrated in Figure 9.6. Thus fluid exchange downstream may oscillate between periods of filtration and transient reabsorption. Another way of looking at this is to say that the functional *mean* capillary pressure, averaged over both time and axial distance, is much lower than the pressure recorded directly in well-perfused capillaries. The functional average is calculated to be very close to venous pressure, so there is only a very small net filtration force over a period of time (perhaps as little as 0.5 mmHg) and a low lymph flow.

Fluid exchange in the low-pressure pulmonary circulation

The lung is an important example where capillary pressure (approximately 10 mmHg) is less than plasma COP (25 mmHg). Although these values might suggest,

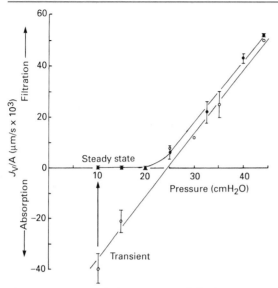

Figure 10.12 Proof of transience of fluid absorption when capillary pressure is lowered. Flow across unit wall area (J_V/A) is plotted against capillary pressure; modified Landis red cell method of Figure 10.2; perfusate COP = 32 cmH$_2$O. When the capillary is perfused with the high-COP test solution for only a few seconds prior to measurement of exchange, the COP drop across the wall is close to perfusate COP. Under these conditions, labelled 'transient' (open circles), a capillary pressure below 25 cmH$_2$O produces absorption. When, however, the capillary was perfused with the high-COP solution for a long period (2–5 min) at a low pressure, to establish a new steady state prior to measurement, absorption was found to have ceased (filled circles, steady-state situation). This is because interstitial COP had increased during the absorption transient. (From Michel, C. C. and Phillips, M. E. (1987) *Journal of Physiology*, **388**, 421–435, by permission)

superficially, that lung capillaries should be absorbing fluid, the lung in fact produces lymph, showing that the capillaries have a net filtration pressure. The reason is that lung interstitial fluid has a high protein concentration (approximately 70% plasma level) with a COP of 16–20 mmHg, which greatly reduces the net absorptive force. The flat part of the steady-state line in Figure 10.12 is probably also an approximate representation of the normal situation in the lung.

Tissues where sustained absorption occurs

Although reabsorption of filtrate from a 'closed' interstitium (one with no other fluid input than capillary filtrate) can only be transient, continuous absorption certainly occurs in renal tubular capillaries, in intestinal mucosal capillaries and probably in lymph node capillaries. This is possible because the interstitial space in these tissues has a second input of fluid, in the form of renal tubule absorbate, gut lumen absorbate or lymph, respectively. This fluid flushes the interstitial space and prevents the accumulation of interstitial plasma protein. In the cat intestine 80% of the water transferred into the lining from the lumen is then absorbed into the microcirculation, while 20% acts as flushing solution and drains into the lymphatic vessels; in the kidney the corresponding figures are around 99% and 1%.

10.7 Transport through interstitial matrix

There are 10–12 litres of fluid in the interstitial compartment of a 70 kg man and this acts as a reservoir for the plasma compartment (3 litres). If the plasma volume is reduced by a haemorrhage, some of the interstitial fluid is absorbed to top up the plasma; conversely, if plasma volume is increased by renal fluid retention or over-infusion, the excess fluid can 'spill over' into the interstitium, raising the interstitial volume and therefore pressure.

The interstitial pressure–volume curve; oedema

Figure 10.13 shows the effect of fluid volume on pressure in subcutaneous interstitium. This tissue is of special interest because it is where peripheral oedema accumulates chiefly. In normally hydrated interstitium, the fluid pressure is slightly subatmospheric, and small changes in volume affect the pressure markedly. The ratio of volume change to pressure change is called 'compliance', and normal interstitial compliance is rather small. This is because any removal of water raises the GAG concentration, which makes the gel swelling pressure more negative and opposes further volume change. The same mechanism operates in reverse during fluid addition, but its range of action is then more limited because a point is soon reached where the swelling pressure is negligible and interstitial pressure is close to atmospheric. Beyond this point, the accumulation of fluid is no longer opposed by changes in GAG swelling pressure: the only opposition comes from the stretching of the collagen and elastin network. Since the subcutaneous network is rather loose and the overlying skin highly distensible, this opposing force is small. Moreover, it decays with time, a process called stress relaxation or delayed compliance. Interstitial compliance therefore increases rather abruptly just above atmospheric pressure, to around 20 times normal. Large volumes of fluid then accumulate with

little opposing rise in pressure, and this creates pools of freely mobile liquid – a condition called oedema. In an oedematous leg, about 98% of the excess fluid is found in the subcutaneous plane and its pressure is only just above atmospheric (Table 10.1). In tissues bounded by an inelastic fibrous capsule, such as the anterolateral muscle compartment of the leg, the pressure-volume curve is steeper and interstitial pressure can reach higher levels.

Interstitial conductivity, pitting and oedema

Although water normally constitutes 65–99% of interstitium by weight (depending on the tissue), it is not easily displaced owing to the low hydraulic conductivity of the interstitial matrix (Section 10.5). The hydraulic conductivity of the interstitial matrix depends on the ratio of the fractional water content (the void volume fraction or 'porosity', ϵ) to the surface

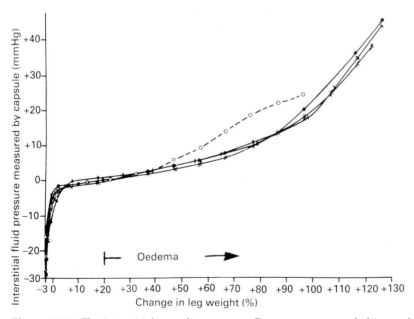

Figure 10.13 The interstitial compliance curve. Pressure was recorded in a subcutaneous capsule in four dog hindlimbs (mean − 6 mmHg). Changes in interstitial volume were assessed by changes in leg weight. Absorption was induced by hyperosmotic dextran solution i.v. and oedema by perfusing with saline at raised venous pressure. Clinical oedema was detected at +20% leg weight, corresponding to an estimated 300% rise in subcutaneous fluid volume. (From Guyton, A. C. (1965) *Circulation Research*, **16**, 452, by permission)

area of the fixed proteoglycan and collagen fibres (S), which are the source of hydraulic resistance. The ratio ϵ/S is called the mean hydraulic radius, and it ranges from 30 nm in Wharton's jelly down to 3 nm in articular cartilage. At normal hydration, interstitial conductivity is between 10^{-10} and 10^{-13} cm^4/s per dyne (depending on tissue), and this is sufficient to allow capillary ultrafiltrate to percolate slowly through the matrix to the lymphatic vessels, under a small pressure gradient.

Interstitial conductivity increases dramatically with hydration especially if pools of free fluid form (oedema). This is illustrated by the clinical test for subcutaneous oedema, the *pitting test*, which is essentially a test of fluid mobility. When a finger is pressed firmly onto normal skin for a minute and then withdrawn, no impression is left behind because interstitial fluid mobility is very low and little fluid is displaced. In oedematous tissue, however, finger pressure leaves behind a distinct pit (see Figure 10.14), indicating that free, abnormally mobile fluid had been present in the interstitium.

Non-pitting forms of oedema also exist. The commonest occurs in chronic lymphoedema (Section 10.10), in which the tissue synthesizes additional collagen and fat. This produces a fibrotic kind of oedema that does not pit easily ('brawny' oedema).

Solute transport through interstitium

Small solutes like oxygen and glucose move easily through the interstitial proteoglycan meshwork, and the diffusional resistance to such solutes is simply related to pathlength (typically 10–20 µm). Larger solutes like albumin, however, experience restricted diffusion and steric exclusion in interstitial matrix (see Section 9.3 for explanation of these terms). Ogston and others have shown that such phenomena also occur in GAG meshworks *in vitro* because the irregular inter-fibre spaces are small enough to partially exclude protein molecules and impede their diffusion. The greater the GAG concentration, the smaller the average inter-fibre

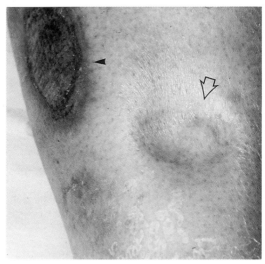

Figure 10.14 Photograph of back of calf (the ankle is off lower edge of picture), to show pitting oedema (arrow), in a patient with cardiac failure. The oedema was exacerbated by immobility and dependency. Note the skin damage (arrowhead, top left) after an oedema blister had stripped the epidermis from the dermis. (Courtesy of Dr P. Mortimer, Department of Dermatology, St. George's Hospital, London)

distance and the greater the amount of space (water) from which the protein is excluded. Indeed, albumin is almost totally excluded from cartilage, the densest of all interstitia. In the less dense interstitia of subcutis and muscle, albumin is excluded from 20–50% of the water volume. As a result, the effective interstitial protein concentration (protein/available water space) is higher than the apparent concentration (protein/total water space).

Convective transport (wash-along or 'solvent drag') by the stream of capillary filtrate largely accounts for protein transport through the interstitial space in the steady state.

10.8 Lymph and the lymphatic system

The anatomy and transport functions of the lymphatic system were explored in the seventeenth century by the Swedish biologist Rudbeck (after whom our yellow-flowered garden annual Rudbeckia is named) and others. The functions of the lymphatic system are as follows:

1. Preservation of fluid balance. Lymph vessels return capillary ultrafiltrate and plasma proteins to the bloodstream at emptying points into the neck veins, and some fluid also returns to the blood in the lymph nodes. This completes the extravascular circulation of fluid and protein (Figure 10.15) and secures the homeostasis of tissue volume. Since the plasma volume circulates in this fashion in less than 24 h, impairment of lymphatic function can lead to a severe protein-rich oedema. The brain and eye, which lack a normal lymphatic system, have unique fluid-draining systems, namely the arachnoid granulations and cribriform-nasal route for cerebrospinal fluid, and the canal of Schlemm for aqueous humour.
2. Nutritional function. Intestinal lymph vessels (lacteals) absorb digested fat in the form of tiny globules or 'chylomicra' and transport them to the plasma.
3. Defence function. Fluid draining out of the interstitial compartment carries with it foreign materials such as soluble anti-gens, bacteria, carbon particles, etc. These are carried in afferent lymph to lymph nodes scattered along the drainage route (Figure 10.16), providing an effective and economical method for the immunosurveillance of virtually the whole body. Particulate matter is filtered out and phagocytosed in the nodes (hence the black mediastinal nodes of smokers and coal miners). Antigens stimulate a defensive lymphocyte response and the activated lymphocytes and plasma cells enter the efferent lymph for transport to the circulation. As a result, efferent lymph has a much higher cell count than afferent lymph.

Structure

Lymphatic capillaries

The lymphatic system begins as a set of lymphatic capillaries (terminal lymphatics, initial lymphatics) which are either blind terminal sacs, as in intestinal villi, or else an anastomosing network of tubes of diameter 10–50 µm (Figure 10.16). The very thin wall consists of a single layer of endothelial cells resting on an incomplete basement membrane. Some of the cell junctions are 14 nm or more wide, so the initial lymphatics are

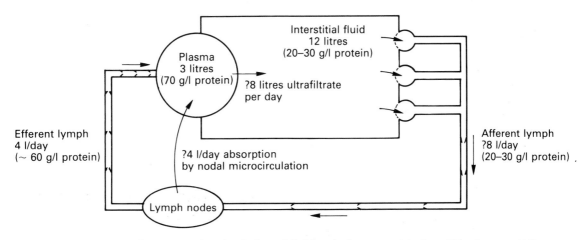

Figure 10.15 Estimate of extravascular circulation of fluid and plasma protein in a 65 kg human. (After Renkin, E. M. (1986) *American Journal of Physiology*, **250**, H706–710)

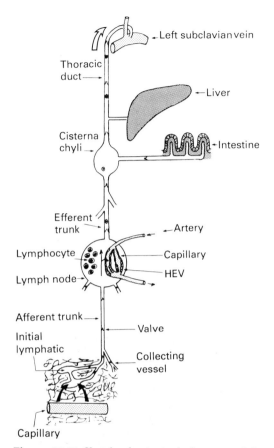

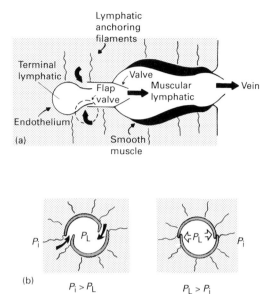

Figure 10.16 Sketch of principal elements of the lymphatic system (not to scale). HEV, high endothelial venule, where lymphocytes re-enter the node from blood. Arrows within node indicate absorption of some water by nodal capillaries

Figure 10.17 Simplified model for lymphatic transport. (a) Interstitial fluid enters the initial lymphatic down a pressure gradient. Each muscular segment or 'lymphangion' pumps lymph into the next one and ultimately into the venous system. (b) Proposed operation of endothelial junctions in the initial lymphatics as flap valves. P_i, interstitial pressure; P_L, lymph pressure. (From Granger, H. J. *et al.* (1984) In *Edema*, pp. 189–228, see Further Reading, by permission)

highly permeable to plasma proteins and even to particulate matter like carbon. The junctions run very obliquely and may function like flap valves, allowing fluid to enter readily but closing to prevent egress when lymph pressure rises above interstitial pressure (Figure 10.17). The outer surface of the wall is tethered to the surrounding tissues by radiating fibrils, the 'anchoring filaments', which may help dilate the vessels in oedematous tissue.

Collecting vessels and afferent lymph trunks

Lymphatic capillaries unite to form collecting vessels which feed into the afferent lymph trunks alongside major vascular bundles like the popliteal vessels. *Semilunar valves* direct the lymph centrally. From the collecting vessels onwards the lymphatics possess a coat of smooth muscle and connective tissue, the muscle element being abundant in man and ruminants but scanty in the dog and rabbit.

Lymph nodes

Several afferent vessels drain into the hilum of each lymph node. The node is a complex cellular body containing maturing lymphocytes in germinal centres, plus many phagocytic cells. The afferent lymph flows through sinuses, which are endothelial tubes with frequent gaps through which mature lymphocytes can enter the lymph. If the afferent lymph presents a foreign antigen to the node, there is a dramatic increase in the release of lymphocytes into postnodal lymph and some lymphocytes develop into 'plasma cells', which secrete gamma-globulin antibodies. The node is supplied with nutrients by a network of continuous capillaries, and these drain into special high-endothelial venules. Lymphocytes in the bloodstream re-enter the node by penetrating the intercellular junctions of the high-endothelial venules, thus completing their own unique circulation.

The major lymphatic ducts

Lymphocyte-rich efferent lymph from the lower limbs and viscera flows into a large lymphatic trunk on the posterior abdominal wall. This possesses a saccular dilatation, the cisterna chyli, which acts as a temporary receptacle for chyle, the fatty lymph arriving from lacteals during absorption of a fatty meal. The ultimate lymphatic trunk, the thoracic duct, receives around three-quarters of the body's efferent lymph and empties into the left subclavian vein at its junction with the jugular vein. The small cervical and right lymphatic trunks have much smaller flows.

How is lymph formed and propelled?

The composition of prenodal lymph indicates that lymph is simply interstitial fluid drawn from the neighbourhood of the lymphatic capillary. But what process drives the interstitial fluid into the lymphatic capillary, where the pressure is slightly higher than interstitial fluid pressure for much of the time? The likely answer is that first the lymphatic capillary empties proximally, either because it is compressed by the surrounding tissue during movement or

because of contractions of the lymphatic wall (Figure 10.18). Then, as the vessel re-expands elastically (probably helped by the anchoring filaments) the pressure inside falls transiently below interstitial fluid pressure, setting up a pressure gradient for filling. (The process may be not unlike the filling of a fountain pen or Pasteur pipette by first squeezing the rubber bulb empty and then allowing its recoil to suck in fluid.) The presence of

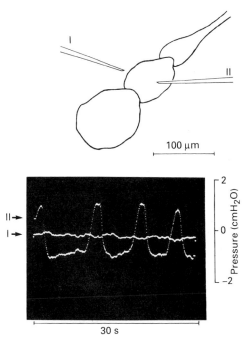

Figure 10.18 Evidence for the lymphatic suction theory of interstitial drainage in the bat wing. Top: Micropipettes were inserted into the interstitium and a contractile terminal lymphatic to assess the interstitium-to-lymph pressure gradient. Bottom: Interstitial pressure (I) exceeded lymph pressure (II) for 43% of the time, because lymph pressure fell to subatmospheric levels during relaxation. Measurements of interstitial pressure at more distant sites revealed a gentle interstitial pressure gradient towards the lymphatic (0.004 cmH$_2$O per µm). Unlike the bat wing, however, most tissues do not have actively contractile terminal lymphatics. (From Hogan, R. D. (1981) In *Interstitial Fluid Pressure and Composition* (ed. Hargens, A. R.), Williams and Wilkins, Baltimore, pp. 155–163, by permission)

lymphatic valves upstream ensures that backflow does not interfere with this process.

Once formed, lymph is moved along by both intrinsic and extrinsic mechanisms. *Intrinsic rhythmic contractions* occur in lymph vessels with abundant smooth muscle, including those in the human leg, and the contraction rate is typically 10–15 per min. Animal studies show that each inter-valve segment, or 'lymphangion', functions as a rhythmic pump and the lymphangion resembles the heart in many of its physiological characteristics: each has a pacemaker, a filling and ejection phase, a stroke volume, contractility that depends on extracellular Ca^{2+}, and even a sympathetic innervation in the larger vessels. Both the frequency and stroke volume of the lymphangion increase with lymph volume and this enables the lymphatic system to respond to increased fluid input by increasing its transport rate.

The chief *extrinsic propulsion* process is intermittent compression during movement. The flow of lymph from the leg of an anaesthetized dog is greatly increased by passive or active flexion, and the flow of mesenteric lymph is enhanced by intestinal peristalsis. Extrinsic propulsion is obviously important for non-contractile vessels. The lymph valves permit lymph pressure to rise stepwise in successive segments so that the lymph finally drains into venous blood at several mmHg above atmospheric pressure.

Fluid exchange in lymph nodes

Lymph nodes, like the popliteal and iliac nodes, modify the volume and protein concentration of lymph; postnodal lymph in the dog and sheep has up to twice the protein concentration of prenodal lymph, due mainly to absorption of water by the node's continuous capillaries. Presumably, capillary pressure is less than plasma COP in such vessels and extravascular accumulation of protein is prevented by the stream of lymph bathing the nodal capillaries. Thus *post*nodal lymph is *not* representative of either interstitial composition or formation

rate. The proportion of human prenodal lymph that gets absorbed is uncertain; Figure 10.15 is based on a plausible estimate, but the exact value probably varies with posture in man, since nodal capillary pressure must increase with dependency.

Regional differences in flow and composition of lymph

Postnodal lymph flow in the human thoracic duct averages 1–3 litres per day. The greatest producer of lymph is the liver which contributes 30–50% of thoracic duct flow (Table 10.2). Due to the discontinuities in hepatic capillaries, hepatic lymph is particularly rich in plasma protein. Intestinal lymph flow is abundant after a meal and makes the second greatest contribution to thoracic duct flow. Renal and lung lymph flows are substantial too. The limbs contribute a variable quantity of lymph depending on the exercise level. The concentration of plasma protein in lymph varies from region to region and depends on the permeability and reflection coefficient of the tissue's exchange vessels, the molecular size and charge of the individual protein and the capillary filtration rate, as described earlier.

Table 10.2 Postnodal lymph flow and composition in man

	Flow*(%)	L/P†
Thoracic duct	(1–3 litres/day)	0.66–0.69
Liver	30–49%	0.66–0.89
Gastrointestinal	~37%	0.50–0.62
Kidney	6–11%	0.47
Lungs	3–15%	0.66–0.69
Limbs and cervical trunks	<10%	0.23–0.58

*Expressed as percentage of total thoracic duct flow. The flows are approximate owing to the difficulty of collection and variability of flow
† Concentration of protein in postnodal lymph relative to plasma. (From Joffey, J. M. and Courtice, F. C. (1970) *Lymphatics, Lymph and the Lymphomyeloid Complex*, Academic Press, London)

10.9 Challenges to fluid balance: posture and exercise

Two physiological events which markedly disturb fluid exchange in man are the adoption of an upright posture and exercise.

Posture and dependent swelling

The rise in capillary pressure below heart level, illustrated in Figure 10.5, increases the filtration rate in dependent tissues. The foot, for example, swells at an initial rate of around 30 ml/h. This is often noticed by people compelled to sit still for hours in aeroplanes and in the cinema, and many find it necessary to unlace their shoes to ease the expanded foot. Taking the circulation as a whole, plasma volume falls by 6–12% during a 40-min period of standing, causing a rise in haematocrit and protein concentration. Plasma COP in students is found to increase from 25 mmHg to 29 mmHg after an 8-h day involving sitting through lectures, reading in the library, etc.

The swelling of dependent tissues and decline in plasma volume would be very much worse but for several compensatory mechanisms.

1. Increase in R_A/R_V. Arteriolar contraction in the dependent tissue increases the pre- to postcapillary resistance ratio (R_A/R_v) and limits the rise in capillary pressure to about two-thirds of the rise in arterial and venous pressures (Figure 10.5). This is a local response, not a baroreceptor reflex, and it involves the myogenic response and/or a local sympathetic axon reflex. Autonomic neuropathy in diabetic patients can abolish the local reflex and this probably explains why leg oedema is common in such patients.
2. The skeletal muscle pump (Section 8.7). Dynamic exercise reduces venous pressure to 30–40 mmHg in the calf during walking, cycling, etc., and this reduces capillary pressure correspondingly. The muscle pump also enhances lymph transport.
3. Reduced blood flow. The dependent vasoconstriction referred to above reduces not only capillary pressure but also blood flow (see Figure 8.5). The low plasma flow, coupled with the increased filtration pressure, raises the filtration fraction enormously, namely to 20–27% in the foot, and the ensuing haemoconcentration raises the COP to 35–44 mmHg in the downstream capillaries. This helps to offset the increased blood pressure there.
4. Reduced capillary filtration capacity. It is possible that the constriction of some terminal arterioles may stop flow completely through capillary modules for short periods, lowering the local filtration capacity. There is evidence of this in intestinal preparations, but rather conflicting evidence in limbs.

Exercise and the swelling of muscle

During exercise, local vasodilatation not only increases muscle blood flow but also increases capillary pressure by reducing R_A/R_V (see Figure 10.4). At the same time, the number of perfused capillaries is increased. As a result the filtration rate rises in exercising muscle and the muscle can swell by 20% over the course of 15 min. Rock-climbers, for example, often notice a marked swelling of the forearm muscles after a 'fingery' ascent. An important additional factor promoting swelling is the release of small solutes like lactate and K^+ by the active muscle fibres, which increases the interstitial osmolarity by 20–30 mOsm/litre (7–10%). Such molecules exert only a fraction of their potential osmotic pressure at the capillary wall because their reflection coefficient is low – perhaps as little as 0.1. Nevertheless an osmotic pressure of 0.1×25 mOsm is 42 mmHg (van't Hoff's law, Section 10.3) and this is a substantial force enhancing filtration. The osmotic pressure of such small solutes is probably exerted mainly across the endothelial cell membrane which has a small but finite permeability to water, rather than across the small pore system.

When exercise involves the whole body, the increased transcapillary filtration can reduce the plasma volume by 16–20%. The decrease in plasma volume (by up to 600 ml in man) is actually less than the increase in muscle volume, which can rise by 1100 ml during strenuous cycling. The difference is due to a compensatory absorption of interstitial fluid into plasma from non-exercising tissues, which minimizes the fall in blood volume.

10.10 Oedema

Oedema is an excess of interstitial fluid, and in clinical practice the two commonest sites for oedema are subcutaneous tissue (peripheral oedema) and the lungs (pulmonary oedema).

In *subcutaneous oedema* the increased fluid volume shifts the tissue onto the flat, unstable part of the compliance curve (see Figure 10.13). Subcutaneous oedema is not detected clinically, however, until the interstitial volume has increased by over 100% (well along the compliance curve), which corresponds to a 10% increase in limb size. The nature of oedematous interstitium was described in Section 10.7. Peripheral oedema has undesirable, albeit non-fatal, effects including impaired cell nutrition (due to increased diffusion distances), skin ulceration, blistering (see Figure 10.14), deformity, discomfort and impairment of limb usage.

Pulmonary oedema is most commonly caused by left ventricular failure, which elevates the left-side filling pressure and therefore pulmonary venous pressure (whereas right ventricular failure causes peripheral, subcutaneous oedema). Pulmonary oedema has serious consequences, partly because the stiff oedematous lung is difficult to inflate, causing dyspnoea (difficulty in breathing), and partly because the gas-to-blood distance increases, slowing down gas exchange and causing hypoxia. If the inter-stitial oedema spills over into the alveolar spaces and floods them, pulmonary oedema can be fatal.

Causes of oedema

Oedema develops when the capillary filtration rate exceeds the lymphatic drainage rate for a sufficient period, i.e. the pathogenesis involves either a high filtration rate or a low lymph flow. Since the factors governing filtration are given in the Starling expression, equation (10.3), the terms of this equation provide a logical classification for oedema.

Raised capillary pressure

Elevation of capillary pressure is usually secondary to chronic elevation of venous pressure caused by ventricular failure or fluid overload (as in over-transfusion and acute glomerulonephritis), or deep venous thrombosis (which raises postcapillary resistance and may later lead to venous valve incompetence). Pressures of 20–40 mmHg can develop in the venous limbs of skin capillaries during right ventricular failure. The oedema fluid in such cases has a reduced protein level, namely 1–10 g/litre, due to the diluting effect of a high filtration rate (see Figure 10.8).

Reduced plasma COP

Hypoproteinaemia raises net capillary filtration rate and lymph flow as shown in Figure 10.19. At the same time, the lymph protein concentration falls (1–6 g/litre), and these changes provide some protection against oedema formation (see later). Clinically, it is found that overt oedema only develops when the protein concentration in plasma falls below 30 g/litre. Hypoproteinaemia can be caused by malnutrition or malabsorption due to intestinal disease, by excessive loss of plasma protein either into urine (nephrotic syndrome) or into the gut lumen (protein-losing enteropathy), or by hepatic failure, the liver being the site of synthesis of the plasma proteins albumin, fibrinogen, α-globulins

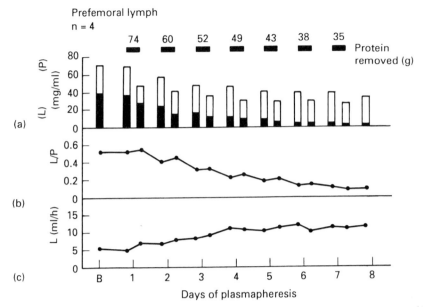

Figure 10.19 Experimental hypoproteinaemia in sheep. (a) Protein was removed by daily plasmapheresis (the removal of blood and replacement of only the cells, water and electrolytes). This caused protein concentration in the plasma to fall (P, white bars). The concentration of protein fell relatively further in postnodal leg lymph (L, black bars), so the L/P ratio fell (b). Lymph flow, an indication of capillary filtration rate, more than doubled (c). These data illustrate the operation of two 'buffers' or *safety factors against oedema formation*, namely dilution of interstitial protein (lowering the pericapillary COP) and increased lymphatic drainage. (From Kramer, G. *et al.* In Renkin, E. M. (1986) *American Journal of Physiology*, **250**, H706–710, by permission)

and β-globulins. The commonest cause of hepatic failure is a fibrotic condition called cirrhosis, which gives rise to abdominal oedema (ascites) by raising portal vein pressure as well as lowering plasma COP. The nephrotic syndrome is characterized by albuminuria due to leakage of albumin through the glomerular membrane, often exceeding 20 g/day.

Changes in capillary permeability (L_p, σ, P)

In inflammation, the properties of the capillary wall itself change: hydraulic conductance and protein permeability increase and the reflection coefficient decreases. This causes a severe high-protein oedema. Inflammation is such a fundamental pathological process that it is described separately in Section 10.11.

Lymphatic insufficiency

Impairment of lymphatic drainage causes the accumulation of both fluid and protein since both enter the interstitial space in substantial amounts over a day. Because lymph is the sole route for returning escaped protein to the plasma, lymphoedema fluid is rich in protein. In limb lymphoedema, the protein content is 30 g/litre or more and the lymph:-plasma ratio is > 0.4, in contrast to the dilute oedemas described above (< 10 g/litre). The condition evokes a fibrotic-fatty overgrowth, so long-standing lymphoedema does not pit easily. In Western countries lymphatic insufficiency is usually due either to poor formation of limb lymph trunks (idiopathic lymphoedema) or to damage to lymph nodes during cancer therapy, as in Figure 10.20. The commonest cause world-wide, however, is filariasis, a nematode worm infestation transmitted by mosquitoes. The nematodes impair lymphatic function in the limbs and scrotum, causing a gross lymphoedema associated with hyperkeratotic elephant-like skin (elephantiasis).

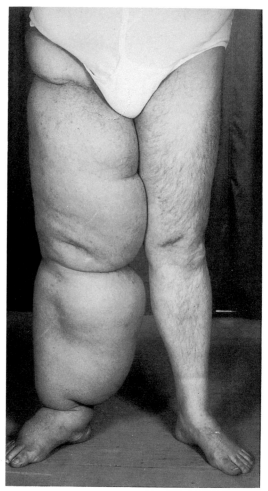

Figure 10.20 Lymphoedema caused by surgery of the groin to treat testicular cancer. (Courtesy of Dr P. Mortimer, Department of Dermatology, St. George's Hospital, London)

The safety margin against oedema

Clinicians have long recognized that clinical oedema does not develop unless plasma COP or venous pressure have changed by at least 15 mmHg. There is thus a margin of safety against oedema of 15 mmHg or there-abouts, and this is due to three buffering factors: changes in interstitial fluid pressure, interstitial COP and lymph flow (Figure 10.21).

1. Rise in interstitial fluid pressure (P_i). When filtration rate is increased the interstitial pressure of normally-hydrated tissue rises markedly for only a very small rise in interstitial volume (see Figure 10.13). This reduces the filtration pressure ($P_c - P_i$). If P_i is normally −2 mmHg and clinical oedema appears at, say, +1 mmHg, the change in P_i gives a safety margin of 3 mmHg. This mechanism fails above 1–2 mmHg in tissues like subcutis where compliance increases sharply.

2. Fall in interstitial COP (π_i). An increase in filtration rate lowers the interstitial protein concentration and COP and thereby increases the absorptive force ($\pi_p - \pi_i$), as shown by the COPs of ankle fluid in Table 10.1. Like mechanism 1, this buffer has a limited capacity, because the ratio of interstitial:plasma protein concentrations can fall no lower than $1 - \sigma$ (see Figure 10.8). Interstitial dilution is most effective as a buffer mechanism in tissues where the interstitial protein concentration is normally high, e.g. the lung. In the limbs, where interstitial COP is 5–10 mmHg, interstitial dilution offers a safety factor of 4.5–9 mmHg.

3. Increased lymph flow. When interstitial volume and pressure increase, the lymph flow from the tissue increases too. In the cat intestine, for example, raising venous pressure to 30 mmHg causes a 20-fold rise in lymph flow. Some workers find, however, that the rise in lymph flow reaches a limit, the maximum rise being equivalent to a 5 mmHg safety factor. The combined effects of the changes in P_i, π_i and lymph flow add up to a total safety margin of around 15 mmHg. The relative importance of P_i and π_i in this process depends on their starting levels but in most tissues π_i seems to be the major

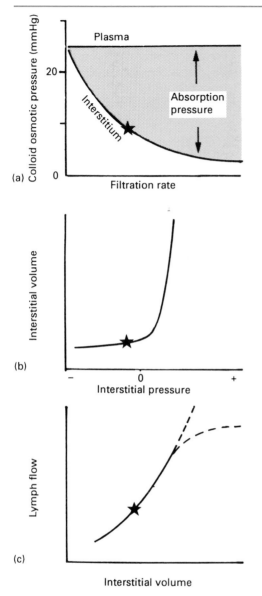

Figure 10.21 Three safety factors against oedema. Stars indicate normal state. (a) When capillary filtration rate increases, the COP difference opposing filtration increases too, owing to the fall in interstitial protein concentration. (b) Change in interstitial pressure with volume in subcutaneous space; compliance is low at subatmospheric pressure so marked pressure changes oppose modest filtration. But compliance is very large above atmospheric pressure, so there is little further rise in pressure. This is essentially Figure 10.13 turned on its side. (c) Lymph flow increases with interstitial hydration, opposing oedema formation. Dashed lines indicate that lymph flow reaches a limit in stationary tissue but may not do so in moving flexed limbs. (After Taylor, A. E. and Townsley, M. I. (1987) *News in Physiological Science*, **2**, 48–52)

buffer. The lung in particular is well protected against oedema by its high interstitial COP.

10.11 Inflammatory swelling

The ancient definition of inflammation by Celsus (30 BC–AD 38) is hard to better: inflam-mation is a combination of redness (rubor), heat (calor), swelling (tumor) and pain (dolor), to which Galen (AD 130–200) added a fifth criterion, loss of function. Some diverse examples include scalded skin, rheumatoid joints, infective peritonitis and disseminated cancer. The redness, heat and swelling all arise from microvascular changes. The redness and heat are due to vasodilatation caused by substances produced locally in response to tissue damage (wounding, infection, ischaemia, etc.). These 'chemical mediators of inflammation' include histamine, bradykinin, prostaglandins, substance P, platelet-activating factor, super-oxide radicals and others. Most of these substances, plus the potent leukotrienes (Section 12.4) and cytokines also initiate a series of changes in the walls of pericytic venules. (Cytokines are mediators of the inflammatory response produced by mono-cytes, endothelial cells and fibroblasts. They include tumour necrosing factor and the interleukin series.) The changes are as follows:

1. The *endothelial surface* becomes attractive to leucocytes. These adhere to the wall (margination) and then push through the intercellular junctions to invade the inflamed tissue (Figure 10.22). They are followed more slowly by migrating lymphocytes and mono-cytes. The process of leucocyte margination–extravasation involves a complex system of recently-discovered adhesion molecules. Histamine and thrombin stimulate the ap-pearance of *P-selectin* on the endothelial cell surface within minutes, while inter-leukin-1 and tumour-necrosing factor act more slowly over several hours to stimulate *E-selectin* production (endothelial–leuco-cyte adhesion molecule, ELAM). The se-lectins render the capillary wall 'sticky' to

white cells, but the captured cells at first continue to roll slowly along the the sticky wall. Tightly binding proteins are then activated, those on the leucocytes being called *integrins* and those on the endothe-lium being intercellular adhesion molecules (ICAMs) and vascular cell adhesion molecules (VCAMs). This binds the leucocyte tightly to the endothelium and halts rolling. Finally, the cell penetrates the intercellular junction, a process that depends on high local concentrations of ICAM-1 and on PECAM (platelet-endothelial cell adhe-sion molecule), an adhesion molecule con-centrated in the junctions. This rolling–attachment–extravasation sequence is illu-strated in Figure 10.22.

2. Quite independently of leucocyte extra-vasation, *gaps* up to 1 μm wide form in the endothelial cell close to the intercellular junction. Gap formation is probably powered by contraction of *actin–myosin filaments*, which are found close to the intercellular junction, and is initiated by a rise in *cytoplasmic* Ca^{2+} concentration (normal con-centration < 0.1 μM). The Ca^{2+} seems to act via calmodulin and myosin light chain kinase, as described under 'Vascular smooth muscle' in the next chapter. The rise in Ca^{2+} is initiated by gap-inducing agonists such as histamine and bradykinin, and occurs in two phases. A few seconds after agonist binding

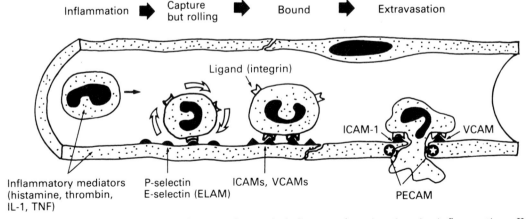

Figure 10.22 White cell capture by venular endothelium and emigration in inflammation. IL-1, interleukin 1. TNF, tumour necrosing factor. For adhesion molecule abbreviations, see text

there is a rapid rise in cytoplasmic $[Ca^{2+}]$, peaking at 1 μM within 30 s. This is followed by a sustained level at about half the peak value. The initial peak is due to release of an intracellular Ca^{2+} store, mediated by a second messenger (inositol trisphosphate, IP_3 – see next chapter). The subsequent lower but sustained level of Ca^{2+} is due to influx of extracellular Ca^{2+} via non-specific cation channels. Gap formation in response to histamine can be reduced by the H_1-receptor antagonist mepyramine and by the β-adrenergic agonists isoprenaline and terbutaline.

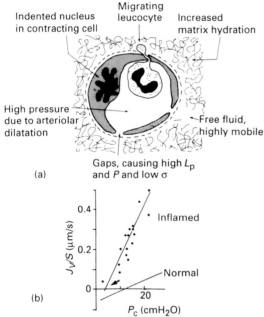

Indented nucleus in contracting cell Migrating leucocyte Increased matrix hydration

High pressure due to arteriolar dilatation

Free fluid, highly mobile

(a) Gaps, causing high L_p and P and low σ

(b) J_V/S (μm/s) 0.4 0.2 0 Inflamed Normal 20 P_c (cmH₂O)

Figure 10.23 (a) Structural and functional changes during acute inflammation. P, permeability to protein (b) Filtration rate per unit surface area of frog mesenteric capillaries, injured by mercuric chloride or alcohol, studied by the red cell method. The perfusate was the frog's own plasma (COP approximately 13 cmH₂O). The 7-fold increase in slope shows that hydraulic conductance (L_p) increases in inflammation. The fall in intercept to 3 cmH₂O (arrow) shows that the effective osmotic gradient across the capillary wall ($\sigma\Delta\pi$) is reduced by inflammation. (After the classic paper of Eugene M. Landis (1927) *American Journal of Physiology*, **82**, 217–238)

The *inflammatory swelling* which ensues is caused partly by the gap formation and partly by changes in net filtration pressure. Capillary pressure rises due to arteriolar vasodilatation and a consequent fall in R_A/R_V. The hydraulic conductance of the wall increases many times, as can be seen from the increased slope in Figure 10.23. The gaps also raise the permeability to plasma protein: this speeds the movement of immunoglobulins into the tissue but at the same time raises the interstitial concentration of plasma proteins, reducing the gradient of COP that opposes filtration. The gaps also lower the protein reflection coefficient to around 0.4, which further reduces the effective COP across the wall (see Figure 10.23b, arrow). The ensuing capillary filtration rate is very rapid because the fall in the COP gradient is aggravated by the fall in σ, and the rise in net filtration force is further amplified by the rise in L_p (equation 10.3). Eventually the combination of a high filtration fraction and adhering leucocytes can lead to plugging of the capillary lumen by a packed column of red cells, a condition called *microvascular stasis*.

Inflammation is a high-permeability disorder and the oedema fluid has a high protein concentration; it is sometimes called an *'exudate'* by way of contrast with the low protein oedema or 'transudate' of venous hypertension and hypoproteinaemia. Large volumes of exudate can form in the peritoneal, pleural, pericardial and synovial cavities during local inflammatory conditions such as peritonitis, pleurisy, pericarditis and rheumatoid arthritis. These exudates contain relatively high concentrations of fibrinogen, owing to the loss of molecular selectivity at the capillary gaps. Fibrin adhesions can then develop and complicate the disease (e.g. intestinal adhesion after peritonitis).

Ischaemia-reperfusion injury is an interesting condition whereby, after a period of poor perfusion due to vascular obstruction, the restoration of blood flow delivers oxygen which is partly converted into toxic superoxide radicals by xanthine oxidase in metabolically-altered tissue. These radicals damage the endothelium, leading to inflammation and impairment of tissue recovery, e.g. after myocardial infarction. (See Section 12.3 for a fuller account.)

10.12 Summary

Fluid transfer across the capillary wall determines the partitioning of extracellular fluid between plasma and interstitial compartments. It also provides a stream of fluid to transport proteins and antigens through the interstitium and into lymph. The fraction of plasma water filtered per transit (the filtration fraction) is very low in continuous capillaries, 0.20–0.3%, but is higher in fenestrated capillaries, e.g. 20% in glomerular capillaries.

The capillary wall acts as a slightly imperfect semipermeable membrane, across which plasma proteins typically exert 80–90% of their potential osmotic pressure (oncotic pressure); the protein reflection coefficient σ is 0.8–0.9. The rate of filtration across unit area of wall depends on its hydraulic conductance and the net pressure acting across the wall, namely the hydraulic pressure drop (i.e. capillary pressure – interstitial fluid pressure) minus the opposing effective absorption pressure across the wall (i.e. $\sigma \times$ {plasma oncotic pressure – interstitial oncotic pressure}). This is the *Starling principle of fluid exchange*.

Capillary pressure, typically 35–12 mmHg at heart level, lies between arterial pressure and venous pressure, and its value within these confines is actively regulated by arteriolar resistance (strictly, the pre- to postcapillary resistance ratio). In this way extracellular fluid partitioning is brought under central nervous control. Capillary pressure is raised in dependent tissue due to the effect of gravity on arterial and venous pressure, so dependent tissue is especially prone to oedema. *Plasma oncotic pressure* is 21–29 mmHg in man. Albumin is the most osmotically important plasma protein. *Interstitial oncotic pressure* is typically one-third or more that of plasma due to escaped plasma proteins. A rise in filtration rate reduces the concentration of these interstitial plasma proteins. The resulting fall in interstitial oncotic pressure limits the filtration rate. Conversely, when fluid is absorbed by capillaries, interstitial oncotic pressure rises, and this opposes further absorption. *Interstitial fluid pressure* is slightly subatmospheric in skin, subcutis, lung and joints but supra-atmospheric in the kidney, contracting muscle and myocardium, and in oedema. The fluid is of gel-like consistency (i.e. does not flow easily) owing to the presence of interstitial glycosaminoglycans. Like interstitial oncotic pressure, interstitial pressure varies with filtration rate, and the pressure-versus-hydration curve (compliance curve) is nonlinear, being steep at physiological values and flat in the oedematous range.

In many tissues the algebraic *sum of the Starling pressures* favours filtration, even in venous capillaries and postcapillary venules at heart level (skin, lung, relaxed muscle). Fluid absorption can occur, transiently, if capillary pressure is reduced by precapillary vasoconstriction or hypovolaemia. The transience of the absorption in most tissues is due to the rise in interstitial oncotic pressure and fall in interstitial fluid pressure that ensues. In certain tissues, however, capillary absorption can be sustained because the interstitium is 'flushed' by a stream of fluid (interstitial mucosa during water absorption, renal peritubular capillaries, lymph node microcirculation).

The capillary filtrate and escaped plasma proteins are removed, in most tissues, by a *lymphatic system* to produce a steady state. The main lymph vessels have smooth muscle and valves; propulsion is by both active contraction and external compression. Impairment of lymph transport results in lymphoedema. In man, over 4 litres of fluid is thought to enter the afferent lymph vessels per day. Some fluid can be reabsorbed by the microcirculation of lymph nodes, while the rest drains via efferent lymph trunks into neck veins.

Fluid filtration rate is raised in dependent limbs, in exercising muscle and in clinical oedema. There is, typically, a 'safety margin' against oedema of about 15 mmHg due to changes in interstitial oncotic pressure, interstitial fluid pressure and lymph flow as filtration rate increases. Clinical oedema arises when the safety margin is exceeded by a sustained rise in capillary pressure (dependent oedema, cardiac failure, deep venous thrombosis, renal failure) or fall in plasma oncotic pressure (malnutrition, hepatic failure, nephrotic syndrome). Inflammatory oedema results from increased capillary permeability to both water and proteins, which is due to the formation of wide gaps near the cell junctions. These leaks are induced by agonists (e.g. histamine) that raise intracellular free Ca^{2+} in the endothelial cell. There is also white cell margination and emigration through endothelial junctions.

Further reading

Reviews and chapters

Aukland, K. and Reed, R. K. (1993) Interstitial-lymphatic mechanisms in the control of extracellular volume. *Physiological Reviews*, **73**, 1–78

Bevilacqua, M. P. (1993) Endothelium-leucocyte adhesion molecules. *Annual Reviews of Immunology*, **11**, 767–804

Comper, W. C. and Laurent, T. C. (1978) Physiological function of connective tissue polysaccharide. *Physiological Reviews*, **58**, 255–315

Curry, F. E. (1992) Modulation of venular microvessel permeability by calcium influx into endothelial cells. *FASEB*, **6**, 2456–2466

Grega, G. J. (1986) (Chairman) Role of endothelial cells in the regulation of microvascular permeability to molecules (Symposium). *Federation Proceedings*, **45**, 75–109

Levick, J. R. (1987) Flow through interstitium and other fibrous matrices. *Quarterly Journal of Experimental Physiology*, **72**, 409–438

Levick, J. R. (1991) Capillary filtration–absorption balance reconsidered in light of dynamic extravascular factors. *Experimental Physiology*, **76**, 825–857

Michel, C. C. (1984) Fluid movement through capillary walls. In *Handbook of Physiology, Cardiovascular System*, Vol. IV, *Microcirculation*, Part 1, American Physiological Society, Baltimore, pp. 375–409

Olszewski, W. C. (1985) *Peripheral Lymph: Formation and Immune Function*, CRC Press, Florida

Staub, N. C., Hogg, J. C. and Hargens, A. R. (1987) (eds) Interstitial-lymphatic liquid and solute movement. In *Advances in Microcirculation 13*, Karger, Basel

Staub, N. C. and Taylor, A. E. (1984) *Edema*, Raven Press, New York

Research papers

Bates, D. O., Levick, J. R. and Mortimer, P. S. (1994) Starling pressures in the human arm and their alteration in postmastectomy oedema. *Journal of Physiology* **477**, 355–363

Neal, C. R. and Michel, C. C. (1992) Transcellular openings through microvascular walls in acutely inflamed frog mesentery. *Experimental Physiology*, **77**, 917–920

Schnittler, H.-J., Wilke, A., Gress, T., Suttorp, N. and Drenckhahn, D. (1990) Role of action and myosin in the control of paracellular permeability in pig, rat and human vascular endothelium. *Journal of Physiology*, **431**, 379–401

Watson, P. D., Garner, R. P. and Ward, D. S. (1993) Water uptake in stimulated cat skeletal muscle. *American Journal of Physiology*, **264**, R790–R796

Chapter 11
Vascular smooth muscle

The tunica media of a blood vessel contains smooth muscle cells arranged in a helical pattern, and the degree of contraction of the muscle controls vessel radius and blood flow. Our knowledge of vascular smooth muscle (VSM) has expanded enormously in recent years, and it is now possible to discuss the ultrastructure, contractile mechanism and electrical behaviour of the VSM cell rather as we did for the myocyte in Chapter 3.

11.1 Structure of the VSM cell

The VSM cell is spindle-shaped, about 20–60 µm long and 4 µm wide at the nuclear region. It contains thick filaments composed of myosin (diameter 15 nm), surrounded by numerous long thin filaments composed of actin (diameter 6 nm; see Figure 11.1). The actin: myosin ratio is about eight times larger than in striated muscle and this is chiefly due to the great length of the actin filaments in smooth muscle. This feature may explain the very high degree of shortening that smooth muscle cells are capable of. The actin filaments insert not into Z lines but into 'dense bands' on the inner surface of the cell, and into 'dense bodies' in the cytoplasm. These structures are composed of α-actinin, the same substance that forms Z-lines in striated muscle. There are no striations in VSM because the contractile units are not aligned in register. A third kind of filament, the intermediate filament, is also abundant in VSM. It is composed of the proteins filamin, actin, α-actinin and desmin, and may have a structural role.

The VSM cell possesses a system of smooth endoplasmic reticulum which forms about 2% of the cell volume and contains a releasable store of calcium ions. The smooth endoplasmic reticulum approaches to within

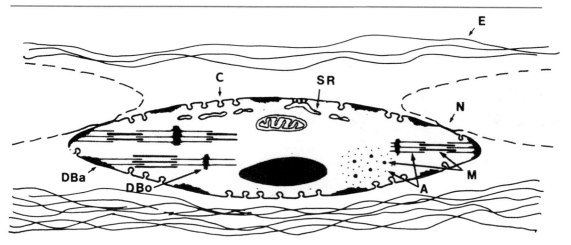

Figure 11.1 Sketch of main elements within a vascular smooth muscle cell. A, actin filaments in longitudinal and transverse view; C, caveola; DBa, DBo, dense band and dense body; E, elastic elements in parallel to cell (collagen and elastin); M, myosin filaments; N, nexus or gap junction, SR, sarcoplasmic reticulum. (After electron micrographs in Gabella, G. (1984) *Physiological Reviews*, **64**, 455–477)

12–20 nm of the cell membrane in places, and is linked to the surface by periodic dark-staining bands which could be involved in excitation–contraction coupling. The cell surface also has numerous tiny invaginations called caveolae, whose function is uncertain. The membranes of adjacent cells are linked by electrically conductive 'gap junctions', which allow depolarization to spread from cell to cell, so the cells form a functional syncytium. The spread is decremental, however, and extends only a millimetre or so along the axis of the vessel.

11.2 Mechanism of contraction

Experiments with calcium-sensitive intracellular indicators show that contraction is initiated by a rise in free Ca^{2+} ions in the cytoplasm, from about 10^{-7} M in the relaxed state to about 6×10^{-7} M in the contracted state. The free calcium derives partly from the sarcoplasmic reticulum store and partly from the extracellular fluid via calcium channels in the cell membrane; this has been proved by electron-probe analysis and electrophysiological methods, respectively. If

extracellular calcium is removed, only a transitory constriction can be elicited, indicating that both internal and external sources of Ca^{2+} are important. The rise in free calcium causes the myosin filaments to form crossbridges with the actin filaments and thereby 'row' themselves into the spaces between the actin filaments, producing shortening and tension. The process in VSM has, however, some important differences from that in myocardium.

1. *Myosin light-chain phosphorylation*. Unlike cardiac or skeletal muscle myosin, VSM myosin can only interact with actin after its light chains have been phosphorylated by ATP. (The light chains are part of the crossbridge head; see Figure 3.3). The phosphorylating enzyme, myosin light-chain kinase, is itself activated by a complex of calcium and calmodulin, calmodulin being a calcium-binding protein closely related to troponin C. Thus a rise in cytoplasmic calcium causes the formation of the calcium–calmodulin complex, which activates myosin light-chain kinase, leading to myosin phosphorylation and crossbridging.

2. The *latch state*. Striated muscle relies on the continuous, rapid making and breaking of crossbridges to maintain tension (crossbridge cycling), and this is an energy-expensive process. VSM, however, can maintain an active tension for just 1/300th of the energy expenditure of striated muscle. This is achieved by the formation of long-lasting crossbridges called 'latch bridges', which cycle only very slowly. It is thought that the latch bridges may be crossbridges that become dephosphorylated yet remain attached.

3. *Sensitivity to cytoplasmic Ca^{2+}*. The sensitivity of the contractile apparatus to Ca^{2+} can be increased or decreased by chemical factors. To be more precise, the sigmoidal relation between contractile force and cytoplasmic $[Ca^{2+}]$ can be shifted to the left (increased sensitivity) or right (decreased sensitivity). Sensitivity is increased by the vasoconstrictor noradrenaline and reduced by the vasodilators isoprenaline (which acts via intracellular cAMP) and hypoxia. This provides another mechanism, supplementary to changes in cytoplasmic $[Ca^{2+}]$, for altering VSM tension.

11.3 Ion channels in VSM

The contractile state of VSM is greatly affected by ion-conducting channels in the cell membrane, because these influence membrane potential and intracellular Ca^{2+} concentration. VSM cells from different blood vessels often differ in the mix of the ion channels present (unfortunately for the non-specialist!), so their electrical behaviour is correspondingly varied.

K^+ channels Resting VSM cells have a negative intracellular potential of -70 to -50 mV. This is due to the resting membrane being more permeable to K^+ ions than any other ion. There is a slight outward flux of K^+ ions through open K^+ channels, driven by the K^+ concentration gradient (Table 11.1), and this leaves behind a net negative charge as described previously for cardiac myocytes (Chapter 3). The high intracellular concentration of K^+ is maintained by an active $3Na^+ - 2K^+$–ATPase pump in the surface membrane (Figure 11.2). Blockage of the electrogenic $3Na^+ - 2K^+$ exchanger by ouabain shows that it contributes at most 11 mV to the resting potential.

There are many subtypes of K^+ channel and the chief ones are listed in Table 11.2, with a brief summary of their key properties and role. It is not necessary for the first-year medical student to know all of these, but two that merit special mention are the calcium-activated K^+ channel (K_{Ca}) and the ATP-dependent K^+ channel (K_{ATP}). The former, K_{Ca} *channels*, are often abundant, and their conductance is increased by a rise in cytoplasmic Ca^{2+} concentration. Their hyperpolarizing effect appears to prevent many VSM cells from generating an action potential, which depends on an inward Ca^{2+} current in VSM cells. Action potentials can often be generated by such cells if the K_{Ca} channels are blocked pharmacologically. K_{ATP} *channels* open when intracellular ATP level falls and ADP and H^+ concentrations rise, as in hypoxic tissue. Their hyperpolarizing effect contributes to ischaemic dilatation in many small vessels (Section 11.7).

Chloride channels Activation of α-adrenoceptors by noradrenaline produces, in some cells, a small depolarization called an excitatory junction potential (EJP, Figure 11.3). If the EJP is large enough it then triggers an action potential, provided that the cell has abundant voltage-operated calcium channels (see below) and not too high a density of K_{Ca} channels. The EJP is due partly to opening of chloride channels. Since the chloride equilibrium potential is about -20 mV (Table 11.1) and the resting membrane potential is about -70 mV, an increase in chloride conductance results in chloride ions leaving the cell, depolarizing it. The chloride channel is not activated directly by the receptor but indirectly via a

Table 11.1 Ionic composition of vascular smooth muscle

Ion	Intracellular (mM)	Extracellular (mM)	Nernst equilibrium potential § (mV)
K⁺	165	5	−89
Na⁺	9	137	+69
Ca²⁺	0.000 1†	1.2‡	+124
pH	7.06	7.40	−20
*Cl⁻	54	134	−23
HCO₃⁻	7.3	15.5	−19

* Chloride ion concentration is unusually high in VSM
† Relaxed state
‡ Plasma calcium is ~2.5 mM but only 1.2 mM is in the ionic form
§ See Chapter 3

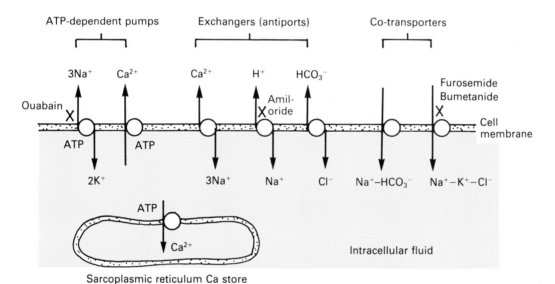

Figure 11.2 Ion pumps and exchangers in surface membrane and sarcoplasmic reticulum of vascular smooth muscle cell. Na^+–HCO_3^- co-transport into cell and Na^+–H^+ exchange help combat intracellular acidosis during sustained contraction. The HCO_3^-–Cl^- exchanger presumably accounts for the unusually high Cl^- concentration in vascular smooth muscle

rise in intracellular Ca^{2+}. The latter probably results from the adrenoceptor–G_s–IP_3–calcium store sequence described in Section 11.5. A further current contributing to the excitatory junction potential is a current of cations through a *non-selective cation channel*.

Voltage-operated channels for Ca^{2+} (VOCs)
The smaller arteries and arterioles are well endowed with channels that conduct divalent cations like Ca^{2+} and Ba^{2+}, and whose probability of opening is greatly increased by depolarization ('voltage-operated' channels). There is a large gradient into the

cell for Ca^{2+} (Table 11.1) so when depolarization causes opening of these channels, extracellular Ca^{2+} enters the cell, leading to contraction. This way of initiating contraction, via depolarization, is called *electromechanical coupling*. Even at resting membrane potential, many of these channels have a finite open-state probability and so allow a small current of Ca^{2+} into the cell, which influences the basal tension in the cell (basal tone). As a result, even small changes in resting membrane potential influence active tension; action potentials are not vital to change the contractile state (in contrast to cardiac and skeletal muscle). For example, if an external stimulus hyperpolarizes the cell (e.g. hypoxia), fewer VOCs open, Ca^{2+} influx falls and the cell relaxes (vasodilatation).

There are various subtypes of VOC-Ca^{2+} channel (Table 11.2). The predominant type in small arteries/arterioles is the L-type channel, which is important for generating action potentials. The L-type channel, and with it the VSM action potential, is blocked by dihydropyridines (calcium channel blockers such as nifedipine). Long-term calcium balance is maintained by Ca^{2+}–ATPase pumps located in the cell membrane (Figure 11.2; cf. mostly Na^+–Ca^{2+} exchange in cardiac cells).

Receptor-operated channels (ROCs) This ion channel is insensitive to voltage but is activated when a chemical agent such as noradrenaline binds to a specific receptor. The open channel is permeable to both Ca^{2+} and Na^+, and entry of the former leads to contraction. This then is an additional, depolarization-independent way by which agents (agonists) such as noradrenaline, vasopressin, angiotensin, 5-hydroxytryptamine and histamine can cause contraction. Since depolarization is not necessary, this is termed *pharmacomechanical coupling*. It is thought that the agonist receptor may be physically connected to the ROC via a special protein called a G protein.

Intracellular Ca^{2+} The concentration of free Ca^{2+} in the cytoplasm represents the balance struck between three processes.

1. Entry of extracellular calcium through VOCs and ROCs.
2. Release of calcium from a store in the sarcoplasmic reticulum (Section 11.5).
3. Removal of cytoplasmic calcium by the Ca^{2+}–ATPase pumps in the cell membrane and sarcoplasmic reticulum.

When the balance tips in favour of a Ca^{2+} rise, tension increases (contraction) and when Ca^{2+} concentration falls, tension decreases (relaxation).

11.4 Neuromuscular excitation

Nearly all arteries and arterioles are innervated by sympathetic vasoconstrictor fibres. The sympathetic fibres run along the adventitial–medial border, and the inner part of the media is not directly innervated, except in veins. The terminal fibres bear a string of swellings (several hundred per fibre) called 'junctional varicosities'– see Figure 12.12. There are up to 6 varicosities per VSM cell at the adventitia–media border. The varicosity lies very close to the VSM cell membrane, the gap being about 75 nm according to serial section reconstructions. Each varicosity contains around 500 small dense-cored vesicles grouped close to the prejunctional membrane, plus a smaller number of large vesicles. The vesicles contain a variable mixture of ATP and noradrenaline. When a sympathetic nerve action potential reaches the varicosity, N-type calcium channels in the varicosity membrane open, leading to a rise in intraneural $[Ca^{2+}]$. This leads to the discharge of a single vesicle into the junctional cleft. Thus neurotransmitter is released as a discrete, uniform-sized packet or quantum (*quantal release*). Recent work indicates that only about 1 in every 100 action potentials actually succeeds, however, in releasing a vesicle. The released neurotransmitter diffuses rapidly across the short neuromuscular cleft and binds to receptors on the VSM cell membrane – see Figure 12.12, next chapter.

Table 11.2 Ion channels present in vascular smooth muscle membrane

Channel	Properties	Role
Potassium		
Inward rectifying	Conductance present at resting potential but reduced on depolarization	Supplies outward current for resting potential
Calcium-activated (K_{Ca})	Open state promoted by Ca_i^{2+} and depolarization. Large conductance and often strongly expressed. Blocked by tetraethyl ammonium (TEA)	Contributes repolarizing outward current after action potential. Can suppress a.p. if abundant
Delayed rectifying	Opens slowly on depolarization ($-30\,mV$) but not calcium dependent. Outward rectifying. Blocked by 4-aminopyridine (4-AP)	Contributes repolarization current after action potential
ATP-dependent (K_{ATP})	Closed by normal [ATP] (5–10 mM). Opens at low ATP coupled with raised ADP and [H^+]. Blocked by glibenclamide. Activated by cromakalim and pinacidil	Probably links vascular tone to metabolic state of tissue
Calcium-conducting		
Voltage-operated (VOC)	L-type is high threshold, long-opening. Abundant in small arteries. Blocked by dihydropyridines	Inward current for action potential. Also modulates resting potential.
	T-type is low threshold, transient-opening	Slight modulation of resting potential.
Receptor-operated (ROC)	Permeable to Na^+ too. Activated by agonists such as NAd	Mediates pharmacomechanical coupling for NAd, angiotensin, vasopressin, 5HT, histamine
Chloride		
Calcium-activated (Cl_{Ca})	Open state promoted by Ca_i^{2+} ($> 0.2\,\mu M$). Latter is raised by noradrenaline	Contributes 'inward' current for EJP (actually an outward current of negative ions)
Other channels		
Non-selective cation channel	Open state promoted by NAd and ATP (may be same as ROC)	Contributes 'inward' current for initial depolarizing effect of NAd and ATP
Stretch-sensitive cation channels	Activated by physical stretch Non-specific cation permeability	May contribute to contractile response of smooth muscle to stretch

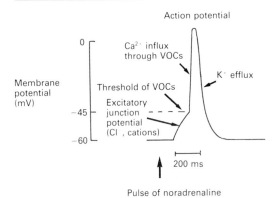

Figure 11.3 Response of a spike-forming vascular smooth muscle cell to application of a brief pulse of noradrenaline from a micropipette. The more complex response to sympathetic nerve stimulation is shown in Figure 11.4. VOC, voltage-operated channel permeable to Ca^{2+} (Courtesy of Dr. W. Large, Dept of Pharmacology, St. George's Hospital Medical School, London)

To understand the effect of the released neurotransmitters, let us first consider the relatively simple case of a VSM cell responding to a brief pulse of noradrenaline alone (no ATP) applied close to the cell via a micropipette. The response of a spike-forming VSM cell is illustrated in Figure 11.3. Activation of post-junctional α-adrenoceptors leads, after some delay, to a sluggish depolarization, the *excitatory junction potential (EJP)*, which is due to an inward current. The 'inward' current is actually composed partly of cations passing into the cell through non-selective cation channels, and partly of Cl^- ions leaving the cell through activated chloride channels. When the EJP reaches a certain threshold depolarization, the increased frequency of opening of voltage-operated calcium channels becomes so great as to produce a positive feedback and trigger an *action potential*. The action potential is a simple spike depolarization of rather variable amplitude and duration, usually 10–100 ms. It is due to an inward current of Ca^{2+} ions from the extracellular fluid through the VOCs. A twitch-like contrac-

tion follows as cytoplasmic $[Ca^{2+}]$ rises. The rise in $[Ca^{2+}]$ is due partly to the Ca^{2+} current of the action potential and partly to Ca^{2+} release from the internal store.

Let us next consider the more complicated response to stimulation of a real sympathetic nerve. Figure 11.4 shows electrical and mechanical responses to *nerve* stimulation that are typical of many small arterial vessels. When the perivascular sympathetic fibres are stimulated briefly and at low intensity, an electrical response with two components is evoked, in contrast to the single component evoked by applying

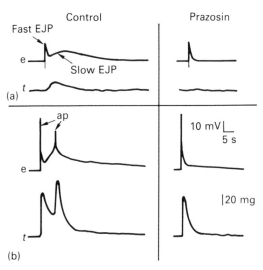

Figure 11.4 Simultaneous records of membrane potential recorded by an intracellular microelectrode (*e*) and tension (*t*) in a rat tail artery. The perivascular nerves were stimulated by a single external pulse in each frame, in the absence (left) or presence (right) of the α-adrenoceptor blocker, prazosin. (a) Medium intensity stimulation produced a fast excitatory junction potential (EJP) and a slower one. Only the latter was blocked by prazosin. Note that contraction precedes the slow EJP. (b) Higher intensity of stimulation evoked larger EJPs, each of which triggered an action potential (ap) and associated twitch contraction. (From Cheung, D. W. (1984) *Pfluger's Archiv*, **400**, 335–337, by permission)

noradrenaline (Figure 11.3). There is a rapid, small depolarization (10 mV, 1 s) followed by a slower, longer-lasting one. Both are excitatory junction potentials (not action potentials). The initial *fast EJP* is not blocked by α-adrenoceptor antagonists such as prazosin, and is due to ATP co-released with noradrenaline from the sympathetic varicosity (see next chapter, Figure 12.13). ATP binds to P_{2X} purinergic receptors to activate non-selective cation channels. The later *slow EJP* is due to noradrenaline, being blocked by prazosin, and is due to both chloride current (outward) and cation current (inward) as described earlier.

The mechanical response, a slow contraction, begins before the slow depolarization and peaks earlier. Although this contraction is blocked by α-adrenoceptor antagonists, it is clear from the time sequence that the contraction is not caused by the slow depolarization; nor is it caused by the fast EJP since the latter is unaffected by α-adrenoceptor antagonists whereas the contraction is. The electrical events are thus *not* the cause of slow contraction: the slow contraction is in fact an example of the *pharmacomechanical coupling* referred to earlier.

If the stimulus strength is increased, the fast EJP becomes larger, reaches the threshold of the voltage-gated calcium channels and triggers an action potential: this elicits a short-latency brief contraction, i.e. twitch (Figure 11.4b). The slow depolarization becomes larger too and triggers another action potential: this produces a second twitch superimposed on the underlying slow contraction. The twitches are examples of *electromechanical coupling*, while the underlying slow contraction reflects pharmacomechanical coupling.

It must be stressed that the response to sympathetic stimulation varies greatly from vessel to vessel, and not all vessels respond as above, although the pattern is a common one. In some vessels, such as the pulmonary artery, slow depolarization and contraction can be elicited without action potentials ever developing (Figure 11.5c).

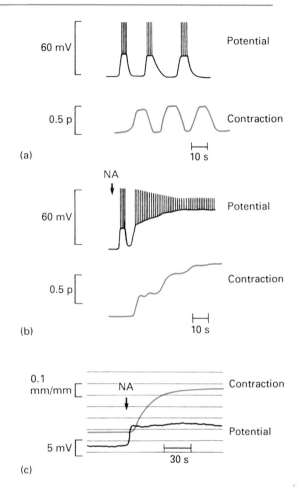

(a)

(b)

(c)

Figure 11.5 Varying characteristics of vascular smooth muscle. (a) Upper trace shows membrane potential in a spontaneously active vessel *in vitro* (guinea pig portal vein), illustrating automaticity. Regular spontaneous slow depolarizations trigger bursts of action potentials, followed after some delay by contraction (lower trace; p is tension). (b) Response of same preparation to addition of noradrenaline (NA, 10^{-6} g/ml) illustrating electromechanical coupling. (c) By contrast, response of sheep carotid artery to superfused noradrenaline demonstrates pharamacomechanical coupling. There is only a small depolarization and no action potentials, yet a sustained contraction occurs. ((a) and (b) From Golenhofen, Hermstein and Lammel (1973) *Microvascular Research*, **5**, 73–80. (c) From Keatinge, W. R. and Harman, C. M. (1980) *Local Mechanisms Controlling Blood Vessels*, Academic Press, London, by permission)

11.5 Pharmacomechanical coupling

Pharmacomechanical coupling is the induction of contraction by a chemical agent (whether released from a local nerve or circulating) without the necessity of a change in membrane potential or the firing of an action potential. Many large vessels, such as the pulmonary artery, do not fire action potentials because they possess relatively few VOC–Ca^{2+} channels, so inward Ca^{2+} current never succeeds in overwhelming the outward K^+ current. In such vessels the superfusion of noradrenaline at a low concentration causes a sustained contraction without any detectable membrane depolarization. Superfusion at higher concentrations or sympathetic nerve stimulation causes a slow sustained depolarization without action potentials (Figure 11.5c). Moreover, even action potential-generating vessels such as the portal vein (Figure 11.5a) can be induced to contract without action potentials if their VOCs are blocked by verapamil. Pharmacomechanical coupling is initiated by activation of the specific receptors in the VSM membrane such as α-receptors. This sets two mechanisms in operation (Figure 11.6), as follows.

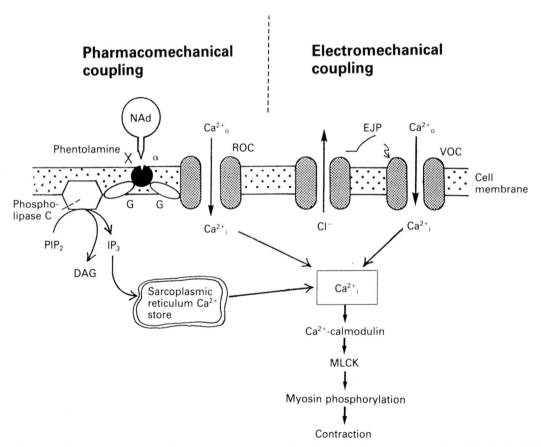

Figure 11.6 Mechanisms underlying vasoconstrictor effect of agonist (here noradrenaline, NAd). G, GTP-binding protein. ROC, receptor-operated cation channel. VOC, voltage-operated calcium channel. EJP, excitatory junction potential. PIP_2, phosphatidyl inositol bisphosphate. IP_3, inositol trisphosphate. DAG, diacylglycerol. MLCK, myosin light chain kinase

One mechanism is the opening of the receptor-operated channels. This allows extracellular calcium ions to flow into the cell and initiate contraction.

The second mechanism involves a chain of biochemical reactions in which a membrane protein called a 'G protein' activates the enzyme phospholipase C. The latter catalyses the breakdown of phosphatidyl inositol bisphosphate (PIP_2) to form an intracellular 'second messenger', inositol trisphosphate (IP_3). This acts on the sarcoplasmic reticulum to induce the release of stored Ca^{2+} (see Appendix II, 'Second messengers'). The other product of PIP_2 breakdown, diacylglycerol, activates a cyptoplasmic enzyme, protein kinase C, which increases the sensitivity of the myofilaments to Ca^{2+}. Because many steps are involved in the G protein–phospholipase–second messenger sequence, there is a delay of 1 s or so between receptor activation and the response.

Contraction in response to noradrenaline thus involves the arrival in the cytoplasm of Ca^{2+} from two sources – the extracellular fluid and the internal store. In keeping with this, it is found that removal of extracellular Ca^{2+} weakens the force of contraction but does not abolish it.

11.6 Automaticity (vasomotion)

In most arteries and veins the VSM cell has a stable resting potential but in some vessels (portal vein, terminal pial arteries and many arterioles) the resting potential is unstable and depolarization occurs spontaneously, triggering action potentials and spontaneous contractions (see Figure 11.5a). The process bears some resemblance to that in SA node cells, though it is less regular. The excitation then spreads from cell to cell via the gap junctions. If most of the VSM cells contract synchronously the vessel undergoes rhythmic variations in calibre, producing the 'vasomotion' often seen in small arterioles. The frequency of the spontaneous discharges

increases up to threefold when an unstable VSM cell is stretched and this probably contributes to the myogenic response described in the next chapter.

11.7 Relaxation (vasodilatation)

Agents that dilate blood vessels do so by reducing the active tension in VSM cells. This can be achieved by three different mechanisms, one involving electromechanical coupling and the other two pharmacomechanical coupling. All three mechanisms reduce cytoplasmic [Ca^{2+}].

Hyperpolarization-mediated vasodilatation
As Figure 11.7 shows, there is a steep relation between the level of the resting membrane

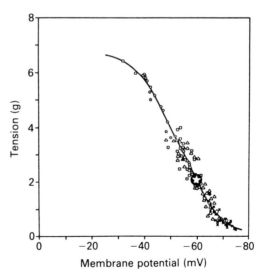

Figure 11.7 Dependency of mechanical tension on the membrane potential in isolated carotid arteries. The membrane potential was changed by varying the extracellular concentration of H^+ ($\triangle$), K^+ ($\square$), Ca^{2+} ($\bullet$), noradrenaline ($\bigcirc$), or prostacyclin ($\diamond$), or by lowering the oxygen tension ($\times$). The star indicates membrane potential and force under control conditions. (After Siegel, G. *et al.* (1991) *Journal of Vascular Medicine and Biology*, **3**, 140–149)

potential and the active force exerted by VSM. Hyperpolarization reduces the probability of the open state for voltage-gated Ca^{2+} channels, leading to a fall in cytoplasmic free Ca^{2+} and relaxation. For example, the dilator drugs *diazoxide, cromakalim* and *pinacidil* activate K^+_{ATP} channels and therefore hyperpolarize the cell, leading to VOC closure, a fall in intracellular Ca^{2+} and vascular relaxation. The important physiological vasodilator factors *hypoxia* and *acidosis* also produce hyperpolarization of the cell (Figure 11.7), as does the sensory nerve neuropeptide *calcitonin-gene related peptide*.

Cyclic AMP-mediated vasodilatation The circulating hormone *adrenaline* causes vasodilatation in certain arterioles with abundant β_2-adrenoceptors, such as those in skeletal muscle (α-adrenoceptor activation by contrast causes vasoconstriction, as described

above). This is because the β_2-adrenoceptor has a different biochemical linkage from the α-adrenoceptor (Figure 11.8). The β_2-adrenoceptor is linked to an intra-membrane G protein, G_s, which activates a membrane-bound enzyme, adenylate cyclase (like the β_1 receptor in the cardiac cell – Chapter 4). Adenylate cyclase catalyses the conversion of ATP to cyclic adenosine monophosphate (cAMP). cAMP causes relaxation chiefly by lowering the free cytoplasmic Ca^{2+} concentration. It probably does this indirectly, via activation of protein kinases that stimulate Ca–ATPase pumps in the surface membrane and sarcoplasmic reticulum, and also inhibit release of stored Ca^{2+}. The vasodilatation induced by activated VIP receptors (*vasoactive intestinal polypeptide*) and *histamine* H_2 receptors likewise operates via G_s–adenylate cyclase–cAMP linkages. VIP also acts partly by activating K^+_{ATP} channels.

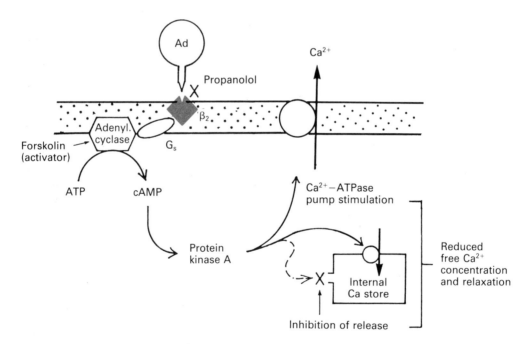

Figure 11.8 Mechanism of β-adrenoceptor mediated vasodilatation. Histamine H_2 receptors and vasoactive intestinal polypeptide receptors likewise activate the cAMP mechanisms. Actions to the right of 'cAMP' in the figure are less clearly understood than those to the left. Forskolin is a drug much used to study cAMP-dependent processes. (After McDaniel, N. L., Rembold, C. M., Richard, H. M. and Murphy, R. A. (1991) *Journal of Physiology*, **439**, 147–160 and Ushio–Fukai, M. *et al.* (1993), see Further Reading)

Cyclic GMP-mediated vasodilatation Another important vasodilator substance, *nitric oxide* (NO, Chapter 12), and NO-releasing vasodilator drugs such as glyceryl trinitrate, act by a third mechanism. NO diffuses into the cytoplasm and there activates the cytoplasmic enzyme guanylate cyclase. This leads to a rise in intracellular cyclic guanosine monophosphate (cGMP), which activates phospholipase G (Fig. 12.5). This probably induces relaxation by phophorylation of other proteins, although the details are unclear. *Atrial natriuretic peptide* operates via the cGMP mechanism too.

As indicated in Section 11.2, there may also be a fourth mechanism, unrelated to changes in $[Ca^{2+}]$, that contributes to vasodilatation in some conditions. This is a reduction in the *sensitivity* of the contractile process to $[Ca^{2+}]$. This may contribute to the vasodilator effect of cAMP and hypoxia.

11.8 Summary

Vascular smooth muscle (VSM) comprises spindle-shaped cells joined by gap junctions that allow limited cell-to-cell spread of electrical excitation. The contractile machinery of VSM comprises interdigitating thin (actin) and thick (myosin) filaments, the former being attached to cytoplasmic dense bodies and to the cell membrane at dense bands. Contraction is initiated by a rise in free intracellular $[Ca^{2+}]$ which, via Ca^{2+}–calmodulin complex, activates myosin light-chain kinase. The latter catalyses phosphorylation of myosin heads by ATP, and this causes myosin–actin crossbridge formation and development of tension. Long-lasting crossbridges allow tension to be maintained with low energy expenditure (the latch state).

Numerous classes of ion channel occur in the VSM cell membrane. *K^+ channels* allow an outward K^+ current that is largely responsible for the negative resting potential and for hyperpolarization-mediated vasodilatation. *Voltage-operated Ca^{2+} channels* (VOCs) open during depolarization, allowing entry of extracellular Ca^{2+} and hence contraction (*electromechanical coupling*). In some but not all vessels, VOCs are sufficiently abundant to generate action potentials. *Receptor-operated cation channels* (ROCs) open when an agonist binds to a receptor that is linked via a G-protein to the channels (e.g. α-adrenoceptors). Entry of extracellular Ca^{2+} through these non-specific cation channels leads to tension development without the necessity of depolarization or action potentials (*pharmacomechanical coupling*). A third mechanism for initiating contraction is the release of Ca^{2+} from an *internal* store in the sarcoplasmic reticulum. This happens when an agonist activates receptors (e.g. histamine H_1 receptors) that are linked via a G-protein to phospholipase C. This leads to formation of the store-releasing compound, IP_3.

Free cytoplasmsic $[Ca^{2+}]$ and tension are determined by the balance between, on the one hand, the state of membrane depolarization (opening VOCs) and agonist–receptor complex density (opening ROCs and releasing internal Ca^{2+} stores) and, on the other, membrane pumps that return Ca^{2+} to the calcium store and extracellular fluid.

Vasoconstriction in the intact animal arises from either sympathetic nerve activity or vasoconstrictor agonist secretion. *Sympathetic terminals* release both noradrenaline and ATP. The noradrenaline produces a slow rise in tension by pharmacomechanical coupling. In some but not all vessels there is also an electrical response; the neurotransmitters activate *Cl^- channels* and *non-selective cation channels* in the VSM cell membrane to produce small depolarizations (*excitatory junction potentials*). If the excitatory junction potential is large enough, sufficient VOCs may open to produce a Ca^{2+} *action potential* and contractile twitch (electromechanical coupling), superimposed on the slow tension rise due to pharmacomechanical coupling. In some arterioles, action potentials arise spontaneously (i.e. without neural drive), leading to rhythmic contractions (*vasomotion*).

Vasodilatation (reduction of active tension) can be induced via at least three distinct mechanisms. (1) *Hyperpolarization*. This reduces the open probability of VOCs, which reduces intracellular Ca^{2+} and so produces relaxation. An important source of hyperpolarization is activation of K_{ATP} channels. These are activated by hypoxia, CGRP and the channel-activating drugs cromakalim and pinacidil. (2) *Cyclic AMP mechanism*. Activation of β-adrenoceptors, histamine H_2 receptors or VIP receptors activates G_s protein, which leads via adenylate cyclase stimulation to production of the second messenger cAMP from ATP. cAMP stimulates Ca^{2+}–ATPase pumps in the cell membrane and sarcoplasmic reticulum membrane to reduce free cytoplasmic $[Ca^{2+}]$, and hence reduce tension. (3) *Cyclic GMP mechanism*. Nitric oxide and atrial natriuretic peptide activate cytoplasmic guanylate cyclase, leading to a rise in cGMP and activation of phospholipase G. This produces relaxation by mechanisms as yet unclear.

Further reading

Reviews and chapters

Bolton, T. B. and Large, W. A. (1986) Are junction potentials essential? Dual mechanism of smooth muscle activation by transmitter release from autonomic nerves. *Quarterly Journal of Experimental Physiology*, **71**, 1–28

Brock, J. A. and Cunnane, T. C. (1993) Neurotransmitter release mechanisms at the sympathetic neuroeffector junction. *Experimental Physiology*, **78**, 591–614

Hirst, G. D. S. and Edwards, F. R. (1989) Sympathetic neuroeffector transmission in arteries and arterioles. *Physiological Reviews*, **69**, 546–604

Khalil, R. A. and Morgan, K. G. (1992) Protein kinase C: a second excitation–contraction coupling pathway in vascular smooth muscle? *News in Physiological Sciences*, **7**, 10–15

Minneman, K. P. (1988) α-Adrenergic receptor subtypes, inositol phosphates and sources of cell Ca^{2+}. *Pharmacological Reviews*, **40**, 87–119

Mulvaney, M. J. and Aalkjaer, C. (1990) Structure and function of small arteries. *Physiological Reviews*, **70**, 922–961

Murphy, R. A. (ed.) (1989) Contraction in smooth muscle cells. *Annual Review of Physiology*, **51**, 275–331

Somlyo, A. P. (1985) Excitation-contraction coupling and the ultrastructure of smooth muscle. *Circulation Research*, **57**, 497–507

Standen, N. B. (1992) Potassium channels, metabolism and muscle. *Experimental Physiology*, **77**, 1–25

Stjärne, L., Bao, J. X., Gonon, F. G., Msghina, M. and Stjärne, E. (1993) A nonstochastic string model of sympathetic neuromuscular transmission. *News in Physiological Sciences*, **8**, 253–260

Research papers

Amédée, T., Benham, C. D., Bolton, T. B., Byrne, N. G. and Large, W. A. (1990) Potassium, chloride and non-selective cation conductances opened by noradrenaline in rabbit ear artery cells. *Journal of Physiology*, **423**, 551–568

Draeger, A., Amos, W. B., Ikebe, M. and Small, J. V. (1990) The cytoskeletal and contractile apparatus of smooth muscle: contraction bands and segmentation of the contractile elements. *Journal of Cell Biology*, **111**, 2463–2473

Smirnov, S. V. and Aaronson, P. I. (1992) Ca^{2+} currents in single myocytes from human mesenteric arteries: evidence for a physiological role of L-type channels. *Journal of Physiology*, **457**, 455–475

Ushio-Fukai, M., Abe, S., Kobayashi, S., Nishimura, J. and Kanaide, H. (1993) Effects of isoprenaline on cytosolic calcium concentrations and on tension in the porcine coronary artery (action of cAMP). *Journal of Physiology*, **462**, 679–696

Chapter 12
Control of blood vessels

12.1 Overview of vascular control

The tunica media of blood vessels contains smooth muscle cells arranged in a predominantly circumferential pattern. The active tension of these cells controls the radius of the vessel. Vasoconstriction is brought about by contraction of the smooth muscle cells. Vasodilatation, by contrast, is a passive, not active process, being powered by blood pressure as vascular smooth muscle relaxes.

What does vessel radius control?

The *arterioles* and terminal arteries are the chief resistance vessels of the systemic circulation and even quite small changes in their radius cause large changes in vascular resistance, owing to the fourth-power term in Poiseuille's law (Section 8.5). This has the following effects. (1) Local arteriolar resistance regulates *blood flow* to the tissue downstream of the arteriole. The range of flows that can be produced is enormous in some organs, as shown in Figure 12.1. As a general rule the flow is varied to match the metabolic activity of the tissue. (2) The total arteriolar resistance, acting in concert with the cardiac output, regulates *arterial blood pressure*. (3) *Capillary recruitment* and capillary *filtration pressure* are both regulated by local arteriolar tone, as shown in Figures 9.16 and 10.4, respectively. Thus, arteriolar radius exerts both local effects (control of nutritive supply

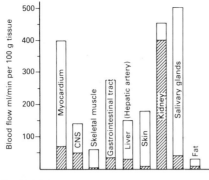

Homo
Rest. blood flow (l/min): 0.21 0.75 0.75 0.7 0.5 0.2 1.2 0.02 0.8 =5.1
Max. blood flow (lmin): 1.2 2.1 18.0 5.5 3.0 3.8 1.4 0.25 3.0 =38
Organ weight (kg): 0.3 1.5 30.0 2.0 1.7 2.1 0.3 0.05 10 =48

Figure 12.1 Range of flows between rest (▨) and maximal function (▢) in the various organs of a 70 kg man. Maximal flow through all organs at the same time is impossible because the total flow would be 38 litres/min, which exceeds the output capacity of the heart. (From Mellander, S. and Johansson, B. (1968) *Pharmacological Reviews*, **20**, 117–196, by permission)

and organ fluid balance) and central effects (homeostasis of blood pressure and plasma volume).

The *veins and venules* normally contain around 60% of the blood volume, and a decrease in the average radius of the peripheral veins and venules can displace a considerable volume of blood into the central veins. Venous smooth muscle can thus influence the *cardiac filling pressure*, and hence stroke volume.

Basal tone and its regulation

The active tension exerted by vascular smooth muscle (VSM) in a segment of wall is called vessel 'tone'. The arterioles and some larger arteries retain a degree of tone (i.e. remain partially contracted) even when their sympathetic innervation is interrupted, and this is called the basal tone. *A high basal tone is vital if a vessel is to be capable of substantial dilatation* because dilatation is simply a reduction in tone: the greater the basal tone the greater the potential ability to

vasodilate. Tissues capable of producing large increases in blood flow, such as skeletal muscle and the salivary gland (Figure 12.1), have a high basal tone. By contrast, basal tone is slight in most veins. Regarding mechanisms, basal tone is the result of a continuous interplay between vasoconstrictor influences that tend to depolarize the cells and open their Ca^{2+} channels, and vasodilator influences such as tonic secretion of nitric oxide by endothelial cells (see later).

The tone of a vessel *in vivo* is actively controlled by numerous factors. These fall into two broad categories: intrinsic control mechanisms and extrinsic control mechanisms (Figure 12.2). *Intrinsic control mechanisms* are local processes located entirely within the organ. They include physical factors (temperature, pressure), the myogenic response, tissue metabolites, locally secreted vasoactive chemicals called autacoids and endothelial secretions such as nitric oxide. The *extrinsic control mechanisms* are the autonomic nerves and circulating endocrine secretions.

12.2 Local control

Local temperature

This is chiefly important in the skin. High ambient temperatures cause cutaneous arterioles and veins to dilate, producing the familiar reddening of a limb immersed in hot water. Conversely, skin temperatures down to 10–15°C cause vasoconstriction which conserves heat and safeguards core temperature. The vasoconstrictor response of skin vessels to cold contrasts with the behaviour of most other tissues, where vessels relax in response to cold. This appears to be related to the relative abundance of α_2-type adrenoceptors in skin vessels, in contrast to α_1 in other tissues. The affinity of α_2-adrenoceptors for noradrenaline, the sympathetic vasoconstrictor neurotransmitter, increases as temperature falls towards 10°C. In support of this explanation, it is found that blockers of α_2-adrenoceptors such as

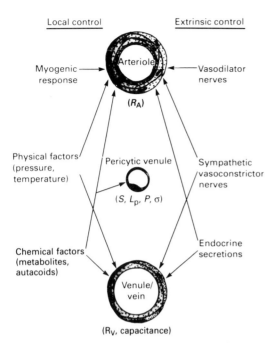

Figure 12.2 Scheme for control of the peripheral vessels. R_A, R_V, pre- and postcapillary resistances respectively; S, perfused area of capillary bed, influenced by metabolites; L_p, P and σ are the microvascular permeability parameters (see Chapter 9) which are altered by the mediators of inflammation

yohimbine and rauwolscine inhibit the cutaneous vasoconstrictor response to cold.

Cooling skin below approximately 12°C, by contrast, leads to paradoxical cold vaso-dilatation (see Chapter 13), which is caused by the impairment of neurotransmitter release and by the release of vasodilator substances like prostaglandins (see later) from the tissue.

Transmural pressure and the myogenic response

A high *external pressure* compresses the vessels and impairs blood flow, as in skeletal muscle and myocardium during their contraction phase (see Figure 12.9,

later). Similarly, flow through the skin is impaired by compression during sitting, kneeling, lying, etc., and should a patient be bedridden by age or paralysis, the prolonged impairment of skin nutrition can result in large ulcerating bed sores over the buttocks and heels.

The immediate mechanical effect of raising *internal pressure* is to distend the vessel slightly and reduce its resistance but most systemic arterioles and some arteries (e.g. cerebral arteries) then react to the distension by contracting, as in Figure 12.3. This is called the *myogenic response*, and was first described by Sir William Bayliss, brother-in-law of Ernest Starling, in 1902. The myogenic response stabilizes blood flow and capillary filtration pressure in the face of changes in blood pressure (see 'Autoregulation', Section 12.3), and also contributes to basal tone.

The immediate cause of the myogenic response in spike-generating vessels, like

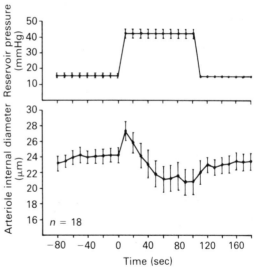

Figure 12.3 Change in arteriolar diameter upon raising the luminal pressure in cat mesentery. The initial diameter increase is due to passive distension. The active myogenic response at about 10 s then reduces the diameter to less than its original value. (From Johnson, P. C. and Intalietta, M. (1976) *American Journal of Physiology*, **231**, 1686–1698, by permission)

the arterioles and portal-mesenteric vein, is that stretch increases the frequency of the spontaneous action potentials resulting in increased active tension. In non-spike-forming arteries, stretch evokes a maintained depolarization that increases the open probability for the VOC–Ca^{2+} channels.

The nature of the stretch sensor is a more difficult issue because the myogenic response is sometimes so strong that vessel radius is actually reduced, as shown in Figure 12.3, i.e. the VSM cell is no longer stretched overall. This has led to the suggestion that a region of VSM membrane in series with the contractile proteins (possibly at the dense bands) might be sensitive to local stress; VSM stress, unlike vessel radius, is increased during the myogenic response (see Figure 8.12). Such a region might initiate depolarization. It is relevant to note that stress-activated calcium-conducting channels have been identified recently in some arterial VSM cells, and these might contribute to the myogenic response. Another possibility is that arterial endothelium may release vasoconstrictor substances in response to mechanical stress (see later). Endothelial stripping abolishes the myogenic response of some large arteries like the basilar and cerebral arteries, but not in most small arteries.

Local metabolites

Many of the chemical by-products of metabolism cause vascular relaxation, so any increase in tissue metabolic rate causes arteriolar dilatation and an automatic increase in local tissue perfusion. This process is called *metabolic vasodilatation* or *functional hyperaemia* and can be seen in Figures 12.8, 12.9 and 13.10. The increase in blood flow is almost linearly proportion to metabolic rate in tissues such as exercising muscle, myocardium and brain. The vasodilator influences include local *hypoxia*; *acidosis* due to the release of carbon dioxide and lactic acid; *breakdown products of ATP*, namely adenosine and inorganic phosphate; *potassium ions* released by contracting muscle or, in the

brain, by active neurons; and a rise in *interstitial osmolarity* due to the release of lactate, K^+ and other small solutes. The relative importance of each factor varies from organ to organ: cerebral vessels for example are particularly sensitive to H^+ and K^+ ions, while coronary resistance vessels are influenced chiefly by hypoxia and/or adenosine.

The mechanisms of action of the vasodilator metabolites are varied and are summarized briefly below. The three basic mechanisms for VSM relaxation (hyperpolarization–Ca^{2+} channel closure, cAMP rise, cGMP rise) were described in Section 11.7.

Local hypoxia Hypoxic *vasodilatation* of arterioles is mediated in some vessels by hyperpolarization, caused by activation of K_{ATP} channels as cell ATP falls and ADP and intracellular {H^+} rise. Adenosine receptor activation also contributes to the K_{ATP} channel activation (see below). In some cases, endothelial secretion of the vasodilator substances nitric oxide and prostacyclin also contributes to hypoxic vasodilatation.

In some *large arteries* such as large coronary arteries, severe hypoxia by contrast causes *vasospasm* which can endanger myocardial function. This seems to be due partly to endothelial secretion of an unidentified vasoconstrictor substance, partly to release of noradrenaline from hypoxic sympathetic nerve terminals and partly to local release of a vasoconstrictor autacoid, PAF (next section).

Adenosine, which is released by hypoxic muscle, acts by several mechanisms. (1) Activation of the purinergic P_1 receptors on vascular smooth muscle stimulates the cAMP pathway leading to relaxation. (2) P_1 receptors are coupled to K_{ATP} channels, leading to hyperpolarization-mediated relaxation. (3) In addition, adenosine acts on sympathetic terminal varicosities to inhibit noradrenaline release (see Figure 12.12). Methylxanthines such as phenyltheophylline block the P_1 receptors and have been used to assess the contribution of adenosine to metabolic vasodilatation. Such work indicates that hypoxia-induced vasodilatation in some tissues, for example skeletal muscle, is partly due to release of adenosine following degradation of ATP.

Carbon dioxide, lactate and local acidosis Acidosis causes hyperpolarization due to increased potassium permeability (see Figure 11.7), which then reduces the open probability for voltage-operated Ca^{2+} channels. Also, in the case of CO_2 much of the vasodilatation, at least in some tissues (brain, mesentery), is endothelium-dependent; hypercapnia is thought to increase the rate of production of the vasodilator NO by endothelial cells (see later).

Extracellular [K^+] This can reach 9 mM in the interstitium of contracting muscle, and 7–8 mM in arterial blood (normal value 4 mM). A small, physiological rise in concentration, to between 5 and 10 mM, causes vasodilatation whereas a large, pharmacological rise (to >20 mM) causes vasoconstriction. The latter is easily understood; the fall in transcellular K^+ gradient lowers the resting membrane potential, i.e. depolarizes it (see Nernst equation, Section 3.1), leading to contraction. The vasodilator effect of small rises in extracellular K^+ *in vivo* is more complex and there is evidence for three mechanisms: (a) stimulation of the electrogenic Na–K exchange pump leading to membrane hyperpolarization, (b) increasing permeability of the VSM membrane to K^+, so that the membrane potential moves closer to the Nernst equilibrium potential for K^+, i.e. hyperpolarization, and (c) release of an endothelium-derived relaxing factor (see later).

Autacoids

Autacoids are vasoactive chemicals that are produced locally, released locally and act locally, unlike endocrine secretions. They include histamine, bradykinin, 5-hydroxy-tryptamine, the prostaglandins, thromboxane, leukotrienes and PAF (platelet activating factor). Autacoids are in effect 'local hormones' and they are involved in local responses such as inflammation and haemostasis.

Histamine This is produced from the amino acid histidine by decarboxylation, and is found in granules within mast cells and basophils. Histamine is one of the chemical mediators of inflammation, being released in response to trauma and certain allergic reactions (urticaria, anaphylaxis, asthma). Histamine dilates arterioles, constricts veins and increases venular permeability. These differences in action depend upon whether the target vessel bears H_1 or H_2 histamine receptors. H_1 receptors activate the phospholipase C – IP_3 pathway (see Figure 11.6) leading to vasoconstriction and venular permeability increases. H_2 receptors activate the adenylate-cyclase–cAMP pathway, leading to vascular relaxation.

Bradykinin Exocrine glands like the salivary gland and sweat glands secrete the enzyme kallikrein into their ducts when stimulated by cholinergic nerves. If kallikrein back-diffuses into the interstitium (e.g. following duct obstruction) it acts on an interstitial plasma globulin, kininogen, to produce a decapeptide, kallidin. This is converted by an aminopeptidase into the 9 amino acid peptide, bradykinin. Bradykinin is also generated in inflamed tissue. Bradykinin is strong vasodilator agent and also increases venular permeability. Its vasodilator effect is mediated via endothelial release of nitric oxide (see below). Its inflammatory effect on venular endothelium is mediated via a rise in endothelial Ca^{2+} concentration (Section 10.11).

5-hydroxytryptamine (serotonin, 5-HT) This derivative of the amino acid tryptophan is found in (1) platelets, (2) the intestinal wall and (3) the central nervous system. (1) 5-HT is released from platelets during clotting and its vasoconstrictor effect on large vessels contributes to haemostatis. Vasoconstriction appears to be brought about by activation of receptor-operated cation channels similar to those described earlier for ATP. (2) In the intestinal tract, 5-HT occurs in argentaffin cells and may be involved in the regulation of local blood flow as well as gastrointestinal smooth muscle. The argentaffin cells occasionally form a tumour (carcinoid tumour). This can release large quantities of 5-HT into the circulation, causing attacks of hypertension and diarrhoea. (3) In the brain, 5-HT occurs in neurons close to cerebral vessels; it markedly potentiates the effect of noradrenaline and may be involved in the vasospasm associated with migraine and subarachnoid haemorrhage. Its action on brain vessels is largely via pharmacomechanical coupling (receptor–phospholipase C – IP_3 – release of stored Ca^{2+}). 5-HT is also a central neurotransmitter, and the hallucinogenic drug lysergic acid diethylamide (LSD) is an antagonist of 5-HT.

Prostaglandins These vasoactive agents are synthesized from a fatty acid precursor, arachidonic acid, via the enzyme cyclooxygenase. Prostaglandins are produced by macrophages, leucocytes, fibroblasts and endothelium. The different prostaglandins have different actions; the *F series (PGF)* are mainly vasoconstrictor agents, while the *E series (PGE)* and *prostacyclin (PGI$_2$)* are vasodilator substances (Figure 12.4). The vasodilator prostaglandins contribute to inflammatory vasodilatation and reactive hyperaemia (see later), and their synthesis is inhibited by the anti-inflammatory drugs aspirin and indomethacin. The related arachidonic-acid derivative, *thromboxane A$_2$*, is a powerful vasoconstrictor substance found in platelets; it is involved in platelet aggregation and haemostatis. A general term for all these arachidonic acid derivatives is 'eicosanoid'.

Leukotrienes This group of vasoactive substances is produced from arachidonic acid by a different pathway, involving the enzyme lipoxygenase. They are synthesized by leucocytes and are important mediators of the inflammatory response. They cause vasoconstriction, leucocyte margination and

emigration, and the formation of gaps in the walls of venules. Their gap-inducing action develops at 1000th the concentration at which histamine acts.

Platelet activating factor (PAF) This vasoactive lipid is misnamed in the sense that it exerts many of its major actions on smooth muscle. It is produced by activated inflammatory cells (polymorphs, macrophages) and contributes to the vascular phenomena of inflammation, namely vasodilatation and increased venular permeability. It is particularly important in the airways of asthmatic subjects, where it also causes bronchoconstriction. It may also contribute to coronary artery spasm in hypoxia.

Contrariness of pulmonary vessels The response of pulmonary resistance vessels to chemical factors is often different from the response of systemic vessels. Alveolar hypoxia, for example, causes pulmonary vasoconstriction, not dilatation. This is physiologically important, for it reduces the perfusion of underventilated regions and thereby helps to maintain a normal ventilation–perfusion ratio. If hypoxia is generalized, as at high altitude, pulmonary hypertension results from this response. The pulmonary vascular response to many other agents too is reversed: histamine and bradykinin, for example, cause pulmonary vasoconstriction rather than dilatation.

Endothelium-dependent relaxation and contraction

In 1980, Furchgott and Zawadski discovered that whereas a normal artery ring relaxes in response to carbachol (a stable analogue of acetylcholine) the response changes to contraction when the endothelial lining is rubbed away. The same is true for human hand veins if their endothelial lining is destroyed by local perfusion with distilled water. The explanation is that arterial and venous endothelium can synthesize a dilator substance, *endothelium-derived relaxing factor*

(EDRF), in response to stimulation by acetylcholine and many other agonists (see Figure 12.4). The EDRF diffuses directly from the endothelial lining into the underlying smooth muscle. There it activates an enzyme, guanylyl cyclase, by reacting with the haem group present in this enzyme. This leads to a rise in the intracellular second messenger cyclic guanosine monophosphate (cGMP) and vasodilatation (Figure 12.5).

Stimuli to EDRF production EDRF is not stored. Its formation is stimulated by agonists that activate endothelial cells, namely thrombin, bradykinin, substance P, ADP, acetylcholine and, in certain tissues or species, histamine. The action of other vasodilators is not endothelium-dependent e.g. adenosine, AMP, isoprenaline, papaverine, nitrodilators. Whether parasympathetic cholinergic dilator nerves act via EDRF stimulation seems open to question (Figure 12.16, legend).

An important physiological stimulus to EDRF production is the *shear stress* exerted on the endothelial cell by the flowing blood (Figure 12.5). This underlies a long-known phenomenon, *'flow-induced vasodilatation'* in arteries. When arterioles dilate, increasing blood flow to a tissue, the artery feeding the tissue also dilates, even when it is some distance outside the tissue. For example, reactive hyperaemia in the human forearm is associated with an increase in brachial artery diameter in the upper arm by as much as 50%.

Flow-induced vasodilatation also occurs when fluid is pumped through isolated arteries. It is endothelium-dependent and is due to increased EDRF production with increased shear stress. The physiological importance is that arterial resistance, which otherwise would significantly limit flow after arteriolar dilatation, is reduced, i.e. EDRF serves to 'couple' arterial resistance to arteriolar resistance.

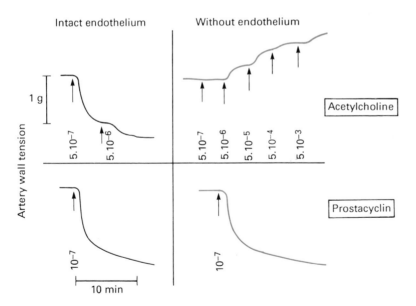

Figure 12.4 Response of canine intrapulmonary arteries *in vitro* to addition of acetycholine and prostacyclin to bathing medium. Artery strips precontracted with 5-hydroxytryptamine, and isometric force recorded. Both agonists produce a potent relaxation when the vessel endothelium is intact. When the endothelium is removed by rubbing, the acetylcholine-induced response changes to contraction. The prostacyclin-induced relaxation, however, is not endothelium-dependent. (From Altura, B. (1988) *Microcirculation Endothelium and Lymphatics*, **4**, 91–110, by permission)

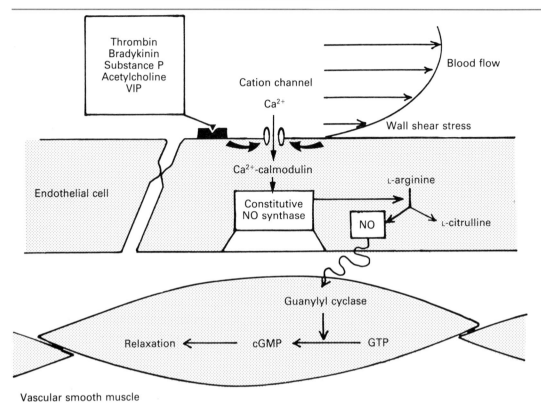

Figure 12.5 Physiological regulation of NO production by endothelial cell

EDRF also inhibits platelet aggregation, so it has an anti-thrombogenic action at the endothelial surface.

Nature and synthesis of EDRF (NO) The half-life of EDRF is only 6 s and along with other clues this led to the discovery that EDRF is an extremely simple, primitive molecule, nitric oxide (NO). NO is produced by cleavage from the amino acid arginine by an endothelial membrane enzyme called *NO synthase*. The activity of this enzyme is regulated by the level of intracellular Ca^{2+}–calmodulin complex, so agents that promote extracellular Ca^{2+} entry into endothelial cells (acetylcholine, etc.) increase the rate of NO synthesis (Figure 12.5). Shear stress is thought to act by opening stress-sensitive cation channels, thereby raising intracellular Ca^{2+} concentration.

NO synthesis can be blocked by various stable analogues of arginine. In intact animals, including man, these blockers produce vasoconstriction (Figure 12.6) and a rise in arterial pressure. From this it is clear that NO production is continuous and exerts a tonic vasodilator influence on the resistance vessels. Thus *vessel tone represents a balance between the opposing effects of NO and vasoconstrictor influences like the myogenic response and sympathetic nerve activity.*

Organic nitrates like glyceryl trinitrate have long been used as vasodilator drugs in the treatment of angina. It is now realized that they act by mimicking EDRF and releasing nitric oxide into the tissue.

Inducible NO synthase and endotoxin shock Endotoxin is a lipopolysaccharide

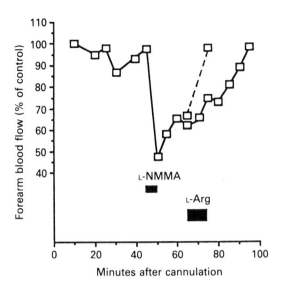

Figure 12.6 Role of NO in regulating vascular resistance in human forearm. N monomethyl-L-arginine (L-NMMA), an inhibitor of nitric oxide production, was infused into the brachial artery while forearm blood flow was measured by venous occlusion plethysmography. The 50% reduction in flow indicated that there is normally a tonic production of the vasodilator NO. Inhibition was reversed by the NO substrate, L-arginine (broken line). (After Vallance, P., Collier, J. and Moncada, S. (1989) *The Lancet*, **ii**, 997–1000)

released by bacteria. Its effect is to produce a severe, intractable hypotension due to vasodilatation ('shock'), which develops over 8 h or so. It was recently discovered that NO synthesis increases greatly over this same period and partly accounts for the hypotension. The NO is produced by newly synthesized NO synthase. The new enzyme is *inducible NO synthase*, which differs from the endogenous or *constitutive* NO synthase in several respects: it is a cytosol enzyme; its activity does not require Ca^{2+}–calmodulin; and it produces NO at a far greater rate than the constitutive endothelial enzyme. It is induced in VSM cells and macrophages as well as endothelium.

Vasoconstrictor products

Endothelium can produce not only dilator substances but also vasoconstrictor compounds. One vasoconstrictor substance appears to be a *prostanoid*, i.e. a product of cyclo-oxygenase; it mediates the contractile response of larger arteries to hypoxia. Another agent discovered recently is a peptide called *endothelin* which causes a strong vasoconstriction lasting 2–3 h. Its physiological role is still unclear. It should be noted that most of the work on endothelium-derived substances has been carried out on large vessel endothelium, and we know much less about endothelial-dependent responses in arterioles, which are the vessels controlling blood flow *in vivo*.

12.3 Circulatory adjustments due to local mechanisms

Several major circulatory adjustments are initiated by the above local mechanisms rather than by extrinsic neural control. The most important examples are autoregulation, metabolic hyperaemia and reactive hyperaemia.

Autoregulation

Autoregulation of flow

The relation between perfusion pressure and blood flow through skeletal muscle, myocardium, intestine, kidney or brain is remarkable because, over a certain range, changes in the perfusion pressure have relatively little effect on blood flow in the steady state, seemingly in defiance of Poiseuille's law (Figures 12.7a and 8.15). The relative constancy of tissue perfusion in the face of pressure changes is called autoregulation. Autoregulation is independent of the nervous system; the resistance vessels respond directly to the changes in arterial pressure. A rise in pressure evokes arteriolar vasoconstriction and increased vascular resistance, while a fall in pressure

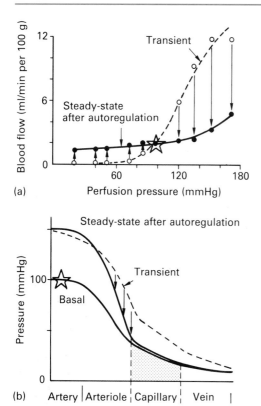

(a)

(b)

Figure 12.7 Autoregulation of blood flow (a) and of capillary pressure (b) in isolated, perfused skeletal muscle. The dashed line in each plot shows the transient flow or pressure immediately after changing perfusion pressure from its control level of 100 mmHg (star). Arteriolar contraction/dilatation (arrows) then adjusts the flow and downstream pressure to a steady-state value (solid curve) that is only slightly different from the control value. ((a) From Jones, R. D. and Berne, R. M. (1964) *Circulation Research*, **14**, 126, by permission)

evokes vasodilatation and reduced resistance. This accounts for the near constancy of the flow. Cerebral blood flow, for example, is well maintained during spinal anaesthesia, despite the concomitant systemic hypotension induced by this procedure. Although autoregulation holds flow almost constant in the steady state, the underlying change in arteriolar radius takes 30–60 s to

develop fully, so there is initially a brief rise in flow with pressure which affords a glimpse of the unregulated pressure–flow relation (Figure 12.7a, dashed line).

Autoregulation of capillary pressure

As well as stabilizing tissue perfusion, autoregulation stabilizes capillary filtration pressure. Capillary pressure depends on the pre- to postcapillary resistance ratio (Section 10.2), and the autoregulatory changes in precapillary resistance protect the capillaries from changes in arterial pressure. In a study in which skeletal muscle was perfused by a pump at various pressures, the pressure in the muscle capillaries changed by only 2 mmHg as the pump pressure was varied between 30 mmHg and 170 mmHg (Figure 12.7b). This autoregulation of capillary pressure assists the homeostasis of plasma and interstitial volumes, and protects the tissue against oedema if arterial pressure rises. Autoregulation of capillary pressure is particularly important in the kidney where it ensures a virtually constant glomerular filtration rate. Autoregulation operates only over a limited range of pressures, however, and cerebral blood flow, renal function, etc., fall off during severe hypotension.

Mechanisms underlying autoregulation

Two mechanisms mediate autoregulation in most organs, namely the myogenic response and vasodilator washout. The *myogenic response* was described in Section 12.2. *'Vasodilator washout'* refers to the effect of blood flow on locally-produced vasodilator substances: if blood flow is increased transiently by a rise in arterial pressure, vasodilator products of tissue metabolism are washed out and their interstitial concentration declines, allowing vessel tone to increase. The relative importance of the myogenic response and vasodilator washout has been estimated by venous congestion. Venous back-pressure stretches the arterioles and should elicit a myogenic constriction; but it also reduces the pressure gradient driving flow, which by temporarily reducing flow and washout of vasodilators should cause vasodilatation. In practice, venous congestion elicits vasoconstriction in the brain, intestine, colon, liver and spleen, indicating a myogenic predominance, while in skin and skeletal muscle the effect is variable, indicating an approximate equipotence of the two mechanisms.

It must be emphasized that while autoregulation is an intrinsic property of most vascular beds (except the lungs), this does not mean that blood flow and capillary pressure are necessarily constant in the intact animal. On the contrary, they are frequently altered by changes in sympathetic drive and changes in local metabolic rate, which reset autoregulation to operate at a new level. This is illustrated in Figure 12.8. Here, increases in

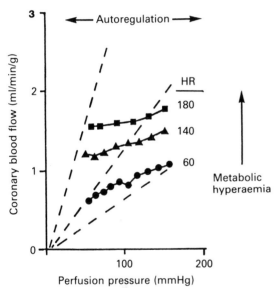

Figure 12.8 Effect of perfusion pressure and metabolic rate on coronary blood flow in dog. Dashed lines are theoretical pressure–flow lines at constant conductance (steepest line, highest conductance). At any given metabolic rate (heart rate, HR), blood flow increases relatively little with pressure and shifts to lower and lower conductance lines (*autoregulation*). At any given perfusion pressure, flow increases with metabolic rate (heart rate); this is *functional or metabolic hyperaemia*. (Data of Laird, in *Cardiac Metabolism*, eds Holland, A. and Noble, M. (1983) Chichester, Wiley, pp. 257–278)

cardiac work (heart rate) are seen to increase myocardial blood flow, yet the pressure–flow relation remains relatively flat, i.e. autoregulation continues at a reset, higher flow.

Metabolic hyperaemia

Blood flow increases almost linearly with metabolic rate in exercising skeletal muscle, myocardium and secreting exocrine glands. The rise in myocardial blood flow with increasing work rates is illustrated in Figure 12.8. This is called metabolic, functional or active hyperaemia. It is caused by a fall in vascular resistance due to the active tissue releasing vasodilator substances, e.g. adenosine, K^+ and H^+ (Section 12.2). As well as acting on the vessel wall, most of these agents inhibit the release of noradrenaline from sympathetic fibres ('neuromodulation', Figure 12.12).

Dilatation of the main conduit artery to the tissue follows dilatation of the resistance vessels due to flow-induced production of EDRF, as described earlier. The feeding arteries dilate too. These are vessels of diameter up to 0.5 mm, located between the conduit artery and the arterioles. Their dilatation involves a phenomenon called 'ascending dilatation', in which the dilatation of the arterioles (caused by vasodilator metabolites) spreads proximally, perhaps due to electrical transmission through the gap junctions between VSM cells. There is thus a *co-ordinated* dilatation of all the elements of the arterial tree to the active tissue.

In *rhythmically* exercising skeletal muscle, mean blood flow is increased but the flow oscillates, decreasing during each contraction as the vessels are compressed (Figure 12.9). Most of the hyperaemia occurs during the resting phases: myoglobin within the muscle fibres provides a small oxygen reserve for the poorly-perfused contraction phase. Figure 12.9 also shows that the hyperaemic response takes a minute or so to develop fully, creating a blood-flow deficit or '*debt*' over

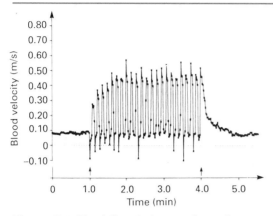

Figure 12.9 Blood flow in human femoral artery during rhythmic quadriceps muscle exercise. Flow was measured by the Doppler ultrasound method. Note the slow build-up to maximum response, creating a nutritional debt; the post-exercise period of hyperaemia repays the nutritional debt. (From Walloe, L. and Wesche, J. (1988) *Journal of Physiology*, **405**, 257–273, by permission)

the first minute. The muscle's store of high-energy creatine phosphate is drawn on during this period, until oxygen supply catches up with demand. When the exercise stops, the hyperaemia takes 2–3 min to die away and this 'post-exercise hyperaemia' repays the metabolic debt.

During *static* exercise, hyperaemia during the active period is less pronounced because the sustained muscle pressure upon the vessels limits their dilatation. Consequently an oxygen debt builds up more rapidly, leading to lactic acidosis and rapid muscle fatigue.

It is worth emphasizing that the sustained vasodilatation in active muscle and myocardium is caused by the locally-produced vasodilator substances and not by vasomotor nerves. It should also be noted that while the increase in blood flow is a local or 'automatic' process, it is not an example of autoregulation, for autoregulation is by definition a relative *constancy* of flow in the face of changes in arterial pressure. The way in which metabolic hyperaemia and true autoregulation can coexist was illustrated in Figure 12.8.

Reactive hyperaemia

If the blood flow to a tissue is stopped for a while by compressing the supplying artery, or is slowed to the point where it is inadequate for tissue nutrition (a state called 'ischaemia'), the blood flow immediately after releasing the compression is much higher than normal, and then decays exponentially (Figure 12.10). This is called reactive hyperaemia or post-ischaemic hyperaemia. It is particularly obvious in the skin, which flushes a bright pink after a period of compression.

The myogenic response probably contributes significantly to the hyperaemia following brief arterial occlusions (<30 s); the arterioles dilate in response to the fall in transmural pressure. With longer periods of occlusion, however, vasodilator metabolites accumulate and after 3 min of occlusion the vasodilatation is near-maximal in human limbs. Prostaglandins are known to contribute too, because the hyperaemia is reduced (but not abolished) by indomethacin. The longer the ischaemic period, the greater is the accumulation of vasodilator substances and the greater the total cumulative blood flow afterwards; as a result, a hyperaemic plateau precedes the exponential decay after long occlusions. The functional importance of reactive hyperaemia lies in resupplying oxygen and nutrients to ischaemic tissue as rapidly as possible.

Oxygen-derived free radicals and ischaemia-reperfusion injury

Surgeons sometimes have to interrupt the blood flow to a limb for very long periods (hours, for example, when repairing an abdominal aortic aneurysm). It is often found that when the clamped vessel is subsequently released, instead of the brisk reactive hyperaemia seen after minutes of occlusion, there is very little hyperaemia and blood flow falls to abnormally low levels within minutes. Thus periods of ischaemia exceeding an hour or so impair

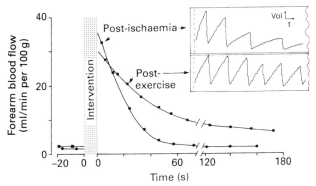

Figure 12.10 Forearm blood flow in a medical student measured by venous occlusion plethysmography (see Section 8.3) after 120 s of ischaemia (brachial artery occlusion) or after 30 s of strenuous forearm exercise. Note that blood flow remains elevated for a longer period after exercise. Insets show typical forearm volume traces during plethysmographic measurements.

reactive hyperaemia, and this is called ischaemia-reperfusion injury.

Reperfusion injury arises as follows. During the prolonged anoxic period the enzyme xanthine dehydrogenase is converted to xanthine oxidase, an enzyme capable of oxidizing hypoxanthine to xanthine when oxygen becomes available. Hypoxanthine itself is formed during the anoxic period as a breakdown product of ATP. Upon reperfusion, oxygen becomes available and the xanthine oxidase catalyses the oxidation of the hypoxanthine; but unfortunately ordinary molecular oxygen is converted into superoxide radicals ($O_2^-\cdot$) and hydroxyl radicals (OH·) during this process. Radicals are highly reactive particles owing to a lone electron in the outer shell, and the hydroxyl radical in particular readily attacks cell membrane lipids, proteins and glycosaminoglycans. This damages the tissue and the capillary wall, causing leucocytes to adhere to the wall and obstruct flow ('no-reflow' phenomenon). Such damage can be attenuated by pretreatment with allopurinol (an inhibitor of xanthine oxidase) or superoxide dismutase (an endogenous enzyme that acts as a superoxide scavenger) or dimethyl sulphoxide (a hydroxyl radical scavenger). Reperfusion injury is thought to contribute to myocardial, intestinal and brain damage after thrombotic episodes, and possibly to joint damage in rheumatoid arthritis.

12.4 Nervous control: sympathetic vasoconstrictor nerves

Local mechanisms serve only local needs. To serve the more general needs of the whole organism, such as the homeostasis of arterial pressure and core temperature, the central nervous system superimposes a sentient control system over the circulation. The efferent limb of the system comprises autonomic vasomotor nerves and endocrine secretions, and the afferent limb involves sensory inputs, described in Chapter 14. The autonomic vasomotor nerves fall into three classes: sympathetic vasoconstrictor fibres, sympathetic vasodilator fibres and parasympathetic vasodilator fibres. The terminology refers to the effect of stimulating (cf. inhibiting) the nerve. Of these the sympathetic vasoconstrictor fibres are the most widespread and important. Students accustomed to associating the sympathetic system with alarm and dilatation should note that the *vast majority of sympathetic vasomotor fibres are in fact vasoconstrictor fibres.*

Anatomy of the sympathetic vasoconstrictor system

The pathway controlling the sympathetic vasoconstrictor fibres begins in the brainstem. From here, descending excitatory and inhibitory fibres called bulbospinal fibres

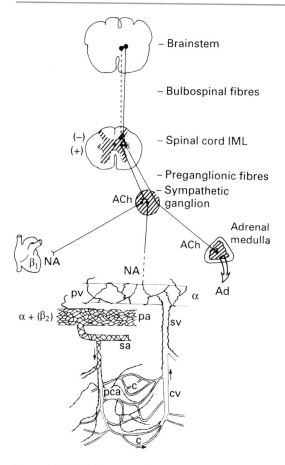

- Brainstem

- Bulbospinal fibres

(-)
(+)

- Spinal cord IML

- Preganglionic fibres
- Sympathetic
ganglion

ACh

Adrenal
ACh   medulla

β₁ NA

NA

Ad

pv

α

α + (β₂)

pa   sv

sa

pca   c   cv

c

Figure 12.11 Schematic diagram of sympathetic innervation of cardiovascular system. α and β refer to predominant adrenoceptors on the end-organs. NA, noradrenaline; Ad, adrenaline; ACh, acetylcholine: cotransmitters not shown; IML, intermediolateral horn of grey matter in segments T1–L3. One descending tract (bulbospinal tract) excites the sympathetic IML cells; other bulbospinal fibres inhibit the cell, but the transmitters involved are complex and are omitted. pa, pv, primary artery and vein to an organ; sa, sv, small artery and vein; pca, precapillary arteriole; c, capillary; cv, collecting venule. (Adapted from Furness, J. B. and Marshall, J. M. (1974) *Journal of Physiology*, **239**, 75–88, by permission)

pass down the spinal cord and synapse with *sympathetic preganglionic neurons* in the intermediolateral columns of the grey matter

in thoracicolumbar segments T1 to L3 (Figure 12.11. The output of the spinal neurons depends on the interplay of excitatory and inhibitory inputs from the bulbospinal fibres, plus local spinal inputs. The sympathetic preganglionic axons travel via the ventral roots of the spinal nerves and white rami communicantes into the sympathetic chains and may travel up or down the chain for several segments before synapsing with postganglionic neurons located in the sympathetic ganglia. Some fibres do not synapse until they reach more distant ganglia (coeliac and hypogastric ganglia) or the adrenal medulla. The preganglionic fibres are mostly cholinergic and the receptors on the cell bodies of the postganglionic neurons are mainly of the nicotinic variety, being blocked by hexamethonium.

The *postganglionic cells* of the sympathetic chain send non-myelinated axons through the grey rami communicantes for distribution in the mixed peripheral nerves. Some fibres also course directly over the major vessels. The terminal fibres run along the outer border of the tunica media but, except in veins, they do not penetrate the inner part, perhaps due to the higher pressure there. Most small arteries and large arterioles are richly innervated, whereas terminal arterioles are poorly innervated and are probably controlled chiefly by local tissue metabolites. This pattern is repeated in the splanchnic venous system, although venous vessels are in general less densely innervated. The venous system of skeletal muscle receives almost no innervation.

Pharmacology of sympathetic vasoconstrictor nerves

Noradrenergic transmission The terminal fibre resembles a string of beads, each bead being a varicosity filled with dense-cored vesicles of neurotransmitter (see Section 11.4). The classical, long-recognized transmitter is noradrenaline (norepinephrine in the American literature). This quickly diffuses across the junctional gap and binds to α-adrenoreceptors on the VSM cell membrane. There are two kinds of α receptor: α_1-receptors are widely distributed over the VSM membrane, while α_2-receptors occur on the nerve fibre as 'prejunctional receptors' (see below) and on certain blood vessels (e.g. human skin arterioles and veins) along with the α_1-receptors (Table 12.1). Activation of the postjunctional receptors elicits vasoconstriction by pharmacomechanical and electromechanical coupling, as described in Chapter 11. About 80% of the noradrenaline is then taken back into the nerve by an active membrane process which terminates its action and restocks the terminal. To a lesser extent, transmitter action is also terminated by diffusion into the nearby capillaries and by postjunctional degrading enzymes, namely catechol-O-methyltransferase and monoamine oxidase (Figure 12.12).

Local modulation of noradrenaline release The amount of neurotransmitter released at the junction depends not just on impulse frequency but also on the chemical environment of the nerve ('neuromodulation'). As mentioned earlier, agents like H^+, K^+ and adenosine act on the nerve membrane to depress the release of transmitter (Figure 12.12), and this contributes to metabolic hyperaemia. Most autacoids have a similar effect. Noradrenaline too binds to prejunctional α_2-receptors ('autoreceptors') and this inhibits further release of noradrenaline. By contrast, angiotensin II facilitates transmitter release and thereby amplifies vasoconstriction.

Non-adrenergic transmission: role of ATP and neuropeptide Y The vasoconstrictor response of the pulmonary artery and

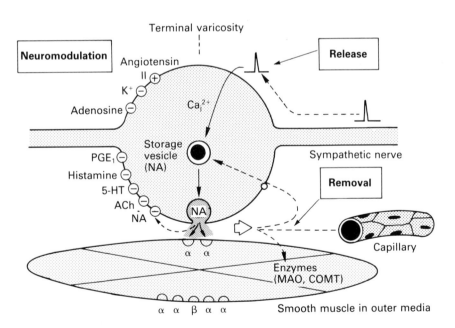

Figure 12.12 Schematic diagram of noradrenergic neurotransmission at the junctional varicosity of a sympathetic vasoconstrictor nerve. Not to scale (the varicosity is 2 μm long × 1 μm wide, the axon 0.1–0.5 μm wide and the smooth muscle cell 4 μm wide at the centre). NA, noradrenaline; for other abbreviations see text. ATP and neuropeptide Y, which act as co-transmitters with NA in some fibres, are omitted for clarity

Table 12.1 Adrenergic receptors in the cardiovascular system

Receptor Subtype	Principal location and effect	Agonist	Antagonist	Medical use of antagonist
α	Vascular smooth muscle: vasoconstriction	Noradrenaline (NA) Adrenaline (Ad)	Ergotamine Phentolamine Phenoxybenzamine	Migraine Raynaud's vasospasm Acute hypertension (phaeochromocytoma)
α_1	Postjunctional receptor of vascular smooth muscle: vasoconstriction	Specific agonist = phenylephrine Also NA and Ad	Prazosin	Anti-hypertension drug
α_2	Prejunctional receptors of nerve varicosity: inhibition of NA release. Also vascular smooth muscle in skin	NA (and Ad) Clonidine	Yohimbine Rauwolscine	—
β	SA node, myocardium and arterioles of coronary, skeletal muscle and liver. Increased heart rate, contractility and vasodilatation	Specific agonist = isoprenaline Also NA and Ad	Propranolol Oxprenolol	Relief of angina by reducing cardiac work Hypertension
β_1	Subtype found in pacemaker and myocardium	NA Ad	Practolol (toxic) Atenolol Metoprolol	Angina relief Hypertension Arrhythmia control
β_2	Arterioles of skeletal muscle, heart and liver: also bronchiole smooth muscle	Ad		

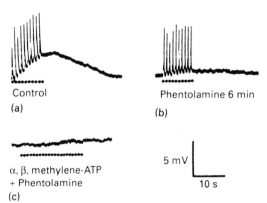

Control
(a)

Phentolamine 6 min
(b)

α, β, methylene-ATP
+ Phentolamine
(c)

5 mV

10 s

Figure 12.13 Evidence for co-transmission by noradrenaline and ATP in sympathetic vasoconstrictor nerves to the rat tail artery. (a) Intracellular potential during sympathetic nerve stimulation at each dot. Each stimulus produces an excitatory junction potential (EJP) (spike) plus a slower depolarization (baseline under the spikes). The spikes are not action potentials (see voltage scale). (b) Phentolamine, an α-adrenoceptor blocker, abolishes the slow response. (c) α, β-methylene ATP, a desensitizer of purinergic receptors, abolishes the fast EJPs. (After Sneddon, P. and Burnstock, G. (1984) *European Journal of Pharmacology*, **106**, 149–152)

most veins to sympathetic stimulation is completely abolished by drugs that block α-adrenoreceptors (e.g. phentolamine, phenoxybenzamine), but the vasoconstrictor response of many systemic arteries and arterioles to sympathetic nerve activity is only partially prevented by α-blockers. This led to the discovery of additional neurotransmitters (*co-transmitters*) in the sympathetic varicosities, namely the purine ATP and the peptide neuropeptide Y (Table 12.2). Their relative abundance and importance vary from tissue to tissue.

ATP is synthesized in the nerve terminal and is released along with the noradrenaline in some large arteries and small mesenteric arteries. It stimulates postjunctional purinergic receptors (P_{2X} receptors) and evokes a fast, brief depolarization by opening cation channels conductive to Ca^{2+} and Na^+ ions (excitatory junction potential), as illustrated in Figure 12.13 and 11.3–11.4.

Neuropeptide Y by contrast is synthesized in the postganglionic cell body and is transported slowly along the axon to the sympathetic terminals where it is probably stored along with noradrenaline in the large

Table 12.2 Main transmitter agents coexisting in perivascular nerves*

Sympathetic vasoconstrictor fibre	Noradrenaline (NA) Adenosine triphosphate (ATP) Neuropeptide Y (NPY)
Parasympathetic dilator fibre	Acetylcholine (ACh) Vasoactive intestinal polypeptide (VIP)
Sensory-dilator axons (C fibre)	Substance P (SP) Calcitonon-gene related peptide (CGRP) ATP

* From Burnstock, G. (1988) *Acta Physiologica Scandinavica*, **133**, Suppl. 571, 53–57. The ratio of transmitter substances within the fibre varies from tissue to tissue

dense-cored vesicles. Neuropeptide Y has been identified in the vasomotor nerves of skeletal muscle, kidney, salivary gland, spleen and nasal mucosa. It is released chiefly in response to high frequency stimulation, which occurs naturally only under stress conditions, and it produces a much slower, more prolonged depolarization than ATP. Neuropeptide Y also appears to sensitize the post-junctional membrane to noradrenaline, and some workers consider this modulatory effect to be its chief action.

Physiological effects of sympathetic activity

Sympathetic vasoconstrictor nerves discharge continually at an average rate of 1 impulse per second or less in resting subjects: the action potentials arrive in bursts rather than uniformly, in reality. The maximum mean frequency is only 8–10 per s *in vivo*. The tonic activity of the system at rest, though low, contributes substantially to vessel tone and if it is interrupted by nerve sectioning or pharmacological blockade vasodilatation ensues. In resting skeletal muscle, for example, interruption of the tonic sympathetic drive increases the blood flow from 2–5 ml min^{-1} 100 g^{-1} to 6–9 ml min^{-1} 100 g^{-1}; the latter flow, however, is far from maximal owing to the persistence of basal tone.

Vasodilatation induced by a *fall in sympathetic activity* is physiologically very important, being part of the baroreceptor reflex which prevents excessive rises in blood pressure (Section 14.1). It is also important in producing cutaneous vasodilatation in the extremities during the regulation of body temperature. Neurogenic tone is in fact especially well developed in the skin of the extremities, and it was the flushing of the rabbit ear upon cutting the cervical sympathetic nerve which led Claude Bernard in 1851 to discover the sympathetic vasomotor nerves.

The effects of *increased sympathetic activity* are illustrated in Figure 12.14.

1. *Local blood flow* is reduced. This can be sustained for hours in some tissues (e.g. skin) but in the intestine the arterioles quickly 'escape' from the vasoconstriction; the veins however do not.
2. *The volume of blood* in an organ is reduced by active venoconstriction, which can displace 28 ml blood per kg in the intestinal tract and liver, and 15 ml per kg in skin. In skeletal muscle, the venous system lacks an effective innervation, but nevertheless up to 7.5 ml/kg can be displaced passively because venous pressure falls secondarily to arteriolar contraction.
3. *Capillary pressure* is reduced by the arteriolar constriction, causing a transient absorption of interstitial fluid into the plasma compartment.
4. If the increase in sympathetic outflow is generalized (which is not inevitably the case), the *total peripheral resistance* and cardiac output rise, altering the arterial blood pressure. The regulation of blood pressure is perhaps the single most important function of the sympathetic vasomotor system.

The above four effects (reduced peripheral flow, reduced peripheral blood volume, fluid translocation and blood pressure

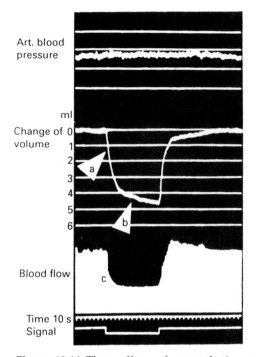

Art. blood pressure

ml
Change of 0
volume 1
2
a
3
4
5
6
b

Blood flow c

Time 10 s
Signal

Figure 12.14 Three effects of sympathetic nerve stimulation in cat hindquarters. Volume of hindquarters was measured by a displacement method (plethysmography), and blood flow by collecting the venous outflow. Lumbar sympathetic nerves were stimulated at just 2 impulses/s (signal). Arrow (a) indicates the decrease in volume due to reduction in capacitance vessel size. This is mostly secondary to a fall in venous pressure induced by arteriolar contraction; skeletal muscle veins have little direct innervation. Arrow (b) indicates the slow fall in volume due to capillary absorption of interstitial fluid, secondary to fall in capillary pressure induced by arteriolar contraction. Letter (c) indicates the fall in blood flow due to contraction of resistance vessels. (From Mellander, S. (1960) *Acta Physiologica Scandinavica*, **50** (Suppl.), 176, by permission)

maintenance) form a life-preserving response in haemorrhage and shock (Chapter 16). It should be noted that changes in sympathetic activity are sometimes widespread, as during a haemorrhage, and sometimes confined to a single tissue (e.g. skin during temperature changes). Activation of the sympathetic system is far from an 'all-or-none' affair.

Sympathetic activity to muscle and gut increases with each inspiration. In conjunction with sinus arrhythmia, this produces small oscillations in blood pressure in phase with respiration, called *Traube–Hering waves*, but these have no known functional significance.

12.5 Vasodilator nerves

In a limited number of tissues, the arterioles are innervated by vasodilator fibres as well as by the ubiquitous sympathetic vasoconstrictor fibres. Vasodilator fibres occur within the sympathetic, parasympathetic and sensory systems and, unlike the vasoconstrictor fibres, they are not tonically active.

Sympathetic vasodilator nerves

Sympathetic cholinergic fibres to muscle vessels in some species: the alerting response

In some species (cat, dog) the arterioles of skeletal muscle are innervated not only by sympathetic vasoconstrictor nerves but also by sympathetic vasodilator nerves whose neurotransmitter is acetylcholine. Selective excitation of the sympathetic cholinergic nerves causes vascular relaxation and increased muscle blood flow.

The sympathetic cholinergic system differs from the vasoconstrictor system in many aspects (Table 12.3). The cholinergic system is controlled by the forebrain and is activated solely as part of the 'alerting response' to fear and danger. The central fibres do not synapse in the brainstem vasomotor regions. The distribution is confined to the skeletal muscle vasculature of certain species. The response is only transient, and the fibres take no part in the baroreflex control of blood pressure.

It is tempting to assume that the increased blood flow 'improves' muscle nutrition, but measurements of microvascular permeability–surface area products (see Chapter 9) show that cholinergic vasodilatation does not increase the permeability–surface area product (unlike metabolic vasodilatation), so the nutritional benefit is limited. Metabolic hyperaemia, by contrast, causes capillary recruitment which facilitates the transfer of all solutes. It cannot be emphasized too strongly that *local metabolic factors, not sympathetic vasodilator nerves, cause the hyperaemia associated with normal, non-emotional exercise.*

Stress-induced vasodilatation in the human forearm muscle

Whether *man* has a sympathetic cholinergic supply to muscle is controversial. Acute mental stress (e.g. mental arithmetic for most of us) causes a marked vasodilatation in human forearm muscle (Figure 12.15), though not in calf muscle. The explanation of the vasodilatation is unclear, because the net discharge frequency in the sympathetic nerves to human forearm muscle is unchanged by mental stress. This could conceivably result from a simultaneous reduction in sympathetic vasoconstrictor fibre discharge and increase in sympathetic vasodilator fibre discharge, if the latter exist in man. The view that cholinergic vasodilator fibres innervate human muscle is based on the partial inhibition of stress-induced vasodilatation by the local infusion of atropine and by unilateral sympathectomy. Another factor contributing to human forearm dilatation in severe stress is the secretion of adrenaline by the adrenal medulla (see later).

Sweating and cutaneous vasodilatation

Human sweat glands are innervated by sympathetic cholinergic nerves. Stimulation of these nerves elicits not only sweating but also marked cutaneous vasodilatation. The vasodilatation is only partially prevented by the cholinergic-blocker atropine and is unaffected by adrenergic blockers. The nerves thus possess a neurotransmitter that is neither acetylcholine nor noradrenaline. The non-adrenergic non-cholinergic (NANC) transmitter seems to be a neuropeptide called vasoactive intestinal polypeptide (VIP). Im-

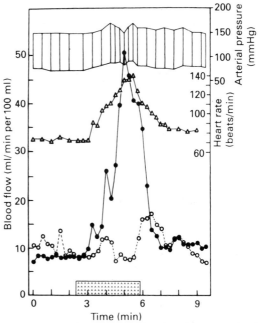

Figure 12.15 Increase in human forearm blood flow in response to stress. Closed circles, forearm blood flow (dominated by skeletal muscle blood flow); open circles, hand blood flow (greater contribution from skin); triangles, heart rate. During the time represented by the rectangle the experimenters alarmed the subject by hinting at a sudden leak and severe blood loss. The increase in forearm flow is comparable with that in severe exercise, and greatly exceeds the maximum flow that withdrawal of sympathetic vasoconstrictor tone can produce. The response is attributed partly to the secretion of adrenaline and perhaps also to the existence of a sympathetic cholinergic innervation (controversial) (From Blair, D. A., Glover, W. E., Greenfield, A. D. M. and Roddie, L. C. (1959) *Journal of Physiology*, **148**, 633–647, by permission)

munocytochemistry confirms that VIP is present in vasomotor fibres close to human sweat glands. It is not clear whether there are separate sudomotor and vasodilator fibres or whether one set of nerves serves both functions. (In the past, sweat-related hyperaemia was attributed to the kallikrein–bradykinin system, as was the analogous hyperaemia in salivary glands and pancreas – see later).

Parasympathetic vasodilator nerves

Parasympathetic preganglionic fibres are much longer than their sympathetic counterparts and leave the central nervous system in two outflows: the cranial nerves (e.g. vagus) and the sacral spinal outflow. Their distribution is less universal than that of sympathetic vasoconstrictor fibres. They innervate the salivary glands and exocrine pancreas, the gastrointestinal mucosa, the genital erectile tissue, and cerebral and coronary arteries. The long preganglionic fibres synapse with postganglionic neurons within the end-organ, and these send short postganglionic fibres to the arterioles. The fibres are not tonically active; they fire only when organ function demands a rise in blood flow.

The postganglionic fibres release the classic neurotransmitter *acetylcholine*. This acts directly on VSM cells in, for example, the lingual artery to cause hyperpolarization after a delay of a second or more, and this leads to relaxation (Figure 12.16). There is strong evidence that the neural effect is *not* mediated by EDRF. Moreover acetylcholine is rapidly locally degraded by cholinesterase in the vessel wall, so is unlikely to survive the long journey from adventitial nerve to endothelium. (By contrast, the vasodilator effect of acetylcholine perfused through an aortic ring is endothelium-dependent and the direct effect of acetylcholine on such VSM is constriction – Figure 12.4.) The slow hyperpolarizing effect is probably due to increased K^+ permeability but the details are unknown.

It has become clear in recent years that most parasympathetic postganglionic fibres can release not only acetylcholine but also *non-adrenergic, non-cholinergic (NANC)* transmitters with a vasodilator action. For example, nerve-induced vasodilatation in the rabbit lingual artery, which supplies the tongue and submandibular salivary gland, is only partially prevented by atropine (see Figure 12.16). The predominant NANC vasodilator transmitter is a neuropeptide, *vasoactive intestinal polypeptide (VIP)*, which also occurs in sympathetic cholinergic fibres.

Dilatation in salivary glands, pancreas and gut

Blood flow to the submandibular gland can be increased tenfold by parasympathetic stimulation (chorda tympani nerve). The increased blood flow supplies the water for saliva formation, which requires an enormous rate of fluid filtration across the gland's fenestrated capillaries; indeed, the gland can secrete up to its own weight of fluid in just 1 minute. The vasodilatation is due partly to acetylcholine, being partially blocked by atropine, and the action of the acetylcholine is independent of endothelial NO production, i.e. is direct. Further vasodilatation at high stimulation frequencies is due to the release of VIP. In addition, a vasodilator neuropeptide called substance P is released from parasympathetic fibres in the rat salivary gland.

Table 12.3 Comparison of sympathetic vasoconstrictor and vasodilator nerves

Feature	Sympathetic constrictor nerve	Sympathetic dilator nerve
Main neurotransmitter	Noradrenaline (and ATP)	Acetylcholine (and VIP)
Distribution	Most organs and tissue	Restricted; e.g., skeletal muscle and sweat glands
Tonically active?	Yes	No
Central control	Brainstem	Forebrain
Involvement in baroreceptor reflex	Major factor governing activity	Negligible
Role in blood pressure homeostasis	Very important	Little
Duration of effect	Mostly well sustained	Transient

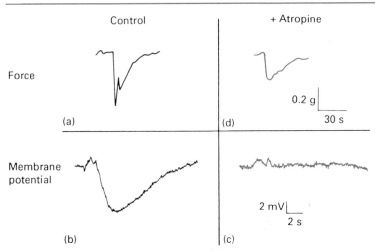

Figure 12.16 Parasympathetic vasodilatation in rabbit lingual artery. Noradrenergic fibres were blocked by guanethidine so perivascular stimulation excited only parasympathetic responses. (a) Mechanical response, showing dilatation. (b) Membrane potential showing slow hyperpolarization (baseline −51 mV). (c) Total abolition of electrical response by atropine, i.e. electrical response is purely cholinergic. (d) Dilatation, however, is only partially blocked by atropine, revealing the existence of non-cholinergic dilator transmitter, whose action does not involve hyperpolarization – possibly vasoactive intestinal polypeptide, acting via cAMP. Removal of the arterial endothelium by rubbing did *not* abolish these responses. (From Brayden, J. E. and Large, W. A. (1986) *British Journal of Pharmacology*, **89**, 163–171, by permission)

In the *pancreas*, VIP seems to be the main parasympathetic transmitter, rather than acetylcholine, i.e. these are true 'peptidergic' vasodilator nerves.

In the *intestinal submucosa*, cholinergic postganglionic fibres cause dilatation by releasing acetylcholine, and this appears to have a direct vasodilator action on the smooth muscle of submucosal arterioles.

In some tissues, nitric oxide may be produced by parasympathetic nerve terminals as a vasodilator neurotransmitter. Such nitroxidergic nerves may exist around mesenteric, cerebral, temporal and possibly coronary arteries.

Role in erectile tissue

Sacral parasympathetic fibres innervate the vasculature of genital erectile tissue and the colonic mucosa. Stimulation of the pelvic nerve in a dog (parasympathetic fibres) causes a profound vasodilatation of the arterioles feeding the corpus cavernosum of the penis, reversing the usual balance of resistances: inflow resistance becomes less than outflow resistance. The sinuses of the corpus therefore fill with blood at a pressure close to the arterial level, creating distension and erection. The vasodilatation is mostly atropine-resistant, implying that transmission is mainly NANC. Immunocytochemistry reveals the presence of VIP in the parasympathetic nerves innervating the penile artery, and assays of the venous effluent show that VIP is released on pelvic nerve stimulation. There is also evidence that some parasympathetic fibres to the corpus cavernosum are nitroxidergic, i.e. secrete NO. Withdrawal of sympathetic vasoconstrictor tone may be a supplementary factor in penile erection. Whatever the exact mechanism, the sacral parasympathetic nerves have been truly essential to the continuation of our species!

Vasodilatation induced by sensory nerves

The curious phenomenon of a sensory nerve having a motor function is illustrated by Lewis's triple response. This is the response of human skin to a mild trauma such as a scratch, investigated by Sir Thomas Lewis in 1927. Three responses are observed: (1) a local redness along the line of the scratch, caused probably by the release of K^+ ions and the vasodilator mediators of inflammation from activated cells; (2) a spreading flare, which is an area of redness that gradually extends laterally from the scratch line for 2–3 cm; and (3) a local swelling or wheal along the scratch line, caused by inflammatory oedema. The flare is mediated by sensory nerves, since it is abolished by local anaesthetics like lignocaine, and by sensory denervation. The ability of sensory nerves to cause cutaneous vasodilatation was demonstrated long ago by Bayliss. He stimulated the spinal nerve dorsal root antidromically, sending action potentials in the 'wrong' direction down the sensory nerves, and found that this elicits cutaneous vasodilatation. Antidromic activity probably explains how infection of a dorsal root by herpes zoster virus causes the segmental cutaneous hyperaemia characteristic of 'shingles'.

The sensory nerves mediating vasodilatation are the nociceptive C fibres, whose terminals contain two vasodilator neuropeptides: *substance P* and *calcitonin-gene related peptide* (CGRP). These are released on nerve activation, whether the fibre is excited antidromically or orthodromically (e.g. by capsaicin, the hot ingredient of chillis). CGRP is

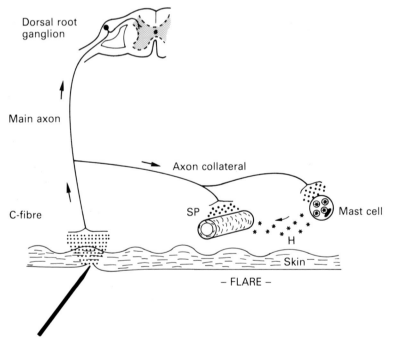

Figure 12.17 Vasodilatation due to release of a neuropeptide, substance P (SP, black dots) from a sensory terminal (nociceptive C fibre). Some fibres end close to mast cells near blood vessels; SP stimulates the mast cell to release the vasodilator histamine (H, shown as asterisks). An 'axon reflex' is believed to cause the lateral 'flare' when skin is traumatized with a needle. Since the axon spreads over only 0.5–1 cm (the receptive field), a flare of 2–3 cm is attributed to histamine triggering adjacent fibres. (After Foreman, J. C. (1987) *Allergy*, **42**, 1–11)

extremely potent and its effect lasts many hours. To explain the rapid lateral spread of the flare in human skin (which does not occur in all species, and which is too fast to be explained by the diffusion of vasodilator), an 'axon reflex' was proposed by Lewis. It is supposed that the C fibre action potential, elicited by trauma in the skin, propagates centrally but also passes antidromically down a side branch of the axon to influence a blood vessel up to a 0.5–1 cm away (Figure 12.17).

Histamine too is involved in mediating the flare. Many of the substance P-containing fibres terminate on mast cells, which possess substance P receptors. Activation of these receptors causes the mast cell to release its granules of histamine, a vasodilator agent. Since histamine also stimulates local C fibres, this could explain the lateral spread of the flare over 2–3 cm.

Substance P and histamine not only cause vasodilatation but also cause a pathological rise in microvascular permeability, leading to plasma exudation and high-protein oedema. This provides an explanation for the *neurogenic inflammation* which is elicited in skin and synovial joints by antidromic stimulation of sensory C fibres.

12.6 Hormonal control of the circulation

Several endocrine secretions have acute effects on the heart and circulation, but these need to be viewed in perspective; in normal healthy animals hormones are of less importance for short-term cardiovascular regulation than is neural control. If, however, neural control is impaired, as in transplanted hearts, or if a pathological event such as haemorrhage arises, then endocrine secretions become very important. Hormones such as *aldosterone* are also of major importance in the long-term regulation of plasma volume. *Oestrogens* have a selective vasodilator effect on certain tissues, e.g. uterus, vagina, mammary gland and skin.

Adrenaline

The adrenal gland is situated at the upper pole of the kidney. Its medulla (core) secretes adrenaline (epinephrine) and noradrenaline (norepinephrine), which are known collectively as the catecholamines: adrenaline is a methylated form of noradrenaline. The medulla develops, embryologically, from postganglionic sympathetic neurons and it retains an innervation by preganglionic sympathetic fibres which run in the splanchnic nerve and control the gland. Although both adrenaline and noradrenaline are secreted, adrenaline forms over three-quarters of the secretion in man. (In diving mammals, by contrast, the secretion is mainly noradrenaline: this induces muscle vasoconstriction during dives and thereby conserves oxygen.) The plasma levels of adrenaline and noradrenaline are 0.1–0.5 nM and 0.5–3.0 nM, respectively, at rest, the higher level of noradrenaline being due to 'spillage' from the tonically active sympathetic terminals rather than glandular secretion.

Catecholamine secretion is increased by exercise, fear–flight–fight situations, hypotension and hypoglycaemia. During exercise the plasma adrenaline level can reach 5 nM and the noradrenaline level 10 nM, the latter again due chiefly to spillover from the increasingly active sympathetic terminals. Adrenaline affects both the heart and vasculature, but these effects are quite small at physiological concentrations compared with the effects of the autonomic nerves and local factors. (The metabolic effects of adrenaline are at least as important as its cardiovascular effects, namely the stimulation of liver glycogenolysis and fat lipolysis, which releases glucose into the bloodstream.)

Adrenaline and noradrenaline show both similarities and differences in their effect on the circulation (Figure 12.18). Both hormones stimulate the cardiac β-adrenoceptors, so their direct action is to increase heart rate and contractility. Both hormones at physiological concentrations cause the arterioles and veins to contract in many tissues, and at high (pharmacological)

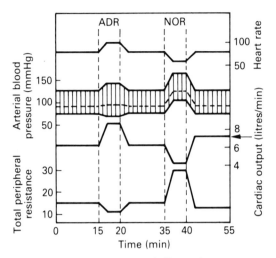

Figure 12.18 Comparison of effects of intravenous adrenaline and noradrenaline on the human circulation in the steady state. For explanation, see text. An initial transient drop in blood pressure that occurs during adrenaline infusion is not shown here. (From the classic monograph of Barcroft, H. and Swan, H. J. C. (1953) *Sympathetic Control of Human Blood Vessels*, Edward Arnold, London, by permission)

concentrations both cause vasoconstriction in all tissues. This is due to activation of the VSM α-adrenoceptors. (Many students have an ingrained belief that adrenaline necessarily causes vasodilatation but this is simply not true.) As an exception to the rule 'catecholamines cause vasoconstriction', adrenaline at physiological concentrations causes vasodilatation in three tissues, namely skeletal muscle, myocardium and liver. This is due to the abundance of β$_2$-adrenoceptors in these tissues, coupled with the high affinity of adrenaline for β$_2$-receptors. After β-blockade by propranolol, adrenaline causes vasoconstriction even in skeletal muscle because it activates α-receptors too. Noradrenaline normally causes vasoconstriction because it has a higher affinity for α-receptors than β-receptors.

Adrenaline and noradrenaline thus have opposite effects on skeletal muscle, which is the single most abundant tissue in the body (approximately 40% body weight). As a result their overall effects on the systemic circulation differ considerably in an intact animal. Intravenous *noradrenaline* causes a generalized vasoconstriction which *raises* the peripheral resistance and blood pressure markedly (Figure 12.18). This elicits a baroreceptor reflex which reduces the sympathetic drive to the heart and increases the parasympathetic drive. These reflexes slow the heart and reduce its output, offsetting the direct stimulatory effect of noradrenaline on the myocardium. Intravenous *adrenaline* by contrast *reduces* the total peripheral resistance slightly, because muscle vasodilatation outweighs vasoconstriction in other tissues. Mean blood pressure therefore changes little, and the direct stimulation of the heart by circulating adrenaline proceeds without significant opposition by the baroreflex. Since adrenaline is the predominant catecholamine secreted by the human medulla, the overall effect of adrenal gland stimulation is to increase cardiac output.

A rare tumour of the adrenal medulla, the phaeochromocytoma, secretes a mixture of catecholamines, causing hypertension. The latter can be treated with α-antagonists like phentolamine (see Table 12.1).

Vasopressin (antidiuretic hormone)

The remaining important hormones all have roles in the regulation of renal fluid excretion as well as vascular tone. Vasopressin is a peptide produced by the magnocellular neurons in the supraoptic and paraventricular nuclei of the hypothalamus. From the cell bodies the vasopressin is transported along the axons, through the pituitary stalk and into the posterior lobe of the pituitary gland. There the vasopressin is released into the bloodstream.

The secretion of vasopressin is regulated partly by hypothalamic cells sensitive to tissue fluid osmolarity (osmoreceptors) and partly by cardiovascular pressure receptors, as illustrated in Figure 12.19. Secretion is

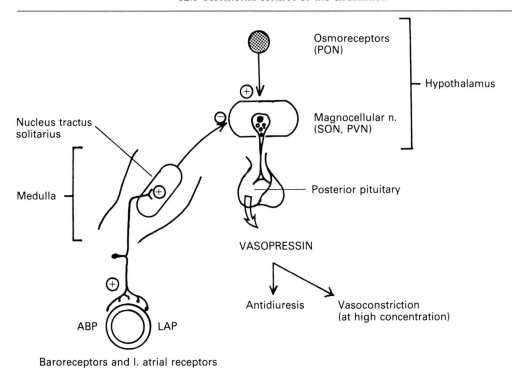

Figure 12.19 Regulation of vasopressin secretion. Relative importance of arterial baroreceptors and left atrial receptors varies between species. ABP, arterial blood pressure; LAP, left atrial pressure; PON, preoptic nucleus; SON, supraoptic nucleus; PVN, paraventricular nucleus

stimulated by a rise in plasma osmolarity (threshold 285 mOs) and by a fall in blood pressure and volume. The sensitivity to osmolarity is much greater than that to blood volume, in that equivalent vasopressin rises are elicited by a 2% rise in osmolarity and 10% fall in blood volume.

The main action of vasopressin at normal plasma levels is to promote water retention by the kidney. The cardiovascular effects of vasopressin are seen at raised concentrations, such as occur during haemorrhagic hypotension, where they are elicited by reduced pressure receptor traffic (see Chapter 14). High concentrations of vasopressin cause a strong vasoconstriction in most tissues which helps to support arterial pressure and contributes to the pallor of the hypovolaemic patient. The cerebral and coronary vessels,

by contrast, respond to vasopressin with an EDRF-mediated dilatation; vasopressin thus produces a redistribution of the cardiac output in favour of the brain and heart, which seems appropriate in hypovolaemia. In dogs with diabetes insipidus and in Brattleboro rats, both of which lack vasopressin, blood pressure is abnormally depressed during dehydration or haemorrhage.

Renin–angiotensin–aldosterone system

Formation of angiotensin II Angiotensin II is a powerful circulating vasconstrictor hormone and is particularly important in hypovolaemia, hypertension and cardiac failure. It is an octapeptide and its production within the bloodstream from a circulating protein precursor is initiated by a proteolytic enzyme, *renin* (pronounced ree-nin). Renin is secreted mainly by the kidneys (although it is also found in the heart). Renin acts on an α_2-globulin in plasma, called angiotensinogen, to cleave off a decapeptide, angiotensin I. Angiotensin I is then cleaved further by an enzyme situated on the surface of endothelial cells (*angiotensin converting enzyme, ACE*) to form the active octapeptide angiotensin II. Conversion takes place mainly in the lungs because this is the first major area of endothelium encountered by venous angiotensin I.

Actions of angiotensin II   The main action at normal plasma concentrations is to stimulate the secretion of the steroid hormone *aldosterone* by the adrenal cortex. Aldosterone acts on renal tubules to promote salt and water retention – for example during hypovolaemia. Angiotensin II at higher concentrations, such as follow a haemorrhage or cardiac failure, causes *vasoconstriction*. It does so by a rather interesting triumvirate of mechanisms. (a) Angiotensin II acts directly on vascular smooth muscle receptors to produce contraction by pharmacomechanical coupling; (b) it activates receptors on the sympathetic terminal varicosities, leading to an increase in the release of noradrenaline from sympathetic varicosities (neuromodulation, see Figure 12.12); (c) it penetrates into the brainstem at a region called the area postrema, where the blood-brain barrier is absent, and increases central drive to the sympathetic system (central action). Another action of angiotensin II is to increase cardiac contractility, which it does partly directly, by enhancing the plateau current of Ca^{2+} ions, and partly indirectly by its central effect on sympathetic outflow.

Control of renin secretion   The level of circulating angiotensin II is determined by the rate of renin secretion. This enzyme is secreted by cells surrounding the afferent arterioles of the renal glomeruli (juxtaglo-

merular cells). The rate of secretion is increased by:

1. A local fall in *afferent arteriolar pressure*, such as occurs in haemorrhagic hypotension. This local effect is responsible for the angiotensin-mediated hypertension that follows renal artery stenosis.
2. *Renal sympathetic nerve* activity and circulating catecholamines raise renin secretion rate by stimulating β_1-adrenoceptors on the juxtaglomerular cells. When hypotension elicits an arterial baroreceptor reflex, there is a reflex, neurally-mediated stimulation of the renin–angiotensin–aldosterone system. Cardiopulmonary receptors can probably initiate this reflex too in man.
3. A decreased load of *NaCl* flowing past the macula densa of the adjacent renal tubule promotes renin secretion. This in turn leads to tubular Na^+ retention via the renin–angiotensin–aldosterone pathway.

Renin and angiotensin II levels are high in haemorrhagic hypotension, cardiac failure and many cases of essential hypertension. In cardiac failure, the various actions of angiotensin II contribute to high levels of sympathetic nerve activity, fluid retention and high cardiac filling pressures (Chapter 16). Angiotensin II levels can be reduced by *ACE inhibitors* (captopril, enalapril), and these are used in the treatment of hypertension and cardiac failure.

Atrial natriuretic peptide (ANP)

This peptide is a relatively recent discovery. It is secreted by specialized myocytes in the atria in response to high cardiac filling pressures. In contrast to vasopressin and the renin–angiotensin–aldosterone system, ANP enhances the renal excretion of salt and water and has a modest relaxing effect on resistance vessels. It also reduces plasma volume to a greater extent than can be accounted for by diuresis alone, which may be due to a rise in capillary pressure and an increase in the hydraulic conductance of the capillary wall.

12.7 Special features of venous control

The venous system has been called 'the Cinderella of the circulation' because it is often neglected. The control of the peripheral capacitance vessels is however important, because these vessels govern the distribution of blood volume between the periphery and thorax. They therefore regulate cardiac filling pressure and thereby influence stroke volume.

Differentiation of the venous system

The venous system may be divided into four parts on the basis of control and function (Figure 12.20): the passive thoracic vessels containing the central blood volume, and three peripheral systems.

Splanchnic veins The veins of the gastro-intestinal tract, liver and spleen contain about 20% of the total blood volume at rest. They are well innervated by sympathetic constrictor nerves and possess α-adreno-receptors. They contract actively during exercise and hypotension due to increased sympathetic activity and circulating catecholamines (as illustrated in Figure 12.21). This helps to maintain CVP at times of circulatory stress.

Skeletal muscle veins The intramuscular veins are very poorly innervated. Their volume is influenced chiefly by body posture (i.e. gravity) and by the muscle pump. Although direct sympathetic control of these veins is almost non-existent, their volume is nevertheless affected indirectly by sympathetic activity because arteriolar constriction

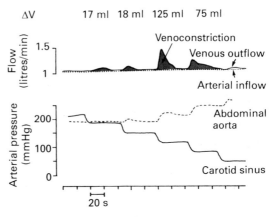

Figure 12.21 Active splanchnic venoconstriction in response to the sympathetic vasoconstrictor nerves in the anaesthetized dog. Step reductions in carotid sinus pressure elicit a reflex increase in sympathetic outflow. Arterial inflow and the outflow from the inferior vena cava were measured. Each transient excess of outflow over inflow marks an episode of venoconstriction. ΔV is the total volume of blood displaced by each venoconstriction. Aortic pressure increases due to a sympathetically-mediated arteriolar constriction. (After Hainsworth, R. and Karim, F. (1976) *Journal of Physiology*, **262**, 659–677, by permission)

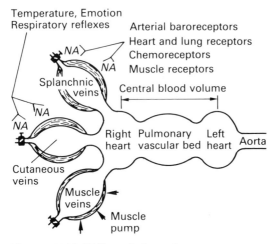

Figure 12.20 Differentiation of venous system. Changes in central blood volume and cardiac filling pressure are brought about by contraction of peripheral veins, especially splanchnic veins. NA, noradrenaline (From Shepherd, J. T. and Vanhoutte, P. M. (1979) *The Human Cardiovascular System, Facts and Concepts*, Raven Press, New York, by permission)

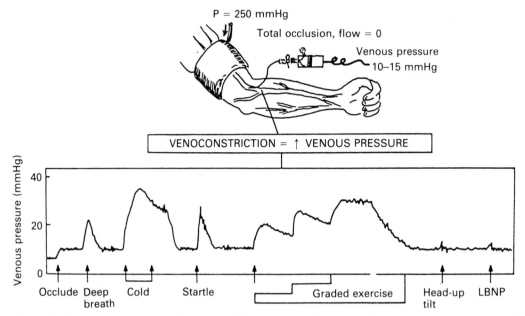

Figure 12.22 Control of venous tone in skin by sympathetic nerves. The pressure in veins when blood flow is halted by a sphygmomanometer cuff is measured as an index of changes in venous smooth muscle tension. LBNP, lower body negative pressure (After Rowell, L. B. (1986) *Human Circulation Regulation During Human Stress*, Oxford University Press, New York)

reduces downstream pressure, allowing the venous system to recoil elastically and displace blood centrally (see Figure 12.14). During exercise the intramuscle venules are dilated by vasodilator metabolites, and this probably helps to buffer the rise in capillary pressure in exercising muscle to some degree.

Cutaneous veins. These are richly innervated by sympathetic noradrenergic fibres. Their tone is greatly influenced by temperature: high core temperatures elicit a reduction in cutaneous sympathetic nerve activity producing venodilatation. Conversely, raised sympathetic activity causes the skin veins to contract strongly, as happens in hypotensive patients. A sympathetic-mediated constriction of the skin veins is also elicited by emotional stress and by deep inspiration (see Figure 12.22).

Comparison between venous control and arteriolar control

Veins respond in the same way as arterioles to many stimuli – in the skin for example both are constricted during hypotension – but there are also differences between venous and arteriolar behaviour. Most veins and venules have little basal tone in the absence of sympathetic activity, unlike arterioles, and they show little myogenic response to stretch (except for the portal vein). The responses to certain hormones, autacoids and drugs also differ. Angiotensin II, for example, has little direct effect on veins but a powerful effect on arterioles. It does, however, act on the sympathetic terminals to potentiate the effect of sympathetic nerves on human veins (neuromodulatory action), and this action contributes to the intense venoconstriction seen in patients with cardiac failure, who commonly have high angiotensin levels. Histamine causes veins to constrict but arterioles to dilate because the receptor population is different in the two kinds of vessel. Glyceryl trinitrate has a greater dilator effect on veins than on arterioles, and its efficacy in relieving angina is due partly to the reduction of cardiac filling pressure (and therefore cardiac work) following venodilatation.

12.8 Summary

Although very complex in detail, the control of blood vessels can be conceptualized fairly simply as a hierarchy of three control systems, each able to override or modify the lower one. The lowest level of control is the Bayliss myogenic response, which generates basal tone in resistance vessels and tends to maintain a constant blood flow and capillary pressure in the face of arterial pressure fluctuations (*autoregulation*).

The second level of control is that exerted by local factors. Vasodilator factors related to local metabolic rate (interstitial P_{O_2}, adenosine, phosphate, P_{CO_2}, lactate, K^+ and osmolarity) reset blood flow and autoregulation to a level that matches the tissue's metabolic activity, as for example in exercising muscle (*functional hyperaemia*). This process is well developed in heart, brain and skeletal muscle. Post-ischaemic or *reactive hyperaemia* is due to a combination of the myogenic response and metabolic accumulation. Other local factors called *autacoids* (e.g. histamine, bradykinin, 5HT, prostaglandins, leukotrienes, PAF) modify local vascular tone in special, often pathological situations, e.g. inflammation. *Nitric oxide* (endothelium-derived relaxing factor) exerts a tonic vasodilator influence and is responsible for flow-induced vasodilatation and for the vasodilator action of certain other substances (e.g. bradykinin, substance P, infused acetylcholine).

The third level of control is the neuroendocrine system, which brings the vasculature under central and reflex control, for the benefit of the organism as a whole and the brain in particular. *Sympathetic vasoconstrictor noradrenergic fibres* to skin, muscle, kidney and gut adjust the tone of resistance vessels to stabilize blood pressure and the partitioning of fluid between plasma and interstitium. They also regulate the tone of capacitance vessels to adjust cardiac filling pressure. In certain tissues and species there are also *vasodilator nerves* (sympathetic, parasympathetic and antidromically activated sensory nerves). *Hormonal control* by adrenaline, angiotensin II and vasopressin is especially important in supporting blood pressure in stressful conditions such as haemorrhage.

Further reading

Reviews and chapters

Burnstock, G. (1986) The changing face of autonomic neurotransmission. *Acta Physiologica Scandinavica*, **126**, 67–91

Calver, A., Collier, J. and Vallance, P. (1993) Nitric oxide and cardiovascular control. *Experimental Physiology*, **78**, 303–326

Furchgott, R. F. and Vanhoutte, P. M. (1989) Endothelium-derived relaxing and contracting factors. *FASEB Journal*, **3**, 2007–2018

Hainsworth, R. (1991) The importance of vascular capacitance in cardiovascular control. *News in Physiological Sciences*, **5**, 250–254

Hill, S. J. (1990) Distribution, properties and functional characteristics of 3 classes of histamine receptor. *Pharmacological Reviews*, 42, 45–83

Lisney, S. J. W. and Bharali, L. A. M. (1989) The axon reflex: an outdated idea or a valid hypothesis? *News in Physiological Sciences*, **4**, 45–48

Lundberg, J. M., Pernow, J. and Lacroix, J. S. (1989) Neuropeptide Y: sympathetic cotransmitter and modulator? *News in Physiological Sciences*, **4**, 13–17

Lundgren, O. (1984) Microcirculation of the gastrointestinal tract and pancreas. In *Handbook of Physiology, Cardiovascular System*, Vol. 4, Part 2, *The Microcirculation* (eds E. M. Renkin and C. C. Michel), American Physiological Society, Bethesda, pp. 799–864

McCord, J. M. (1985) Oxygen radicals in ischaemic injury. *New England Journal of Medicine*, **312**, 159–163

Meininger, G. A. and Davis, M. J. (1992) Cellular mechanisms involved in the vascular myogenic response. *American Journal of Physiology*, **263**, H647–659

Moncada, S. (1992) The L-arginine : nitric oxide pathway. *Acta Physiologica Scandinavica*, **145**, 201–227

Nilius, B. (1991) Regulation of transmembrane calcium fluxes in endothelium. *News in Physiological Sciences*, **6**, 110–114

Renkin, E. M. (1984) The control of the microcirculation. In *Handbook of Physiology, Cardiovascular System*, Vol. 4, Part 2, *The Microcirculation* (eds E. M. Renkin and C. C. Michel), American Physiological Society, Bethesda, pp. 627–688

Rothe, C. F. (1983) Venous system; physiology of the capacitance vessels. In *Handbook of Physiology, Cardiovascular System*, Vol. 3, *Peripheral Circulation*, Part 1 (eds J. T. Shepherd and F. M. Abboud), American Physiology Society, Bethesda, pp. 397–452

Share, L. (1988) Role of vasopressin in cardiovascular regulation. *Physiological Reviews*, **68**, 1248–1284

Smiesko, V. and Johnson, P. C. (1993) The arterial lumen is controlled by flow-related shear stress. *News in Physiological Sciences*, **8**, 34–38

Soloviev, A. I. and Braquet, P. (1992) Platelet-activating factor – a potent endogenous mediator responsible for coronary vasospasm (hypoxic vasoconstriction). *News in Physiological Sciences*, **7**, 166–172

Wallin, B. G. and Fagius, J. (1988) Peripheral sympathetic neural activity in conscious humans. *Annual Reviews in Physiology*, **50**, 565–576

Research papers

Carr, P., Graves, J. and Poston, L. (1993) Carbon dioxide induced relaxation in rat mesenteric arteries in small arteries precontracted with noradrenaline is endothelium dependent and mediated by nitric oxide. *Pflügers Archives*, **423**, 343–345

Edwards, A. V. and Garrett, J. R. (1993) Nitric oxide-related vasodilator responses to parasympathetic stimulation of the submandibular gland in the cat. *Journal of Physiology*, **464**, 379–392

Langton, P. D. (1993) Calcium channel currents recorded from isolated myocytes of rat basilar artery are stretch sensitive. *Journal of Physiology*, **471**, 1–11

McCarron, J. G. and Halpern, W. (1990) Potassium dilates rat cerebral arteries by two independent mechanisms. *American Journal of Physiology*, **259**, H902–908

Mian, R. and Marshall, J. M. (1991) Role of adenosine in dilator responses induced in arterioles and venules of rat skeletal muscle by systemic hypoxia. *Journal of Physiology*, **443**, 499–511

Wennmalm, Å. and Sandgren, G. (1991) Metabolic and myogenic components of reactive hyperaemia in the human calf. *Acta Physiologica Scandinavica*, **142**, 529–530

Chapter 13
Specialization in individual circulations

A catalogue of all the factors controlling the circulation is long and daunting, but fortunately rather fewer factors predominate in the day-to-day regulation of individual circulations, and one function of this chapter is to highlight which factors predominate in which tissue. Each tissue has its own special function, and this often calls for specialized vascular control. The skin for example regulates body heat, and its blood flow is controlled largely by temperature. In the heart, by contrast, metabolic rate dominates vascular control. Five circulations are covered here (heart, skeletal muscle, skin, brain and lung), these being selected partly for their physiological importance and partly for their contrasting characteristics. Space prevents the inclusion of other major circulations (renal, hepatic, splenic and gastrointestinal). To unify the topic, the same approach is adopted for each system. First, the special tasks imposed by the tissue on its circulation are outlined. How these tasks are accom-

plished is considered under the headings 'Structural adaptation' and 'Functional adaptation'. Special vascular problems presented by the organ are assessed, and finally the measurement of blood flow in man is described briefly.

13.1 Coronary circulation

Flow during basal cardiac output:
70–80 ml min^{-1} 100 g^{-1}
Flow during maximal cardiac work:
300–400 ml min^{-1} 100 g^{-1}

The right and left coronary arteries arise from the aorta immediately above the cusps of the aortic valve, the left coronary artery supplying mainly the left ventricle and septum and the right artery mainly the right ventricle – though this distribution is somewhat variable in man. Most of the venous blood drains via the coronary sinus directly into the right atrium (95%) and the rest drains into the cardiac chambers via the anterior coronary and Thebesian veins. Some of the Thebesian veins drain into the *left* side of the heart and contribute to a slight de-arterialization of the blood; aortic P_{O_2} is slightly less than that in blood leaving the lungs. The coronary circulation is the shortest in the body, the mean transit time of the coronary blood being only 6–8 s in a resting man.

Special tasks

The coronary circulation must deliver oxygen at a high rate to keep pace with cardiac demand. Even in a resting subject the myocardial oxygen consumption is very high: approximately 8 ml of oxygen per min per 100 g. This is 20 times greater than in resting skeletal muscle. In exercise, where cardiac work rate can increase over fivefold, the coronary circulation must increase its delivery of oxygen correspondingly.

Structural adaptation

Myocardial capillary density is very high, there being 3000–5000 capillaries per mm^2 cross-section, or roughly one capillary per myocyte (Figure 13.1). This facilitates the efficient delivery of oxygen and nutrients to the cell, partly by creating a very large endothelial area for exchange and partly by reducing the maximum diffusion distance to only 9 µm (the myocyte being approximately 18 µm wide). Oxygen transport is also enhanced by the presence of myoglobin in the cardiac myocytes (3.4 g/litre), as described in Section 9.10.

Functional adaptation

High basal flow and high oxygen extraction
In a resting subject, the blood flow per unit weight of myocardium is roughly 10 times

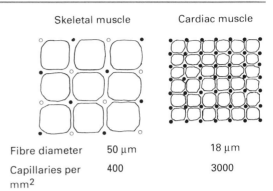

	Skeletal muscle	Cardiac muscle
Fibre diameter	50 µm	18 µm
Capillaries per mm^2	400	3000

Figure 13.1 Density of capillaries in skeletal and cardiac muscle on same scale. Each tissue has approximately 1 capillary per fibre but since the myocardial fibres are smaller, the capillary density is greater in myocardium and the diffusion distances are shorter. Open circles in skeletal muscle represent capillaries not perfused with blood at any given moment in resting muscle. (From Renkin, E. M. (1967) In *International Symposium on Coronary Circulation* (eds. Marchetti, G. and Taccardi, B.), Karger, Basel, pp. 18–30, by permission)

the average value for the whole body. Even so, the myocardium extracts 65–75% of the oxygen from the coronary blood, in contrast to the whole body average of 25% at rest (see Figure 13.2). The high extraction reduces the oxygen content from 195 ml/litre in arterial blood to only 50–70 ml/litre in coronary sinus blood. The corresponding oxygen pressure (P_{O_2}) in coronary venous blood is only 20 mmHg, and in the myocardial fibre itself the P_{O_2} is only about 6 mmHg, falling further during exercise. In heavy exercise, coronary oxygen extraction can rise to 90% leaving just 20 ml oxygen in each litre of venous blood at a P_{O_2} of only 10 mmHg. The extraction of fatty acid from coronary blood is also high (40–70%), but glucose extraction is usually low (2–3%), reflecting the substrate preference of myocardium.

As in many other circulations, NO is produced continuously by the endothelium, helping to maintain basal flow. Blockage of NO production by arginine analogues reduces myocardial blood flow by 60%.

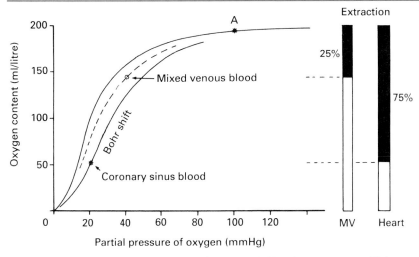

Figure 13.2 Oxygen carriage curves for arterial blood (P_{CO_2} 40 mmHg), mixed venous blood (P_{CO_2} 46 mmHg) and coronary sinus blood (P_{CO_2} 58 mmHg). Carbon dioxide displaces the oxyhaemoglobin dissociation curve to the right (the Bohr shift): this markedly enhances oxygen unloading in myocardium. A, arterial point; MV, mixed venous blood. Oxygen extraction from mixed venous blood and from coronary blood are compared on right (subject at rest)

Metabolic hyperaemia, the dominant control process The extra oxygen required at high work rates is supplied chiefly by an increase in blood flow rather than extraction; the latter can increase only modestly. Coronary blood flow increases in almost linear proportion to myocardial oxygen consumption at light to moderate work rates (see Figure 13.3), while at high work rates the flow increase lags a little and oxygen extraction rises. Myocardial metabolism evidently generates vasodilator messages in a quantitative manner – in other words this is a fine example of metabolic hyperaemia (Section 12.2). The nature of the vasodilator substance(s) however 'remains a well-sought but carefully guarded secret of nature'. The major contenders for the role are *interstitial hypoxia* (acting directly on VSM cells via the hyperpolarization mechanism; Section 11.7) and *adenosine* released by myocytes following ATP degradation. Both candidates dilate coronary arterioles, and the adenosine *versus* hypoxia controversy is not fully unresolved. However, there is growing evidence that adenosine release increases only at very low P_{O_2}s and may be important in ischaemic or

flow-limited myocardium, rather than normal tissue. In healthy hearts a modest fall in myocardial P_{O_2} and rise in P_{CO_2} with increased cardiac work are estimated to account for about 40% of coronary metabolic hyperaemia. The role of endothelial NO is under investigation.

Autoregulation is well developed in the coronary circulation and is reset by metabolic vasodilatation to operate at a higher flow, as illustrated in Figure 12.8. Autoregulation protects myocardium against underperfusion during periods of low blood pressure, though only down to about 50 mmHg.

Coronary vasomotor nerves Myocardial arteries and arterioles are well innervated by sympathetic vasoconstrictor fibres, whose tonic discharge contributes to the arteriolar tone. This effect is partially overcome, in a graded fashion, during metabolic vasodilatation. If all the sympathetic fibres to the heart are excited, including those to the pacemaker and myocytes, the ensuing increase in heart rate and contractility raises the cardiac work and the concomitant metabolic vasodilatation outweighs the increased vasoconstrictor

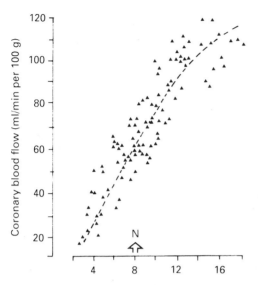

Figure 13.3 Effect of cardiac metabolic rate, as measured by myocardial oxygen consumption, on coronary blood flow in the dog. Arrow (N) marks normal values at resting cardiac output. Cardiac work was either increased above this point by intravenous infusions of adrenaline or reduced below normal by haemorrhage. The dashed line was fitted by eye to highlight the curvilinear tendency at high oxygen consumptions. (From Berne, R. M. and Rubio, R. (1979), see Further Reading, by permission)

nerve activity: blood flow increases. This metabolic 'overriding' of vasoconstriction ensures that any generalized activation of the sympathetic system does not imperil blood flow to this vital organ. Adrenaline, secreted at times of stress, reinforces the coronary hyperaemia by preferentially activating β_2-adrenoreceptors on the coronary VSM, causing dilatation. There is some evidence that parasympathetic cholinergic fibres too can dilate coronary arteries but this is not thought to be important in exercise.

Coronary flow can be affected by neural reflexes. Anger for example leads, after a transient dilatation, to prolonged sympathetic-mediated coronary constriction in dogs – sufficient even to produce ECG evidence of ischaemia. Severe cold can induce reflex sympathetic-mediated coronary constriction in human hearts with ischaemic disease (but not normal hearts), provoking angina.

Special problems

Mechanical obstruction during systole The branches of the coronary arteries within the myocardium are compressed during each systole. This effect is at its worst in the left ventricle during isovolumetric contraction when pressure within the ventricular wall reaches approximately 240 mmHg and coronary blood pressure is simultaneously at its nadir (approximately 80 mmHg). The reversal of the transmural pressure gradient across the coronary vessels transiently closes them so that coronary blood flow ceases briefly and even reverses in early systole (see Figure 13.4). A modest coronary flow is restored during the ejection phase as stress in the ventricle wall eases and arterial pressure rises, but flow is only restored fully during diastole. Roughly 80% of coronary flow occurs in diastole at basal heart rates.

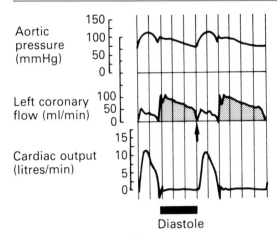

Figure 13.4 Flow in left coronary artery monitored by an electromagnetic flow meter in a conscious dog. Note the sharp curtailment of flow at the onset of systole (arrow); most coronary flow occurs during diastole (shaded area). Time lines 0.1 s. (After Khouris, E. M., Gregg, D. E. and Rayford, C. R. (1965) *Circulation Research*, **17**, 427–437)

Functional end-arteries, myocardial infarction and angina

Sudden obstruction Although cross-connections exist between the branches of the coronary arteries, they are few in number and small in diameter in man (35–500 µm), and can transmit only a low flow. Consequently, when an atheromatous artery is suddenly blocked by thrombosis, the residual blood flow to the tissue downstream is less than 10% of normal, which is insufficient to support normal contraction and metabolism (ischaemia). Human coronary arteries have therefore been called 'functional' end-arteries. The ischaemic myocardium becomes acidotic, causing severe cardiac pain and impaired contractility. Arrhythmias are frequently triggered (Section 5.8). The residual flow may be so low that myocytes begin to die after a few hours (necrosis, see Figure 1.2). This sequence of events is called myocardial infarction or a 'heart attack', and is the single commonest cause of death in the West. Myocardial infarcts are most frequent and largest in the subendocardium

(inner tissue) because the wall stress during systole is greatest here. This selectively curtails endocardial blood flow at low perfusion pressures.

Slow obstruction If an atheromatous narrowing develops gradually, without abrupt thrombosis, the small anastomoses have time to enlarge and maintain a precarious nutritional flow. These vessels cannot, however, supply the additional flow needed during exercise or emotional stress, and such events trigger local ischaemia leading to acidosis and chest pain (angina pectoris). Angina can be relieved by nitrodilator drugs like glyceryl trinitrate which causes peripheral venodilatation and vasodilatation; this lowers the filling pressure and arterial pressure, which together reduce cardiac work and oxygen demand. β-adrenergic blockers like propranolol reduce oxygen demand by reducing heart rate and contractility.

Assessment of the human coronary circulation

The site of an atheromatous obstruction in a major coronary artery can be located by arteriography (coronary angiography), usually as a preliminary to vascular surgery. Blood flow can be measured more quantitatively by the coronary sinus thermodilution method, in which the sinus is cannulated, a bolus of cold saline injected and temperature recorded downstream (see Section 6.2 for thermodilution principle). To assess the evenness of myocardial perfusion, a γ-emitting isotope such as thallium is injected at the root of the aorta and the isotope's appearance in myocardium is followed by an external γ-camera. Images of slices across the isotope-laden myocardium (tomograms) can be generated with this technique. Positron emission tomography (PET) is another method for imaging myocardial perfusion, but it is available in very few centres. A summary of the coronary circulation is given in Table 13.1.

Table 13.1 Summary of coronary circulation

Special tasks
Maintain a high basal oxygen supply.
Oxygen supply must keep pace with cardiac work

Structural adaptation
High capillary density, short diffusion path

Functional adaptation
High oxygen extraction (>60%).
Metabolic vasodilatation dominant controlling factor

Special problems
Functional end-arteries, so risk of infarction and angina
Mechanical interference during systole

Measurement in man
Coronary angiography for sites of stenosis
Coronary sinus thermal dilution method for absolute flow
Isotope imaging for distribution of perfusion

13.2 Circulation through skeletal muscle

Flow in resting tonic (postural) muscle:
about $15\,\mathrm{ml\,min^{-1}\,100\,g^{-1}}$
Flow in resting phasic muscle:
3–$5\,\mathrm{ml\,min^{-1}\,100\,g^{-1}}$
Maximal flow during phasic exercise:
>100–$200\,\mathrm{ml\,min^{-1}\,100\,g^{-1}}$

The circulations of skeletal muscle and cardiac muscle have much in common, for example the predominance of metabolic control, but there are also some marked differences, such as the greater role of cardiovascular reflexes in the regulation of resting skeletal muscle flow.

Special tasks

1. During exercise, the circulation must deliver oxygen and glucose to the muscle fibres at an increased rate and remove waste products and heat at an increased rate.
2. The regulation of arterial pressure is a less obvious but very important duty of the skeletal muscle vasculature. Skeletal muscle constitutes about 40% of the adult body mass, and the resistance of this large vascular bed has a substantial effect on blood pressure.

Structural adaptation

Most human muscle fibres are phasically-active white fibres (twitch fibres), as in the forearm and gastrocnemius muscles. About 15% of human fibres, however, are tonically-active red fibres (slow fibres), and these predominate in postural muscles like the soleus. They are continuously active during the maintenance of posture and have a higher blood flow and capillary density than phasic muscle.

Functional adaptation

Importance of sympathetic vasoconstrictor innervation Skeletal muscle arterioles are richly innervated by sympathetic vasoconstrictor fibres whose tonic discharge enhances arteriolar tone in resting muscle. Muscle blood flow doubles after sympathetic denervation, but can increase 20 times or more during functional hyperaemia. This difference shows that there is a very high level of basal tone of non-neural origin. A high arteriolar tone is of course a prerequisite if dilatation (loss of tone) is to be possible. The vasoconstrictor nerve activity is controlled reflexly by blood pressure receptors in the thorax and neck (see Chapter 14), and when vasoconstrictor activity is increased by these reflexes (as in orthostasis and hypovolaemia) the resistance of the muscle circulation increases. Aided by similar changes in the splanchnic and renal circulations this is important for the regulation of arterial pressure. After a severe haemorrhage the vasoconstrictor discharge to skeletal muscle reaches its maximum rate, namely 6–10 per s, and flow is reduced to around one-fifth the normal level – an exceedingly low perfusion indeed.

Dominance of metabolic vasodilatation during exercise During strenuous exercise the mean flow through phasic muscle can increase more than 20-fold. In some muscle groups maximal flow can exceed 2 litres/kg; indeed, if all the muscle groups were maximally vasodilated at the same time the output capacity of the heart would be greatly exceeded. During strenuous exercise the muscle blood flow accounts for up to 80–90% of the cardiac output (cf. 18% at rest). The muscle hyperaemia is due almost entirely to a fall in vascular resistance occasioned by metabolic vasodilatation, rather than to the relatively modest rise in arterial pressure. The concomittant dilatation of the conduit and feeding arteries is covered in Section 12.3.

As in myocardium, the flow increases almost linearly with local metabolic rate, and the nature of the vasodilator agents is again controversial. During the first few minutes of exercise, *potassium ions* released by the contracting muscle raise the interstitial potassium concentration to as much as 9 mM, which can produce near maximal vasodilatation in some muscles (see Section 12.2 for mechanisms). The clearance of potassium into the blood stream causes a gradual rise in arterial plasma potassium from approximately 4 mM (rest) to as high as 7 mM in intense exercise. A rise in interstitial *osmolarity* contributes to vasodilatation in the early stages of exercise; the venous effluent osmolarity can increase by 20–30 mOsm. Inorganic *phosphate* is released by contracting muscle too and contributes to the hyperaemia. The vasodilator effect of these factors is potentiated by local *hypoxia*. Together these various factors (K^+, phosphate, osmolarity and local hypoxia) probably account for much of the early hyperaemia of exercise. Osmolarity falls again during prolonged exercise, however, and there are conflicting reports on the potassium levels over long periods, so it is far from clear what maintains the vasodilata-

tion during prolonged exercise. A possible contribution by *adenosine* is controversial.

Only about a third of the capillaries in resting skeletal muscle is well perfused at any one instant (Figure 13.1). Metabolic vasodilatation increases the well-perfused fraction by dilating the terminal arterioles. This 'capillary recruitment' shortens the extravascular diffusion distances and thus speeds up the exchange process (see Figure 9.16 for the Krogh cylinder model of this process).

Variable oxygen extraction and 'oxygen debt' Resting skeletal muscle extracts only 25–30% of the oxygen from blood, whereas in severe exercise the extraction can reach 80–90%. The extraction is helped by the presence of myoglobin in muscle fibres, as described in Section 9.10. Intracellular oxygen tension, which is 20 mmHg or less even at rest, falls so low in severe exercise that anaerobic glycolysis begins to predominate and lactic acid production increases. The quantity of lactate formed is an index of the deficit in oxygen supply and this 'oxygen debt' can reach several litres. The local lactic acidosis stimulates nociceptive C fibres, as also does the increased interstitial K^+ concentration, causing pain and the termination of violent exercise. The lactate also stimulates muscle 'work receptors' involved in the reflex control of the circulation (see Chapter 14). At the end of the exercise a period of post exercise hyperaemia resupplies the muscle with oxygen (which takes only seconds) and more gradually washes out the accumulated lactate and other vasodilator substances (see Figure 12.10). Only a little of the lactate is oxidized locally; most diffuses into the bloodstream, as a result of which plasma lactate can increase from 0.5 mM (resting level) to as much as 20 mM in extreme exercise, lowering plasma pH from 7.4 to 6.9. The circulating lactate is then either taken up by the liver for resynthesis into glycogen or by the heart as a primary substrate.

The skeletal muscle pump Although exercise hyperaemia is due chiefly to a fall in vascular resistance, the massaging effect of rhythmic muscle contraction on the deep veins assists limb perfusion, particularly in the calf. In a standing, stationary adult the arterial and venous pressures in the calf are each elevated by approximately 70 mmHg (effect of gravity), to approximately 165 mmHg and 80 mmHg, respectively, giving a calf perfusion pressure (pressure difference) of 85 mmHg. During walking, etc., the muscle pump lowers the venous pressure to approximately 35 mmHg (Figure 13.5), which increases the pressure drop driving flow to 130 mmHg (i.e. 165 − 35), an increase of over 50%.

Two other special adaptations of the skeletal muscle circulation are the sympathetic vasodilator nerves found in certain species (see Section 12.5), and the vasodilator response of skeletal muscle arterioles to adrenaline (Section 12.6).

Special problems

Mechanical interference When skeletal muscle contracts at more than 30–70% of its maximum voluntary force, it compresses the intramuscular vessels sufficiently to impair the blood flow. In rhythmic exercise such as walking, this causes blood flow to oscillate (see Figure 12.9). In a sustained strong contraction, however, the impairment of flow is maintained. Since the store of oxygen

in the muscle's myoglobin is only sufficient for 5–10 s, the fibres quickly become hypoxic and lactate accumulates, leading to pain and fatigue. The rapid loss of strength during a strong sustained contraction will be familiar to anyone who has struggled along with a heavy suitcase.

Fluid translocation across capillaries The problem of fluid translocation across capillaries in exercising muscle, leading to a 10–15% fall in plasma volume, was described in Section 10.9.

Measurement of human muscle blood flow

The soft tissue of a human limb is mainly skeletal muscle, and the limb blood flow can be measured by venous occlusion plethysmography (Figures 8.4 and 12.10) or by a Doppler velocity meter over the principal artery (as in Figure 12.9). Local capillary perfusion rate can be estimated by the Kety tissue clearance method (see Figure 8.5) following an intramuscular injection of xenon-133. A summary of the circulation through skeletal muscle is given in Table 13.2.

13.3 Cutaneous circulation

Flow in a thermoneutral environment (27°C): 10–20 ml min^{-1} 100 g^{-1}
Minimal flow: 1 ml min^{-1} 100 g^{-1}
Maximal flow: 150–200 ml min^{-1} 100 g^{-1}

The skin of a human adult weighs 2–3 kg; its area is approximately 1.8 m^2 and its thickness 1–2 mm (epidermis and dermis combined). In contrast to the coronary circulation where metabolic rate dominates blood flow, the skin's metabolic requirements are modest, and blood flow is primarily controlled by sympathetic fibres whose activity is linked to temperature regulation.

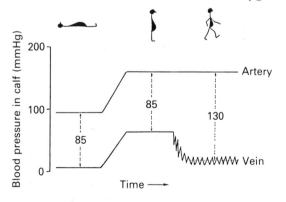

Figure 13.5 Effect of posture and muscle pump on pressure gradient driving blood through calf

Table 13.2 Summary of circulation through skeletal muscle

Special tasks
    Delivery of oxygen and nutrients in proportion to exercise intensity
    Contributes to homeostasis of arterial pressure

Structural adaptation
    High capillary density in tonic (postural) muscle

Functional adaptation
    Participates in vascular reflexes
    Metabolic vasodilatation dominant during exercise
    Vasodilator response to adrenaline
    Skeletal muscle pump
    Variable oxygen extraction

Special problems
    Mechanical interference during contraction
    Increased capillary filtration in exercise

Measurement in man
    Venous occlusion plethysmography
    Doppler velocity meter
    Kety's isotope clearance method

In a thermoneutral environment, namely 27–28°C for a naked man, skin temperature is around 33°C and core temperature is 37–37.5°C. Under these comfortable conditions the blood vessels of the *hands and feet* are subject to a high degree of tonic, sympathetic vasoconstrictor tone. In the skin of the *limbs and trunk*, by contrast, there is only very slight sympathetic vasoconstrictor activity when the subject is comfortably warm. This is proved by the hyperaemia of the extremities but not the limbs that follow surgical sympathectomy or a local nerve block.

Special tasks

1. Regulation of internal temperature. The temperature of the human 'core' (brain, thoracic and abdominal organs) is normally kept within a degree or so of 37°C.

This is achieved by balancing the internal heat production with the heat loss from the surface. The surface in question depends on the species: it is the skin in man, the tongue in dogs and the ears in rabbits. Heat is lost by four processes: radiation, conduction, convection and evaporation (Figure 13.6). With *radiation*, the rate of heat loss is proportional to the difference between ambient temperature and skin temperature. Skin temperature is influenced by the rate at which blood delivers heat from the core, i.e. by blood flow. In *conduction–convection*, warm skin heats up the adjacent air by conduction, and the warmed air is removed by convection (air currents). Again the rate of heat loss increases as a function of skin temperature. In the *evaporation of sweat*, 2.4 kJ of heat energy are consumed per gram of water evaporated (latent heat of evaporation), and both the water and heat are delivered to the skin by the blood. Cutaneous blood flow is thus a key factor in each case. The skin itself is a poikilothermic (variable temperature) not homeothermic tissue, and over short periods it can tolerate temperatures as extreme as 0°C and 45°C without damage.

2. Protection against the environment is the other major role of skin, and the circulation plays a part here too by dilating in response to trauma.

Structural adaptation: the arteriovenous anastomosis

Certain areas termed 'acral skin' possess abundant direct connections between dermal arterioles and venules. These are called arteriovenous anastomoses (AVAs, Figure 13.6). They occur at exposed sites with a high surface area/volume ratio, namely the fingers and toes, palm and sole, lips, nose, ears and, in panting animals, the tongue. AVAs, which were first discovered in the rabbit ear by R. T. Grant in 1930, are coiled, muscular-walled vessels of average diameter 35 μm. They have little basal tone

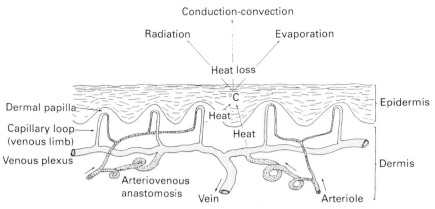

Figure 13.6 Sketch illustrating dermal vasculature and heat flux in an extremity. Arterial system stippled. See text for details

and are controlled almost exclusively by sympathetic vasoconstrictor fibres, whose activity is controlled by a temperature-regulating centre in the hypothalamus. When core temperature is high, vasomotor drive is reduced and the AVAs dilate. Being much wider than the terminal arterioles or capillaries, the dilated AVAs offer a low-resistance shunt pathway, which increases the cutaneous blood flow and delivers more heat to the skin. Heat readily crosses the walls of the dermal venous plexus that is fed by the AVAs, so skin temperature rises and heat loss increases. Conversely, AVAs are constricted to conserve heat under cold conditions. It is worth reiterating that the *dilatation* of AVAs *increases* heat loss, since students sometimes believe the opposite. The following 'aide memoire' might well have been sung by the mud-loving hippopotamus in Flanders and Swan's famous song:

A – V – A's, let 'em flood,
Nothing quite like them
For cooling the blood.
So dilate them widely,
Let's lose heat right blithely –
But close them up tightly
When chill is the mud.

Functional adaptation

The response of skin blood flow to temperature is mediated by several different mechanisms: (1) ambient temperature influences skin temperature, which directly influences cutaneous vessel tone, (2) ambient temperature alters the activity of skin temperature receptors and this initiates a weak spinal reflex evoking changes in sympathetic vasoconstrictor activity to the skin, and (3) core temperature is sensed by receptors in the brain, which powerfully modulate the sympathetic discharge to the skin.

Direct responsiveness to ambient temperature Local heating of the skin causes dilatation of the cutaneous arterioles, venules and small veins, and the skin reddens due to an increase on the volume of well-oxygenated blood in the dermal venular plexus. Conversely, local cooling to 10–15°C causes vasoconstriction and venoconstriction, which conserves heat (Figure 13.7a). The underlying mechanisms were described in Section 12.2.

The constriction of the large vein on the back of the hand in cold weather is easily seen, and this superficial venoconstriction diverts returning blood away from the cold surface into the deep veins. In the flippers of whales and the feet of wading birds, this is developed into

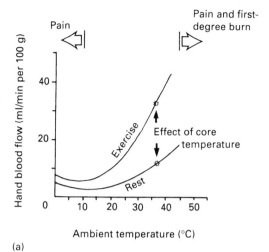

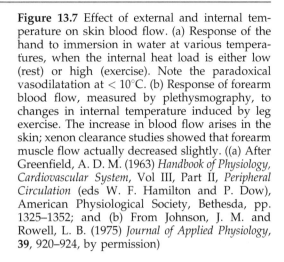

(a)

Figure 13.7 Effect of external and internal temperature on skin blood flow. (a) Response of the hand to immersion in water at various temperatures, when the internal heat load is either low (rest) or high (exercise). Note the paradoxical vasodilatation at < 10°C. (b) Response of forearm blood flow, measured by plethysmography, to changes in internal temperature induced by leg exercise. The increase in blood flow arises in the skin; xenon clearance studies showed that forearm muscle flow actually decreased slightly. ((a) After Greenfield, A. D. M. (1963) *Handbook of Physiology, Cardiovascular System*, Vol III, Part II, *Peripheral Circulation* (eds W. F. Hamilton and P. Dow), American Physiological Society, Bethesda, pp. 1325–1352; and (b) From Johnson, J. M. and Rowell, L. B. (1975) *Journal of Applied Physiology*, **39**, 920–924, by permission)

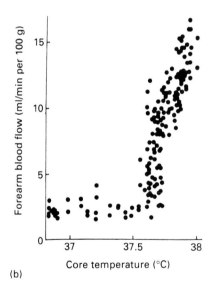

(b)

an elaborate countercurrent heat-conserving mechanism. The cool cutaneous blood from the extremity drains into deep veins, and the deep veins ramify around the limb artery so that heat can pass directly from the warm arterial blood into the cool venous blood. The extremity is thus fed precooled arterial blood, and heat-loss is reduced. The same short-circuiting of heat occurs in human limbs too, though to a lesser degree.

When the hand is placed in water at 10°C or less there is an initial cold-induced vasoconstriction followed by an increasingly painful sensation. After 5–10 min a dilatation sets in, with reddening of the skin and relief of pain – the 'paradox' of cold-induced vasodilatation (see Figure 13.7a). *Paradoxical cold vasodilatation* occurs in regions rich in AVAs and accounts for the cold, red noses and hands seen in frosty weather. The cause of the vasodilatation is thought to be a paralysis of noradrenergic transmission. Its value lies in preventing skin damage during prolonged exposure to cold, and the response is particularly well developed in manual workers in cold climates such as

Arctic Indians and Norwegian fishermen. If the exposure to cold persists, vasoconstriction recurs after a while and cutaneous perfusion oscillates with a 15–20 min cycle time (the 'hunting reaction').

Vasomotor reflexes initiated by skin temperature receptors If skin blood flow is measured in one hand while the opposite hand is immersed in cold water, a modest vasoconstriction is observed in the unimmersed hand. This is a sympathetically-mediated spinal reflex initiated by temperature receptors in the immersed hand.

Regulation of cutaneous perfusion by the hypothalamic temperature-regulating centre The activity of cutaneous vasomotor nerves is to a large extent governed by core temperature. Core temperature is sensed by warmth receptors in the anterior hypothalamus, and these hypothalamic neurons influence the brainstem neurons that control sympathetic vasomotor discharge to the skin. They also control the neurons governing sweating, i.e. the sympathetic cholinergic sudomotor nerves. In this way, a rise in core temperature leads to cutaneous vasodilatation (see Figure 13.7b) and sweating.

In regions containing AVAs, vasodilatation is due mainly to inhibition of sympathetic vasoconstrictor discharge to the AVAs. (Sympathetic vasoconstrictor drive is high in these regions at normal core temperature.) In regions lacking AVAs, namely the limbs, trunk and scalp, sympathetic vasoconstrictor drive is negligible at normal core temperature. Here dilatation is associated with sweating and is due mainly to an active sympathetic vasodilator discharge, for it is abolished by local nerve block (Figure 13.8). This 'active' vasodilatation is impaired but not abolished by atropine, and is probably mediated partly by VIP. Thus the effector side of the core temperature reflex is mediated in acral regions (e.g. hand) by adjustment of sympathetic vasoconstrictor activity and in other regions (e.g. forearm) mainly by adjustment of sympathetic vasodilator activity.

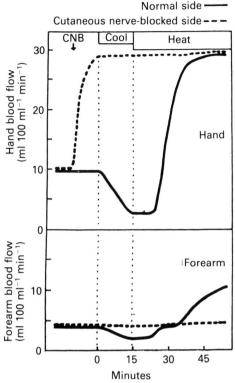

Figure 13.8 Contrast between cutaneous vascular control in human hand and arm. Dashed line shows effect of cutaneous vasomotor nerve block by local anaesthetic (CNB). Cooling or heating was indirect (legs in cold/hot water), with the upper limbs exposed to room temperature. In the forearm, the main vasodilatation evoked by a rise in core temperature is delayed and associated with onset of sweating. See text for explanation. (After Roddie, I. C. (1983), see Further Reading)

Overall, the cutaneous response is finely graded: small central heat-loads lead to hyperaemia chiefly in the hands, feet and facial extremities, while higher heat loads (core temperatures above 37.5°C) recruit the skin of the limbs and trunk. Maximum cutaneous vasodilatation produces blood flows in excess of 5 litres/min in a 70 kg man. This necessitates a substantial rise in cardiac output and also a compensatory vasoconstriction in the splanchnic, renal and skeletal muscle circulations (to maintain blood pressure). If strenuous exercise is undertaken in a hot environment, the massive hyperaemia in both skin and muscle lowers the peripheral resistance greatly, and at the same time plasma volume declines due to sweating and fluid filtration into exercising muscle. As a result, the capacity of the heart to maintain blood pressure can be exceeded leading to hypotension and collapse (*heat exhaustion*).

In a cold environment, by contrast, cutaneous blood flow falls as low as approximately $1\,\text{ml/min}^{-1}\,100\,\text{g}^{-1}$, which is only $20\,\text{ml/min}$ for the entire body surface. This allows the full insulating action of the subcutaneous fat to operate, and protects the core temperature. If the vasoconstrictor response is prevented by inflammatory vasodilatation, as can happen with severe eczema and psoriasis, temperature regulation becomes very unstable and can even necessitate hospitalization.

Role in regulation of arterial pressure and CVP The cutaneous circulation participates in many cardiovascular reflexes. *Hypotension*, caused by hypovolaemia or acute cardiac failure (shock), elicits a constriction of the cutaneous veins and arterioles producing the pale, cold skin characteristic of shock. The vasoconstriction is due to neural reflexes and to the hormones angiotensin, vasopressin and adrenaline (which causes constriction, not dilatation, in skin). The rise in cutaneous vascular resistance helps to support arterial pressure, while the venoconstriction displaces blood centrally and helps to support central venous pressure. The life-preserving value of these responses became clear on the battlefields of France during World War I, when it was noticed that wounded men who were rescued quickly and warmed in blankets (producing cutaneous dilatation) survived severe haemorrhages less successfully than the men who could not be reached for some time and were allowed, inadvertently, to retain their natural cutaneous vasoconstriction.

Exercise initially evokes a sympathetically mediated vasoconstriction in skin, but this later can change to dilatation if core temperature rises. Stimuli that elicit a *defence*

(alerting) response, such as mental arithmetic, cause a transient cutaneous vasoconstriction. So too does *deep inspiration.*

Dependency below heart level causes a strong vasoconstriction in the dependent skin (see Figures 8.5 and 10.5); cutaneous blood flow in the dependent foot falls to under a third of the supine value. The vasoconstriction seems to be caused by local rather than central mechanisms, namely the myogenic response and perhaps also a 'sympathetic axon reflex'. The latter view arose from the finding that dependent vasoconstriction is greatly reduced by sympathectomy and by local anaesthesia.

Reduction of *intra-thoracic blood volume* (by lower-body negative pressure in the laboratory) evokes a reflex sympathetic-mediated vasoconstriction in skin. The sensors might be the cardiopulmonary group of stretch receptors (next chapter). Whether arterial baroreceptors are involved is controversial, because direct recording from human cutaneous sympathetic nerves shows no change in activity upon stimulating the baroreceptor nerve in the neck.

Skin, mirror of the soul Poets and playwrights have long emphasized the responsiveness of the skin to emotion – we blush with embarrassment and blanch in response to stress or fear (defence response, above)*. Blushing is ill-understood because it is difficult to produce on demand. Folkow and Neil in their classic text *The Circulation*, recall how they were unable to make a

---

*Juliet was evidently a blusher. Her nurse, announcing Romeo's desire to marry her, remarked:

There stays a husband to make you a wife:
Now comes the wanton blood up in your cheeks,
They'll be in scarlet straight at any news.
(Romeo and Juliet, Act 2, Sc. 5)

Emotional trauma has the opposite effect; when Salisbury tells King Richard of his army's desertion, the King pales, crying:

But now the blood of twenty thousand men
Did triumph in my face, and they are fled;
And, till so much blood thither comes again,
Have I not reason to look pale and dead?
(Richard II, Act 3, Sc. 2)

habitual blusher blush in a laboratory setting, either by insults or rude jokes, but when they disconnected their equipment and thanked the subject, she blushed violently. Blushing is often associated with emotional sweating, so it might be mediated by a similar mechanism, namely activation of sympathetic vasodilator fibres. A hyperaemic response to emotional stimuli is not confined to skin, having been observed in the gastric and colonic mucosa too.

Response to injury The Lewis triple response (Section 12.5) illustrates the cutaneous vascular response to trauma. The ensuing hyperaemia and increased capillary permeability enhance the delivery of the defensive elements (white cells and immunoglobulins) to the injured tissue.

Special problems

Mechanical interference Skin gets sat on, stood on and leaned on for long periods, and such compression impairs its blood flow. Ischaemic damage is normally prevented by the high tolerance of skin to hypoxia, combined with *reactive hyperaemia* on removal of the external stress, plus the onset of restlessness. The urge to shift position is attributed to metabolites accumulating and stimulating skin nociceptors. The involvement of nociceptive nerves (which contain the vasodilators substance P and CGRP) may also explain why reactive hyperaemia is greatly reduced after applying local anaesthetic cream to the skin. Relief of pressure by movement fails to operate, however, in certain categories of patient, namely paraplegics, the elderly, the enfeebled and the comatose. If such patients are not turned regularly they can develop severe ischaemic necrosis of the skin in the weight-bearing area (*bed sores*).

Problems during hot weather Dilatation of cutaneous veins in a hot environment can lower the central venous pressure and thereby predispose the subject to postural fainting, the classic example being the guardsman who faints while standing at attention in hot weather. Cutaneous vasodilatation also increases the local capillary filtration pressure leading to interstitial swelling. This is why a ring often feels tighter on the finger during hot weather.

Measurement of human cutaneous blood flow

Measurements of skin surface temperature (thermography) have been used as an index of flow but this is unreliable, because skin temperature depends on ambient temperature as well as blood flow. Venous occlusion plethysmography of a digit is often used as a measure of skin blood flow. Kety's isotope clearance technique can be used to measure nutritive flow, and the new laser-Doppler method is gaining popularity as a rapid semi-quantitative measurement of superficial flow. A summary of the cutaneous circulation is given in Table 13.3.

Table 13.3 Summary of cutaneous circulation

Special tasks
  Temperature regulation
  Response to trauma

Structural adaptation
  Arteriovenous anastomoses in extremities

Functional adaptation
  Sympathetic control dominant and regulated by core temperature receptors
  Vessel tone also directly sensitive to local temperature
  Dependent vasoconstriction by local mechanisms
  Reflex vaso- and venoconstriction in response to hypotensive shock
  Triple response to cutaneous trauma

Special problems
  Compression when weight-bearing; bed sores
  Hot weather causes local swelling and venodilatation, aggravating postural hypotension

Measurement in man
  Digital plethysmography
  Kety's isotope clearance method
  Laser-Doppler flow probe

13.4 Cerebral circulation

> Average flow (whole brain): 55 ml min^{-1} 100 g^{-1}
> Basal flow to grey matter: 100 ml min^{-1} 100 g^{-1}

The adult human brain forms about 2% of the body mass and consists of 40% grey matter (mostly neurons) and 60% white matter (mostly myelinated tracts). The brain receives 14% of the resting cardiac output and most of this goes to the grey matter. One peculiarity of the cerebral circulation is that the arterioles are rather short and the arteries account for an unusually high proportion of the vascular resistance, namely 40–50%. These arteries receive a rich autonomic innervation.

Special tasks

1. Need for a totally secure oxygen supply. Grey matter has a very high rate of oxidative metabolism, and its oxygen consumption (approximately 7 ml min^{-1} 100 g^{-1}) accounts for nearly 20% of human oxygen consumption at rest. Grey matter is exquisitely sensitive to hypoxia and in man consciousness is lost after just a few seconds of cerebral ischaemia, with irreversible cell damage following within minutes. The primary task of the cerebral circulation, and indeed of the entire cardiovascular system, is therefore to secure an uninterrupted delivery of oxygen to the brain.
2. Adjustment of local supply to local demand. Many mental functions are localized in well-defined regions; for example, visual interpretation is located in the occipital visual cortex. External monitoring of the uptake of radiolabelled glucose and oxygen in the human brain has proved that local neuronal activity increases the local metabolic rate. Illumination of the retina, for example, increases the metabolic rate of the occipital visual cortex. The cerebral circulation must therefore be capable of regional adjustment to meet the varying metabolic rate of each region.

Structural adaptation

1. The circle of Willis. The arteries that enter the cranial cavity (the basilar and internal carotid arteries) anastomose around the optic chiasma to form a complete arterial circle, called the circle of Willis. (The young assistant employed by Thomas Willis to illustrate the circle later designed St. Paul's cathedral in London, being Christopher Wren.) The anterior, middle and posterior cerebral arteries all arise from the circle of Willis, and this arrangement ought in principle to preserve cerebral perfusion even when one carotid artery becomes obstructed. This is so in young subjects, but in elderly subjects the anastomoses are less effective. The main cerebral arteries divide into pial arteries running over the surface of the brain from where finer arteries penetrate into the parenchyma and give rise to the short arterioles.
2. High capillary density. Grey matter contains on average 3000–4000 capillaries per mm^2 cross-section (similar to myocardium). This provides a large exchange area and minimizes the extravascular diffusion distance.

Functional adaptation

High basal blood flow The grey matter receives about 100 ml blood min^{-1} 100 g^{-1}, more than 10 times the average for the whole body, and it extracts about 35% of the delivered oxygen.

Protection of cerebral blood flow by reflex control of other circulations Cerebral blood flow, like that to other tissues, depends on vascular conductance and arterial pressure. Unlike any other organ, however, the brain is able to safeguard its own blood supply by controlling the cardiac output and the vascular resistance of other organs via its autonomic outflow. Perfusion of peripheral organs (except the heart) is sacrificed to preserve cerebral perfusion, when necessary.

Cerebral autoregulation Autoregulation is very well developed in the brain; a fall in blood pressure causes the resistance vessels to dilate and thereby maintain flow (Figure 13.9). Below approximately 50 mmHg, however, autoregulation fails and cerebral blood flow declines steeply, leading to mental confusion and syncope. The upper limit of autoregulation is probably around 175 mmHg. Cerebral autoregulation seems to involve both myogenic and metabolic mechanisms (Section 12.3).

Sensitivity to arterial carbon dioxide and hypoxia Cerebral vessels have a well-developed response to arterial carbon dioxide: hypercapnia causes vasodilatation and hypocapnia vasoconstriction (Figure 13.9). If

arterial P_{CO_2} is reduced to 15 mmHg by hyperventilation (normal value is 40 mmHg), cerebral blood flow halves and vasoconstriction can be observed directly in the retina, the retina being embryologically an extension of the brain. Owing to the vasoconstriction, hysterical hyperventilation in adults, or hyperventilation 'for fun' by children, can lead to disturbed vision, dizziness and even fainting. The traditional remedy is to hold the opening of a paper bag (not plastic) in front of the mouth and so compel rebreathing of expired carbon dioxide.

Cerebral vessels dilate in response to local hypoxia, but if the arterial blood is hypoxic it stimulates ventilation too, and the ensuing hypocapnia causes vasoconstriction.

There is recent evidence that cerebral vasodilatation by hypercapnia and hypoxia is mediated to a large extent by endothelial NO formation. Hypercapnia may also act to some degree by raising interstitial H^+ concentration (carbonic acid) in the vessel walls. The lack of effect of lactic acid has been attributed to its inability to cross the blood-brain barrier.

Regional functional hyperaemia in the brain It has long been known that shining a light onto one retina causes a rise in temperature in the corresponding occipital cortex. This was an early clue that neuronal activation may evoke a local increase in blood flow. Deeper parts of the visual pathway, such as the lateral geniculate body, also display active hyperaemia. More recently, computer-assisted isotope imaging techniques have greatly extended our knowledge of active hyperaemia in the human cortex. Radioactive xenon-133 solution is injected into the internal carotid artery and its arrival and washout in the brain are monitored externally by an array of over 200 gamma-counters, each covering $1\,cm^2$ of skull. The rate of arrival and washout of the xenon is proportional to the local cortical blood flow, and the local counts can be converted by computer into a colour-coded map of regional flow. This has not only enabled

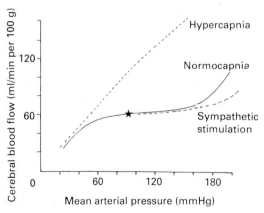

Figure 13.9 Autoregulation of brain blood flow at normal arterial P_{CO_2} (solid line); star represents normal operating point. Flow in the autoregulated range changes by only approximately 6% per 10 mmHg. High carbon dioxide tension causes vasodilatation (upper dashed line). Sympathetic nerve stimulation only affects flow significantly when arterial pressure is abnormally high (lower dashed line). (After Heistad, D. D. and Kontos, H. A. (1983), see Further Reading)

flow to be studied but has also led to the localization of sites of mental function in the conscious human brain (Figure 13.10).

The cause of cortical metabolic hyperaemia is in part an increase in interstitial K^+ concentration, which can rise from its normal level of 3 mM to as much as 10 mM owing to outward currents from the active neurons. The mechanism of action of K^+ was described in Section 12.2. Other causative factors include a rise in interstitial H^+ concentration and adenosine concentration, secondary to increased neuronal metabolism.

Nervous innervation of intracerebral and extracerebral vessels The intracerebral arterioles are innervated rather poorly, whereas the cerebral arteries outside the substance of the brain are well innervated by sympathetic vasoconstrictor nerves. Participation of brain vessels in the baroreceptor reflex is, however, negligible, which is clearly a 'good thing' teleologically. The maximal cerebral response to cervical sympathetic stimulation in anaesthetized humans is a mere 37% rise in vascular resistance (cf. 500–600% in skeletal muscle). The cerebral vessels have a few α-adrenoreceptors and respond only weakly to noradrenaline. Sympathetic vasoconstriction is probably mediated chiefly by neuropeptide Y, which is abundant in cerebral sympathetic fibres. The role of the vasoconstrictor innervation may be to protect the blood-brain barrier against disruption should arterial pressure rise suddenly.

Perivascular nerve fibres also contain 5-hydroxytryptamine, possibly co-stored with noradrenaline. 5HT has a powerful vasoconstrictor effect on cerebral arteries and, along with a high K^+ level, is thought to contribute to the vasospasm that follows a subarachnoid haemorrhage. Release of 5HT is also thought to be the initial event in a migraine attack (see below).

Cerebral arteries are innervated by dilator fibres, probably of parasympathetic origin. They contain acetylcholine and VIP but their role is obscure. There are also abundant perivascular sensory fibres, which are

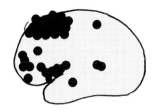

(a) Control:rest

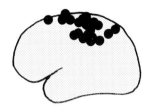

(b) Hand movement

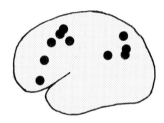

(c) Reasoning

Figure 13.10 Active hyperaemia in human cortex revealed by the xenon-133 imaging method (see text). The filled circles on the computer-calculated images show flows 20% above mean. In the resting, pensive subject (a) there is frontal lobe hyperaemia. On moving the contralateral hand voluntarily (b), there is hyperaemia of the hand area of the upper motor, premotor and sensory cortex. The reasoning test (c) evokes hyperaemia in the precentral and postcentral areas. (From Ingvar, D. H. (1976) *Brain Research*, **107**, 181–197 and Lassen, N. A. *et al.* (1978) see Further Reading, by permission)

thought to be the nociceptor fibres responsible for the vascular headache pain that accompanies strokes and migraines. The sensory fibres contain the vasodilator neuropeptides substance P and calcitonin-gene related peptide (CGRP), which in skin are implicated in antidromic vasodilatation (Section 12.5). Their role in the brain is unclear.

Blood–brain barrier Lipid-soluble molecules like oxygen, carbon dioxide and xenon diffuse freely between the plasma and brain interstitium, but ionic solutes like the dye Evans blue fail to penetrate from plasma into most regions of the brain, demonstrating the existence of a barrier to lipid-insoluble solutes (see Section 9.9). Because of the blood–brain barrier, the neuronal environment is the most tightly-controlled cellular environment in the body, and the neurons are protected from the fluctuating levels of ions (e.g. K^+) and catecholamines in the bloodstream. As J. Barcroft eloquently wrote in his book, *Architecture of Physiological Function*, 'To look for high intellectual development in a milieu whose properties have not become stabilized is to seek music among the crashings of a rudimentary wireless, or ripple patterns on the surface of the stormy Atlantic'. Another function of the barrier may be to conserve neuropeptides, which might otherwise partially wash away after release. The blood–brain barrier can be disrupted experimentally by hyperosmotic infusions, and is disrupted clinically by acute hypertension or cerebral ischaemia. There are a few regions where the barrier is normally absent, these being regions where plasma solutes have access to receptors (e.g. to the osmoreceptors in the circumventricular region and to vomiting-reflex chemosensors in the area postrema).

Special problems

Effect of gravity Gravity has no direct effect on cerebral flow during orthostasis because the cerebral circulation behaves like an inverted U-tube and the drag of gravity on the arterial limb is offset by the drag on the venous limb and on the cerebrospinal fluid (see Figure 8.19). Gravity does, however, influence cerebral blood flow indir-ectly, because central venous pressure and stroke volume are reduced in the upright posture. The ensuing postural hypotension can reduce cerebral flow to the point of dizziness or fainting (postural syncope) in the absence of brisk autonomic reflexes (see Chapter 15).

Effect of encasement in a rigid cranium Except in the neonate the brain is enclosed in a rigid box. Any space-occupying lesion, such as a cerebral tumour or haemorrhage, raises the intracranial pressure and forces the brainstem down into the foramen magnum (the large opening in the base of the skull admitting the spinal cord). As the brainstem becomes compressed, local neuronal activity causes a rise in sympathetic vasomotor drive, and thus a rise in arterial blood pressure (Cushing's reflex). The rise in blood pressure maintains the cerebral blood flow for a while, despite the raised intracranial pressure. The elevated blood pressure also evokes a bradycardia via the baroreceptor reflex, and the combination of bradycardia and acute hypertension is recognized by neurologists as the hallmark of a large, space-occupying lesion.

Migraine This condition is still not fully understood, but vascular changes are clearly an important feature. A visual prodroma (flickering wavy lines in part of the visual field) often precedes the headache and is caused by constriction of intracerebral vessels in the visual pathway. This is probably due to excessive local release of 5-hydroxytryptamine. The subsequent prolonged, severe headache is associated with dilatation of a large extracerebral vessel, such as the middle cerebral artery, and inflammation around it. Release of substance P, CGRP (present in perivascular sensory fibres) and prostaglandins coupled with local depletion of 5HT are thought to contribute to the dilatation. Substance P and 5HT both stimulate pain fibres.

Measurement of human cerebral blood flow

The qualitative technique of carotid angiography (arteriography) is widely used to assess the patency and course of major cerebral vessels. A transcranial Doppler velocity meter is on trial for more quantitative measurement of flow in major cerebral arteries. SPECT imaging (single photon emission compound tomography) is a recent development of the xenon-imaging method for assessing regional perfusion. A lipophilic, high energy γ-emitting isotope is injected into the arterial supply and is distributed within the brain in proportion to local blood flow. Owing to a chemical reaction within the brain, the radiolabelled solute is then trapped in the brain tissue for 4–6 h, thus 'freezing' a representation of the flow distribution. The pattern of distribution can then be mapped by using a large number of short-focus γ-cameras. This enables images of 'slices' through the brain to be generated (tomograms). A summary of cerebral circulation is given by Table 13.4.

13.5 Pulmonary circulation

The lung circulation differs very substantially from the various systemic circulations. The entire output of the right ventricle normally flows through the alveoli, so perfusion vastly exceeds their nutritional needs and metabolic factors exert no influence on flow. The metabolic needs of the bronchi are met by an independent systemic, bronchial circulation. There is only a low basal tone in the pulmonary circulation and no autoregulation. Sympathetic Vasomotor nerves exist but have no well-defined physiological role. The features of importance are as follows.

Very high capillary density

The density of the capillary network in the walls of alveoli is extraordinarily high; in-

Table 13.4 Summary of cerebral circulation

Special tasks
  Maintain oxygen supply to hypoxia-intolerant grey matter
  Adapt local perfusion to local activity

Structural adaptation
  Circle of Willis
  High capillary density
  Tight endothelial junctions (blood-brain barrier)

Functional adaptation
  High basal blood flow
  Brain controls heart and peripheral resistance to maintain its perfusion pressure
  Cerebral vessels 'excused' from baroreflex vasoconstriction
  Good autoregulation in face of pressure changes; sensitive to $P\text{CO}_2$
  Local metabolic hyperaemia in response to local cortical activity
  Blood-brain barrier provides a highly stable neuronal environment

Special problems
  Postural syncope if baroreflex impaired
  Space-occupying lesions lead to bulbar ischaemia

Measurement in man
  Carotid angiography
  Transcranial Dopplerimetry
  Xenon-133 uptake method
  SPECT imaging

spection of an exposed alveolus through the microscope reveals an almost continuous sheet of blood flowing through the septum, with very little tissue separating individual capillaries. The resulting huge capillary surface area (estimates go as high as 90–126 m² in an adult's lung), coupled with a diffusion distance of only 0.3 μm from the alveolar surface to plasma, produces a very high oxygen diffusion capacity. As a result, gas exchange in the lung normally falls into the category of 'flow-limited exchange' (Section 9.10), i.e. raising the pulmonary blood flow increases the rate of oxygen uptake in direct proportion to the rise in flow.

The volume of the adult pulmonary capillary bed is about 100 ml and blood traverses the pulmonary capillary in 0.8 s on average, at a cardiac output of 4800 ml/min. Because of the high diffusion capacity, this is more than enough time to allow equilibration of the blood gases with alveolar oxygen and carbon dioxide. This is true even in exercise in most individuals, despite a fall in capillary residence time to around 0.3 s. In some athletes performing extreme exercise, however, residence time in some pulmonary capillaries can fall to the point where diffusion -limited exchange is reached, leading to arterial hypoxaemia.

The extreme thinness of the blood–alveolar barrier, which is so essential to rapid gas exchange, is not without its disadvantages and even dangers. The physical stresses in the barrier are high due its extreme thinness, and if these are raised further by abnormally high pulmonary capillary pressures (as in mitral stenosis), disruption can occur, resulting in pulmonary oedema with alveolar haemorrhage. In the modern racehorse, pulmonary pressure rises to extreme values during racing (because of the very high cardiac output), namely 120 mmHg pulmonary arterial pressure and 70 mmHg left atrial pressure, which can lead to exercise-induced pulmonary haemorrhage.

Low vascular resistance and pressures

Pulmonary vascular resistance is about an eighth that of the systemic circulation so the pulmonary arterial pressure is normally low, typically 20–25 mmHg in systole and 8–12 mmHg in diastole. Pulmonary arteries and arterioles are shorter and have thinner, less muscular walls than systemic vessels. Consequently, although arterioles dominate vascular resistance in most systemic organs, resistance in the lungs is shared between the arterial vessels (30%), microvasculature (arterioles to venules, 50%) and veins (20%). The capillary pressure (8–11 mmHg) is therefore roughly midway between mean pulmonary arterial pressure (12–15 mmHg) and left atrial pressure (5–8 mmHg). The effect of the low capillary pressure on fluid balance was described in Section 10.6. Elevation of

the left atrial pressure to 20–25 mmHg raises capillary pressure sufficiently to create pulmonary oedema, but smaller rises are within the safety margin against oedema (Section 10.10).

Vertical distribution of blood flow

Blood flow is distributed unevenly in the lung of an upright subject (Figure 13.11). The mean pulmonary arterial pressure at heart level is around 15 mmHg, but owing to the effect of gravity the mean arterial pressure falls to about 3 mmHg at the apex of the lung and rises to 21 mmHg at the base of the lung. The high basal pressure distends the thin-walled vessels lowering their resistance and thus increasing flow through the base. Conversely, vessels at the apex actually collapse during diastole because diastolic pressure at heart level is only approximately 9 mmHg (13 cmH$_2$O) and this is insufficient to distend the apical vessels; the apex is typically 16 cm above heart level. Apical perfusion therefore occurs during systole and the mean apical flow is about a tenth the basal flow at rest. This is an important point, because the efficiency of oxygen transfer in the alveoli depends on the *ventilation/perfusion ratio*, which should ideally be 0.8–1.0. Although ventilation too is greater at the base than at the apex, the vertical variation in ventilation does not fully compensate for the vertical variation in flow. A standing subject, therefore, has a higher ventilation/perfusion ratio at the apex than the base, and this ventilation/perfusion mismatch slightly impairs the efficiency of blood oxygenation in the upright, resting subject. In addition the capillary blood flow is pulsatile, especially at the apex, so oxygen uptake is pulsatile. When a subject is supine, the apex-to-base gradients are abolished and the ventilation/perfusion ratio becomes more even throughout the lung.

Vasoconstrictor response to airway hypoxia

The lungs possess a mechanism that helps to optimize local ventilation/perfusion ratios. If

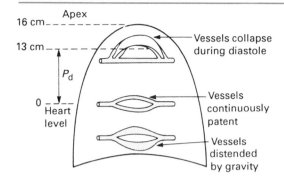

Figure 13.11 Vertical gradient of perfusion in an adult lung in the upright position. Scale on left shows vertical distance above heart level. Diastolic arterial pressure (P_d, 13 cmH$_2$O at heart level) falls to atmospheric pressure at 13 cm above heart level. Vessels higher than this are only perfused during systole. The vertical gradient has been demonstrated by injecting a radioisotope (xenon-133 or labelled microspheres) into the right heart and monitoring its arrival or deposition at various vertical positions by external gamma-counting

the ventilation to a local region falls or if local blood flow is increased, alveolar P_{O_2} falls and P_{CO_2} increases. Small pulmonary arteries pass close to the surface of the small airways and they respond to hypoxia by vasoconstriction, while the bronchiolar smooth muscle responds to airway hypercapnia by relaxation. Together these changes maintain a ventilation/perfusion ratio close to ideal.

Pulmonary hypoxic vasoconstriction is unusual, in that hypoxia has the opposite effect, dilatation, on systematic resistance vessels. The mechanism is not yet clear, but it has been found recently that (1) the slow, sustained contractile response of isolated pulmonary arteries to hypoxia is abolished by removal of endothelium. The endothelial factor involved appears to be neither NO nor a prostanoid nor endothelin. (An initial transient constriction to hypoxia shows less endothelium dependence but is likely to be of lesser importance.) Also, (2), pulmonary hypoxic vasoconstriction is substantially reduced by the adenosine antagonist, 8-phenyltheophylline, in rat lungs *in vivo*. Adenosine can produce vasoconstriction

rather than vasodilatation in the lung. Pulmonary hypoxic vasoconstriction may therefore turn out to be multifactorial. The phenomenon is important not only in minimizing ventilation/perfusion mismatch but also in medicine, where chronic hypoxia leads to pulmonary hypertension, as shown in Figure 13.12(b). Chronic pulmonary hypertension often leads to right heart failure.

Pressure–flow curve and the effect of exercise

Pulmonary vessels are essentially passive conduits and the downstream vessels in particular are distensible. When the pressure driving fluid through an isolated, perfused lung is raised, with pulmonary venous pressure set at left atrial level, the pressure–flow curve is slightly concave (Figure 13.12a, right-hand curve). This indicates that vascular conductance increases with perfusion pressure, due presumably to vessel distension. If airway pressure is above venous pressure, the curvature is more marked (left-hand curve). This is probably due to the opening up ('recruitment') by pressure of some venous vessels that were initially closed by the airway pressure.

In human subjects, the pressure–flow relation has been investigated during *supine exercise*. A supine posture ensures perfusion of the lung apices even at rest; any change in vascular conductance in supine exercise is therefore not due to recruitment of the apical vessels as pressure rises (as happens in upright exercise). Nevertheless, in fit but elderly subjects, the supine curve reveals an increase in vascular conductance as pressure rises during exercise (Figure 13.12b). This is attributed to the distending effect of the increase in pulmonary venous pressure that these subjects develop during the exercise. In younger subjects, by contrast, left atrial pressure remains nearly constant during moderate supine exerise, and the pulmonary pressure–flow relation is virtually a straight line that projects almost through the origin. This indicates that changes in pulmonary vascular resistance with cardiac output are not very great in supine exercise. Physical

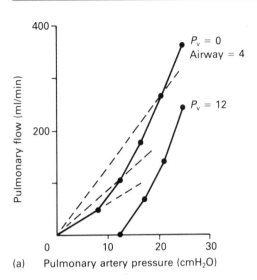

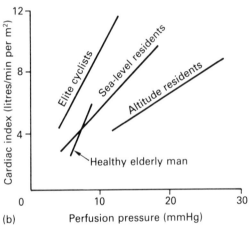

Figure 13.12 Pressure–flow relations for lung. (a) Isolated cat lung perfused with a plasma-dextran solution at varying arterial perfusion pressures. Venous pressure (P_v) was zero or $12\,cmH_2O$, and airway pressure was $4\,cmH_2O$. Dashed lines are lines of constant conductance; the lung curve cuts across lines of increasing conductance. (b) Conscious human subjects during 10-min periods of supine exercise. Perfusion pressure here means pulmonary artery pressure minus left atrial pressure. Venous pressures were greater than zero and airway pressure close to zero (atmospheric). For explanation, see text ((a) From Banister, R. J. and Torrance, R. W. (1960) *Quarterly Journal of Experimental Physiology*, **45**, 352–357 and (b) from Grover, R. F. *et al.* (1983), see Further Reading, by permission)

training by endurance athletes (top cyclists) produces a chronic increase in pulmonary vascular conductance.

During *upright exercise*, a modest rise in pulmonary artery pressure is beneficial, as it improves the perfusion of the apices and thereby increases the area of capillaries available for gas exchange. Exercise can increase the oxygen transfer capacity of the lungs by around 70%, partly due to a rise in the perfused capillary area (by up to 40%, to $90\,m^2$ in the adult lung), and partly due to an increase in capillary blood volume (from approximately 85 ml to approximately 180 ml). Increased capillary volume also prevents the blood's residence time in the capillary from becoming too brief – too brief, that is, for equilibration with alveolar gas.

Capacitance function of pulmonary vessels

Pulmonary blood volume is about 600 ml in a recumbent man. Because the pulmonary vessels are thin-walled, their compliance is high. If intrathoracic airway pressure is raised by a forced expiration against a closed glottis (the Valsalva manoeuvre), the external pressure on the vessels can expel up to half of the blood content. Conversely, forced inspiration, which lowers intrathoracic pressure, can increase the human pulmonary blood volume to about 1 litre. The high capacitance of the pulmonary circulation allows it to act as a variable blood reservoir; for example, the pulmonary capacitance vessels act as a transient source of blood for the left ventricle when output begins to increase at the start of exercise. The capacitance may be influenced by sympathetic vasoconstrictor nerve activity.

Metabolic functions of pulmonary endothelium

The entire cardiac output passes through the lungs and is therefore exposed to up to 90–$126\,m^2$ of endothelium. This provides the ideal opportunity for not only gas exchange but also the transformation or removal of vasoactive substances that have entered venous blood. The conversion of angiotensin

I to *angiotensin II* by ACE (angiotensin-converting enzyme) on the endothelial surface was described in Chapter 12. The same enzyme is responsible for the accelerated removal of *bradykinin* in the lung. A wide variety of other locally-acting vasoactive substances that leak into the venous blood are largely removed by the lungs; for example, *5-hydroxytryptamine* is 98% removed in a single pass, *prostaglandin E* and *leukotrienes* are removed, and *noradrenaline* is 30% removed during a single pass. True circulating hormones on the other hand, such as adrenaline and vasopressin, are not removed. There is also active, tonic production of NO by the endothelium.

Table 13.5 Summary of pulmonary circulation

Special tasks
  Respiratory gas exchange
  Metabolic conversion of circulating vasoactive
    substances by endothelium

Structural adaptation
  Extremely high capillary density and very short
    diffusion distance
  Low vascular resistance, so only modest rises in
    pulmonary vascular pressure when
    pulmonary flow (i.e. cardiac output) increases

Functional adaptation
  Hypoxic vasoconstriction helps match regional
    perfusion to regional ventilation

Special problems
  Because pulmonary arterial pressure is low,
    lung apices are poorly perfused in upright
    subject
  At extreme cardiac outputs (athletes), residence
    time in capillary can be 0.3 s or less
  Chronic hypoxic vasoconstriction can lead to
    right-sided cardiac failure
  Very thin capillary–alveolar barrier can become
    leaky, e.g. mitral stenosis

Measurement in man
  As for measurement of cardiac output, e.g. Fick
    principle, thermal dilution method

Further reading

Reviews and chapters

Bahkle, Y. S. (1990) Pharmacokinetic and metabolic properties of the lung. *British Journal of Anaesthesia*, **65**, 79

Berne, R. M. and Rubio, R. (1977) Coronary circulation. In *Handbook of Physiology, Cardiovascular System*, Vol. 1, *The Heart* (eds R. M. Berne and N. Sperelakis), American Physiological Society, Bethesda, pp 873–952

Edvinsson, L. (1985) Functional role of perivascular peptides in the control of cerebral circulation. *Trends in Neurosciences*, **8**, 126–131

Faraci, F. M. and Heistad, D. D. (1990) Regulation of large cerebral arteries and cerebral microvascular pressures. *Circulation Research*, **66**, 8–17

Feigl, E. O. (1983) Coronary physiology. *Physiological Reviews*, **63**, 1–205

Flanahan, N. A. (1991) The role of α-adrenoceptors as cutaneous thermosensors. *News in Physiological Sciences*, **6**, 251–255

Gorman, M. W. and Sparks, H. V. (1991) The unanswered question. (What is the dilator substance in exercise hyperaemia?) *News in Physiological Sciences*, **6**, 191–193

Grover, R. F., Wagner, W. W., McMurty, I. F. and Reeves, J. T. (1983) Pulmonary circulation. In *Handbook of Physiology, Cardiovascular System*, Vol. 3, *Peripheral Circulation* (eds J. T. Shepherd and F. M. Abboud), American Physiological Society, Bethesda, pp. 103–136

Heistad, D. D. and Kontos, H. A. (1983) Cerebral circulation. In *Handbook of Physiology, Cardiovascular System*, Vol. 3, *Peripheral Circulation*, Part 1 (eds J. T. Shepherd and F. M. Abboud), American Physiological Society, Bethesda, pp. 137–181

Hudlická, O. (1985) Regulation of muscle blood flow. *Clinical Physiology*, **5**, 201–229

Johnson, J. M., Brengelmann, G. L., Hales, J. R. S., Vanhoutte, P. M. and Wenger, C. B. (1986) Regulation of the cutaneous circulation. *Federal Proceedings*, **45**, 2841–2850

Lassen, N. A., Ingvar, D. H. and Skinhoj, E. (1978) Brain function and blood flow. *Scientific American*, **239**(4), 50–59

Mary, D. A. S. G. (1992) Reflex effects on the coronary circulation. *Experimental Physiology*, **77**, 243–270

Roddie, I. C. (1983) Circulation to skin and adipose tissue. In *Handbook of Physiology, Cardiovascular System*, Vol. 3, *Peripheral Circulation* (eds J. T. Shepherd and F. M. Abboud), American Physiological Society, Bethesda, pp. 285–317

Shepherd, J. T. (1983) Circulation to skeletal muscle. In *Handbook of Physiology, Cardiovascular System*, Vol. 3, *Peripheral Circulation*, Part 1 (eds J. T. Shepherd and F. M. Abboud), American Phsyiological Society, Bethesda, pp. 319–370

Sobel, B. E. (1988) Coronary artery and ischemic heart disease. In *Cardiovascular Pathophysiology* (ed. G. G. Ahumada), Oxford University Press, Oxford

West, J. B. and Mathieu-Costello, O. (1993) Pulmonary

blood-gas barrier : a physiological dilemma. *News in Physiological Sciences*, **8**, 249–253

Research papers

Beckenrath, N., Cyrys, S., Dischner, A. and Daut, J. (1991). Hypoxic vasodilatation in isolated perfused guinea-pig heart: an analysis of the underlying mechanism. *Journal of Physiology*, **442**, 297–319

Broten, T. P., Romson, J. L., Fullerton, D. A., Van Winkle, D. M. and Feigl, E. O. (1991) Synergistic action of myocardial O_2 and CO_2 in controlling coronary blood flow. *Circulation Research*, **68**, 531–542

Modin, A., Pernow, J. and Lundberg, J. M. (1993) Sympathetic regulation of skeletal muscle blood flow in the pig : a non-adrenergic component likely to be mediated by neuropeptide Y. *Acta Physiologica Scandinavica*, **148**, 1–11

Sahlin, K. and Broberg, S. (1989) Release of K^+ from muscle during prolonged exercise. *Acta Physiologica Scandinavica*, **136**, 293–294

Schelbert, H. R. and Buxton, D. (1988) Insights into coronary artery disease gained from metabolic imaging. *Circulation Research*, **78**, 496–505

Chapter 14

Cardiovascular receptors, reflexes and central control

14.1 **Arterial baroreceptors and the baroreflex**

14.2 **Cardiac and pulmonary receptors**

14.3 **Excitatory inputs: arterial chemoreceptors and muscle receptors**

14.4 **Central pathways**

14.5 **Summary**

Overview

The heart and blood vessels are controlled by sympathetic and parasympathetic nerves. The activity of these nerves is regulated and coordinated by the brain. The brain itself is guided by sensory information from peripheral receptors located both within the circulation and outside it. The three elements, namely afferent (sensory) fibres, central relays and efferent fibres, form reflex arcs, as illustrated in Figure 14.1. The two most important groups of sensors are pressure receptors around the walls of systemic arteries and pressure receptors within the walls of the heart. Together, the afferent fibres transmit information about arterial pressure and cardiac filling to the brainstem, where it is integrated with information from other sensors such as chemoreceptors and muscle receptors. The process of integration and the computation of an appropriate cardiovascular response involves considerable up-and-down traffic between the brainstem, hypothalamus, cerebellum and cortex. Sympathetic and parasympathetic outflows then initiate appropriate responses in the heart and blood vessels and these responses are often (but not inevitably) directed at stabilizing blood pressure. The reflex response to a rise in blood pressure, for example, is bradycardia and peripheral vasodilatation which tends to lower the blood pressure back to its control level.

14.1 Arterial baroreceptors and the baroreflex

The prefix 'baro-' means pressure. Baroreceptors are sprays of non-encapsulated nerve

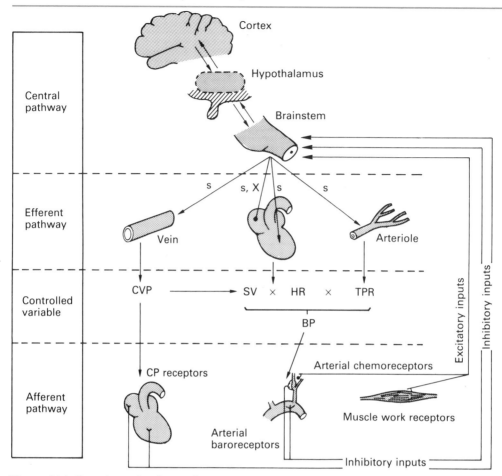

Figure 14.1 Overview of reflex and central control of the circulation. CP, cardiopulmonary receptor group (heterogeneous); CVP, central venous pressure; SV, stroke volume; HR, heart rate; TPR, total peripheral resistance; BP, arterial blood pressure; s, sympathetic fibres (noradrenergic); X, vagal cardiac fibres (cholinergic). Neuroendocrine reflexes and cerebellar relay are not shown. Terms 'inhibitory inputs' and 'excitatory inputs' refer to net effect of receptor activation on cardiac output and blood pressure

endings, packed with mitochondria. They are found in the adventitial layer of arteries at two main locations: the aortic arch and the carotid sinus (Figure 14.2). The *carotid sinus* is a thin-walled dilatation at the bottom of the internal carotid artery. The afferent fibres form the fine carotid sinus nerve and then ascend in the glossopharyngeal nerve (IXth cranial nerve) to the petrous ganglion, where the parent cells are located. Like all afferent neurons, the petrous ganglion cells are bipolar and their centrally-directed axons continue with the glossopharyngeal nerve to enter the brainstem, where they terminate in the nucleus tractus solitarius (see later). The *aortic baroreceptors* are located mainly around the transverse arch of the aorta and their fibres form the aortic or 'depressor' nerve (in some species) before ascending in the vagus (Xth cranial nerve). The cell bodies lie in the nodose ganglion and the central axons again terminate in the nucleus tractus solitarius.

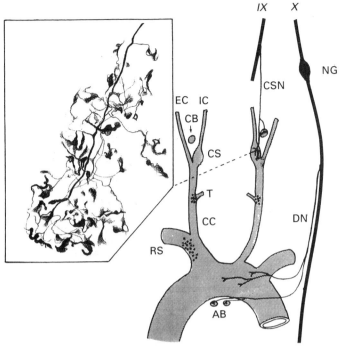

Figure 14.2 Sketch of the arterial reflexogenic areas. CS, carotid sinus; CB, carotid body; AB, aortic bodies. Fibres are shown innervating the two major receptor areas (left side only shown). Minor receptor areas are represented by dots. Nerves are shown only for the left side: CSN, carotid sinus nerve (nerve of Hering); DN, aortic nerve (depressor nerve); IX, glossopharyngeal; X, vagus; NG, nodose ganglion. Arteries: RS, right subclavian; CC, common carotid; IC, internal carotid; EC, external carotid. T, thyroid artery. Inset shows extensive ramification of a single baroreceptor fibre-ending in the human carotid sinus, ×300. (Inset from Abraham, A. (1969) *Microscopic Innervation of the Heart and Blood Vessels in Vertebrates including Man*, Pergamon Press, Oxford)

Receptor properties: dynamic sensitivity, threshold and range

The term *receptor* in the neurophysiological sense has, of course, a completely different meaning from the pharmocological sense of a drug-binding site. The baroreceptors are actually mechanoreceptors; they respond to stretch rather than pressure, and if stretch is prevented by applying a plaster cast around the artery the baroreceptors no longer respond to pressure. Normally, however, a rise in arterial pressure causes arterial distension which in turn excites the mechanoreceptors. In the carotid sinus the transduction of the pressure signal into

stretch is enhanced by the thinness of the tunica media: this makes the wall stretchy and allows a 15% change in diameter for a normal pulse pressure.

Static and dynamic responses When the carotid sinus is distended by a controlled, sustained rise in blood pressure, as in Figure 14.3 (fibre 1) an individual baroreceptor fibre fires an initial burst of action potentials as the pressure is changing (the dynamic response), and this signals the rate of change of pressure. The activity then falls back somewhat and settles down to a sustained rate (the adapted response) signalling the new pressure level. The fast adaptation has often

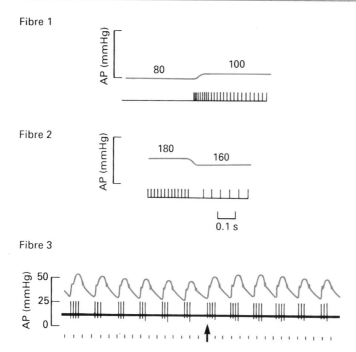

Fibre 1

Fibre 2

Fibre 3

Figure 14.3 Characteristics of baroreceptor afferent fibres. Fibres 1 and
2. Action potentials in myelinated
afferents of cat carotid sinus when
non-pulsatile arterial pressure (AP,
mmHg) is raised (fibre 1) or reduced
(fibre 2). Fibre 3. Single baroreceptor
fibre from rabbit aorta subjected to a
normal pulsatile pressure. There are
4 impulses per pulse when blood
pressure is high (inspiration, arrow)
and 3 when it is lower (expiration).
Time intervals 0.1 s. (Fibres 1 and 2
after Landgren, S. (1952) *Acta Physiologica Scandinavica*, **26**, 1–34 and
fibre 3 from Downing, S. E. (1960)
Journal of Physiology, **150**, 210–213,
by permission)

been ascribed to mechanical 'creep' of the
receptor within its viscoelastic environment.
A recent discovery, however, suggests an
additional mechanism: fast adaptation is
largely prevented by the K^+-channel blocker
4-aminopyridine. This implicates opening of
K^+ channels and hyperpolarization as a
factor in fast adaptation.

Baroreceptors are also dynamically sensitive to a fall in pressure; they transiently fall
silent when pressure is reduced, then resume
activity at a new slower rate (fibre 2). As a
result of this dynamic sensitivity many
baroreceptors *in vivo* fall silent during diastole and their normal activity pattern consists of bursts of action potentials during
systole (fibre 3).

There are two principal types of baroreceptor fibre: *A fibres* with large myelinated
axons and large spikes, and *C fibres* with
small-diameter unmyelinated axons and
small spikes. C fibres are much more
numerous than A fibres. The properties of
the receptor in which each fibre ends differ in
detail.

Threshold This refers to the pressure at
which afferent fibres first begin to fire action
potentials. In the dog carotid sinus, the
threshold for A and C fibres is around 60–
70 mm Hg. The C fibres tend to have higher
thresholds than A fibres. In general carotid
sinus A fibres have lower thresholds than
aortic ones, perhaps becauseof the greater
distensibility of the thin-walled sinus.

Sensitivity The response curve for C fibres
(plot of spike frequency *versus* pressure) is
sigmoidal. The maximum sensitivity of C
fibres, i.e. change in discharge per mmHg
change in pressure, is less than that of A
fibres. Also, maximum sensitivity and saturation occur at higher pressures for C fibres. It
is thought that these characteristics make C
fibres best suited to monitoring high blood
pressures. The A fibres have greater sensitivity but over a narrower range and at lower
pressure. They may be better suited to
monitor onset of hypotension and sudden
changes in pressure.

Range Each individual afferent fibre only responds over a limited pressure range; for example, over 60 mmHg for A fibres in the dog carotid sinus, 100 mmHg for C fibres. The baroreceptor nerve trunk, however, has a wider operating range because it contains numerous individual A and C fibres. When pressure rises, fibres of progressively higher threshold are 'recruited' and this extends the range of pressures signalled in the nerve trunk (Figure 14.4(a)). The effective range of the entire baroreceptor reflex (cf. receptor range) can be defined as the steep part of the stimulus–response curve. Examples of stimulus–response curves for blood pressure and heart rate are given in Figures 14.4(b) and 14.6, respectively.

Importance of pulse pressure Carotid baroreceptors are sensitive to the pulse pressure as well as to mean pressure: the greater the oscillation in pressure about a mean, the greater the aggregate activity in the nerve trunk at that pressure (Figure 14.4(a)), and the greater the ensuing depressor reflex (Figure 14.4(b)). This is partly due to the dynamic sensitivity of the individual receptors and partly to recruitment of high-threshold fibres during each systole. The signalling of pulse pressure is probably very important during orthostasis and during small haemorrhages, when there is often a fall in pulse pressure (due to a reduced stroke volume) without any fall in mean arterial pressure.

The baroreceptor reflex and short-term homeostasis of blood pressure

Reflex response to baroreceptor stimulation The key features of the reflex evoked by baroreceptor activation (the baroreflex) were discovered by Ludwig and Cyon in 1886. They found that stimulating the aortic nerve caused a reflex depression of heart rate and blood pressure. Hering later observed the same reflex changes on stimulating the carotid sinus nerve (Figure 14.5). In the intact animal any acute rise in arterial pressure

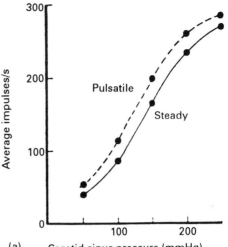

(a)

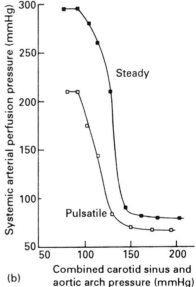

(b)

Figure 14.4 Effect of perfusion pressure on baroreceptor traffic and evoked reflex in anaesthetized dogs. (a) Average rate of discharge in a multifibre preparation of the carotid sinus nerve when sinus pressure is varied. Pulsatile pressure evokes a higher net activity than a steady pressure. (b) Reflex fall in systemic pressure (due to bradycardia and vasodilatation) when pressure in a vascularly-isolated perfused baroreceptor region is increased. Pulsatility strengthens the reflex. ((a) From Korner, P. I. (1971) *Physiological Reviews*, **51**, 312–367 and (b) from Angell-James, J. E. and De Burgh Daly, M. (1970) *Journal of Physiology*, **209**, 257–293, by permission)

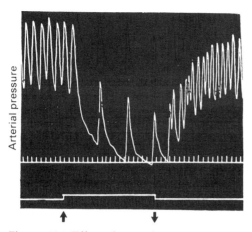

Figure 14.5 Effect of carotid sinus nerve activity on blood pressure and heart rate in the dog. Electrical stimulation of the carotid sinus nerve between the two arrows elicited a reflex hypotension and bradycardia. This classic smoked-drum recording is taken from the work of Hering, who discovered the carotid baroreflex in 1923. Time intervals approximately 0.2 s.

increases the baroreceptor discharge rate and this, via a polysynaptic central pathway, enhances the vagal output to the heart and inhibits the sympathetic outflow to both the heart and the vasculature. Multifibre recordings from sympathetic nerves to human muscle vessels normally show regular bursts of sympathetic activity, but these disappear completely if blood pressure is rapidly raised above 150/90 mmHg. The reduced activity in sympathetic vasoconstrictor nerves leads to vasodilatation and a fall in peripheral resistance. Also, increased vagal activity and reduced cardiac sympathetic nerve activity cause a bradycardia and reduced contractility. Since blood pressure is the product of cardiac output and peripheral resistance, these changes together tend to return arterial pressure to normal (see Figure 14.1). The baroreflex thus functions as a 'buffer', stabilizing the blood pressure against acute change.

The buffering of blood pressure by the baroreflex is very rapid. The latency between baroreceptor stimulation and onset of vagal bradycardia is 0.5 s or less, and the latency

for changes in vascular resistance is about 1.5 s.

Reflex response to baroreceptor unloading
From a clinical point of view, the baroreflex to a fall in pressure is perhaps more important than the response to a rise, since acute hypotension is a common medical emergency. As an experimental manoeuvre in man, external compression of the common carotid arteries is often used to reduce pressure in the carotid sinuses (which lie higher in the neck, close to the angle of the jaw). This reduces the baroreceptor input to the brainstem, as does hypotension in clinical situations (Fig. 16.2), and the reflex effects are as follows.

Tachycardia, and probably increased myocardial *contractility*. Heart rate increases due to reduced vagal inhibition of the pacemaker and increased sympathetic activity.

Arteriolar constriction. In most laboratory animals, the baroreflex elicits a sympathetically mediated vasoconstriction involving the skeletal muscle, skin, kidneys and the splanchnic vasculature: this raises peripheral resistance. In man, compression of the common carotid artery causes a strong reflex vasoconstriction in the splanchnic and renal circulations but a relatively small change in the forearm and none in the calf. Direct stimulation of the human carotid sinus nerve has been found to inhibit directly-recorded activity in sympathetic nerves to muscle but sympathetic activity to the skin is unchanged. It seems, therefore, that carotid sinus baroreceptors exert some reflex control over human muscle vessels but not skin. (The sympathetic output to human skin is probably influenced by cardiopulmonary receptors–see later).

Splanchnic venoconstriction. Reflex venoconstriction actively displaces blood from the gut and liver into the central veins, as illustrated in Figure 12.21. This enhances stroke volume via the Frank–Starling mechanism. In skeletal muscle, the volume of blood in the veins (which are poorly innervated) declines secondarily to the fall in venous pressure caused by arteriolar contraction (see Figure 12.14). Both skin and muscle veins can also be constricted by reflexly secreted adrenaline, vasopressin and angiotensin.

Adrenaline is secreted by the adrenal medulla in response to increased splanchnic nerve activity. Adrenaline stimulates the heart and enhances glycogenolysis (Section 12.6).

Effects on extracellular fluid volume. The baroreflex affects fluid volume and distribution by several mechanisms:

(a) Arteriolar vasoconstriction lowers capillary pressure, producing an absorption of interstitial fluid and expansion of the plasma volume (Fig 12.14).
(b) Increased renal sympathetic nerve activity stimulates renin secretion, activating the angiotensin–aldosterone system (Section 12.6). This contributes to generalized vascular contraction (angiotensin II) and renal retention of salt and water (aldosterone).
(c) In primates, a fall in baroreceptor traffic evokes the release of vasopressin (ADH) from the posterior pituitary gland, producing an antidiuresis and contributing to peripheral vasoconstriction.

The net result of the baroreflex during acute hypotension is thus to stimulate cardiac output, raise TPR, promote fluid retention and enhance plasma volume, thereby countering the hypotension.

Sensitivity and 'setting' of the baroreflex

In animal experiments the sensitivity of the baroreflex can be assessed by isolating the carotid sinus and/or aortic arch and measuring the reflex change in heart rate or systemic pressure in response to controlled distension of the baroreceptors. In human subjects, baroreceptor activity can be altered by injecting the vasoconstrictor drug, phenylephrine in order to raise arterial pressure, reflex changes in heart rate being then monitored. Alternatively, suction can be

applied to a rigid cuff around the neck to distend the carotid sinus directly (but not the aortic region) and reflex changes in arterial pressure as well as heart rate can then be monitored. From such measurements, stimulus–response curves can be constructed, like those in Figures 14.4(b) and 14.6. The responses prove to be sigmoidal functions of the applied pressure change and the maximum slope of the response curve gives the optimal *sensitivity or 'gain'* of the reflex. In man, the sensitivity declines with age and with chronic hypertension, due to a fall in artery wall distensibility. The pressure which the reflex strives to maintain is called its *setting or set point*, and this can be altered either by neural interactions within the central nervous system ('central resetting') or by physical changes in the receptor region ('peripheral resetting'). The advantages and disadvantages of resetting are as follows.

Central resetting *Exercise* offers an example of central resetting. The moderate rise in arterial pressure during exercise does not reduce the heart rate because the reflex is reset centrally to operate around a higher pressure. Thus the cardiac output is not suppressed, yet blood pressure is still buffered around the new level, as can be seen in the upper curve of Figure 14.6. Central modulation also occurs during the *defence response* (see later), which involves a sharp rise in blood pressure and suppression of the baroreflex. *Sinus arrhythmia* (see Figure 5.9) is an example of regular central modulation of the baroreflex: the brainstem neurons that drive inspiration also inhibit the cardiac vagal motor neurons, rendering them temporarily unresponsive to the baroreceptor input (see input 'I' in Figure 14.13). The resulting fall in vagal activity largely explains the tachycardia associated with each inspiration.

Peripheral resetting When pressure is raised for many minutes, the baroreceptor threshold rises to a new, higher pressure over 15 min or so. This shifts the whole stimulus–response curve to the right, and in

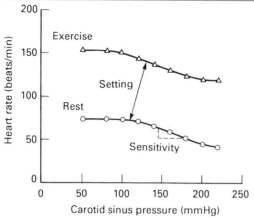

Figure 14.6 The baroreflex in a dog during mild exercise (5 km/h, 7% gradient). The carotid sinus was vascularly-isolated from the rest of the circulation and perfused at controlled, steady pressures to explore the response curve at rest and during exercise. The level of the baroreflex is reset in exercise, whereas its sensitivity (slope) changes little. Systemic arterial pressure increased by approximately 10 mmHg during the exercise. (From Melcher, A. and Donald, D. E. (1981) *American Journal of Physiology*, **241**, H838–849, by permission)

Short-term role of the baroreflex

The baroreflex is important chiefly in buffering *acute* changes in arterial pressure in the short term, rather than regulating the absolute pressure in the long term. If the baroreceptor nerves of a dog are cut under anaesthesia and the dog allowed to recover, it is hypertensive for a few days but the average blood pressure then settles down to a level that is only 11 mmHg above normal, indicating that arterial baroreceptors are not vital for the long-term setting of blood pressure. But while the pressure averaged over a period of time returns to near normal, the pressure is nevertheless very unstable from minute to minute in the denervated animal, fluctuating over a much wider range than normal (see Figure 14.7a). Walking up a 21-degree incline, for example, raises a normal dog's arterial pressure by approximately 10 mmHg, whereas the baroreceptor-deprived dog experiences a 50 mmHg rise in pressure. *The major role of the baroreflex is thus to buffer short-term fluctuations in arterial pressure.*

this way the receptors regain a position on the steep part of the stimulus–response curve where they can operate most effectively. Although this extends the pressure range over which the reflex can effectively buffer sudden pressure fluctuations, it also means that the baroreceptors cannot, over long periods, provide the brain with reliable information about the absolute blood pressure: the new pressure may produce the same signal as the old pressure, after resetting has occurred. The ambiguity of the baroreceptor signal over the long term is exacerbated further by sympathetic motor nerves that innervate the carotid sinus and can enhance the baroreceptor activity. Because the baroreceptors do not transmit unambiguous information about the absolute blood pressure to the brain, they cannot control absolute pressure in the long term.

14.2 Cardiac receptors

The heart and pulmonary artery are richly innervated by afferent fibres, as shown in Figure 14.8. Cardiac deafferentation studies indicate that these fibres have, *overall*, a tonic inhibitory effect on heart rate and peripheral vascular tone. Thus, stimulation of cardiac receptors by an injection of veratridine causes a profound reflex bradycardia, vasodilatation and hypotension (the *Bezold–Jarisch response*). This kind of mass, unphysiological stimulation, however, takes no account of the fact that there are several classes of receptor in the heart, with differing reflex effects.

The cardiopulmonary afferents can be divided into three main functional classes, namely (1) mechanoreceptors around the right and left veno-atrial junctions,

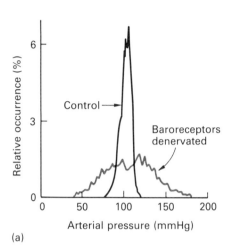

(a)

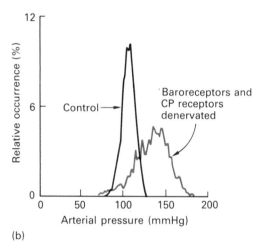

(b)

Figure 14.7 Frequency distribution for arterial pressure. (a) Effect of chronic arterial baroreceptor denervation in dogs. After some days mean pressure has not changed much but the fluctuations about the mean increase, i.e. pressure is less stable. (b) Both the cardiopulmonary and arterial baroreceptors were denervated. There is now a marked increase in mean pressure, as well as pressure instability. ((a) From Cowley, A. W., Liard, J. F. and Guyton, A. C (1973) *Circ. Res.*, **32**, 564–578; (b) Persson, P. B., Ehmke, H., and Kirchheim, H. R. (1989) *NIPS*, **4**, 56–59, by permission)

connected to myelinated vagal fibres, (2) mechanoreceptors that are scattered diffusely throughout the atria, ventricles and pulmonary artery and are served by non-myelinated fibres travelling in the vagus and cardiac sympathetic nerves, and (3) chemosensitive fibres travelling in the vagus and cardiac sympathetic nerves. (Both the vagus and cardiac sympathetic nerves are 'mixed nerves' carrying both motor and sensory fibres.) Of these, the veno-atrial receptors are normally the most active in dogs. Information is lacking in man.

1. The veno-atrial stretch receptors

These are branched, non-encapsulated nerve endings located in the endocardium at the junctions of the great veins and both atria. They are served by large myelinated vagal afferents and the endings resemble the baroreceptor spray illustrated in Figure 14.2. As Figure 14.8 shows, the receptor discharge coincides with either atrial systole (type A pattern) or with the V wave of atrial filling (type B pattern), or with both (intermediate pattern, not illustrated). Receptors with type B activity signal atrial volume and hence provide information about central venous pressure and cardiac distension.

If the veno-atrial receptors are stimulated experimentally by inflating small balloons at the veno-atrial junction, they elicit a reflex tachycardia and a modest increase in urine flow. The *tachycardia* is unusual in that it is brought about by a selective increase in sympathetic outflow to the pacemaker, leaving myocardial contractility unaltered. Vagal efferent activity is unaltered too. This reflex probably contributes to the '*Bainbridge effect*' (discovered in 1915), which is a tachycardia induced by a large, rapid infusion of saline into a dog's venous system. The *reflex diuresis and natriuresis* (salt excretion) are still something of a puzzle. Reduced renal sympathetic nerve activity mediates a reflex renal vasodilatation and natriuresis, but does not explain the diuresis fully. A hormone appears to be involved, because blood from a

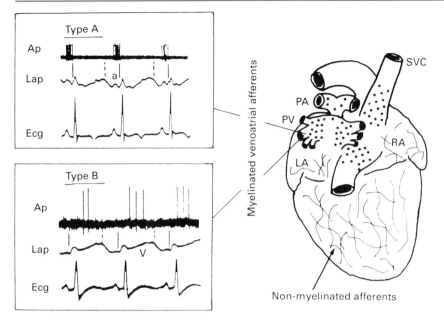

Figure 14.8 Posterior view of heart to illustrate the distribution of cardiopulmonary receptors. Position of venoatrial receptors is indicated by small asterisks. LA, RA, left and right atrium; PA, PV, pulmonary artery and vein; SVC, superior vena cava. The relation between the veno-atrial fibre action potentials (Ap) and left atrial pressure (Lap) is shown on the insets for type A and type B receptors. (Canine recordings from Kappagoda, C. T., Linden, R. J. and Sivananthan, N. (1979) *Journal of Physiology*, **291**, 393–412, by permission)

dog subjected to atrial distension can induce diuresis in a denervated kidney or even an insect Malpighian tubule. Vasopressin (antidiuretic hormone) may be involved in those species where its release can be inhibited by an atrial receptor reflex, as well as by the baroreflex (see earlier). Changes in plasma vasopressin do not, however, seem to explain the reflex diuresis in dogs fully. Some atrial muscle cells secrete a natriuretic hormone (atrial natriuretic peptide, ANP; Section 11.6) as a direct response to stretch: but this is not a neural reflex, and plasma ANP concentration does not correlate well with the reflex natriuresis. It is possible therefore that a further diuretic hormone awaits discovery.

The *function* of the reflex tachycardia may be to help regulate cardiac size, blood being pumped at a faster rate out of the venous

system (see Figure 7.10). The reflex diuresis contributes to the control of plasma volume.

2. Unmyelinated mechanoreceptor fibres

Around 80% of the cardiac vagal afferents are small-diameter, unmyelinated fibres, and many of these subserve mechanoreception: similar fibres also travel in the cardiac sympathetic nerves. Such mechanoreceptors form a network of fine fibres in both atria, and in the left ventricle (mainly). There are also vagal mechanoreceptors (myelinated) close to the walls of the coronary arteries. The mechanoreceptors in the atria respond to substantial distension. They fire sparsely during the 'V' wave of atrial diastole, but only during inspiration, when atrial filling is greatest. Many left ventricular fibres, by contrast, fire during ventricular systole, monitoring the speed and force of contraction, and their level of activity is increased by a rise in end-diastolic pressure. The net effect of these atrial and ventricular mechanoreceptors is depressor, i.e. they induce a reflex bradycardia and peripheral vasodilatation. This contrasts with the excitatory reflex tachycardia evoked by the myelinated veno-atrial group.

The functional significance of the depressor reflex from the atrial non-myelinated afferents is presently unclear. The left ventricular and coronary mechanoreceptors are influenced by arterial pressure via its effects on ventricular and coronary pressures, and their vasodilator reflex probably assists the arterial baroreflex in stabilizing blood pressure. Unlike the arterial baroreceptors, however, they have little effect on heart rate.

3. Chemosensitive fibres

Some unmyelinated vagal afferents are chemosensitive, and discharge in response to capsaicin, bradykinin and prostaglandins, the last two of which are known to be released by ischaemic myocardium. Some unmyelinated sympathetic afferents are chemosensitive too, responding to bradykinin and to other substances released directly by hypoxic myocardium, such as lactic acid and K^+ ions. The sympathetic chemosensitive afferents are thought to mediate the *pain of angina and myocardial infarction*, because surgical interruption of the cardiac sympathetic pathway relieves chronic ischaemic pain from the heart. The sympathetic afferents ascend the spinal cord in the spinothalamic tract, in which there is considerable convergence with somatic afferent fibres, and this convergence could explain why cardiac pain is usually experienced as emanating from the chest wall and arms ('referred pain'). The reflex effect of the sympathetic afferents is mainly excitatory, producing a rise in blood pressure.

Combined action of cardiac and arterial receptors in long-term regulation of mean arterial pressure

As indicated earlier, non-myelinated atrial and ventricular mechanoreceptors can reflexly influence peripheral vascular tone. The arterial baroreceptors reflexly regulate both vascular tone and heart rate. The total, combined input from these receptors seems to be important for the long-term regulation of mean blood pressure. Mean blood pressure alters only a little if the input from one receptor group alone is interrupted. This is illustrated for arterial baroreceptor denervation in Figure 14.7(a), and is also true if the cardiopulmonary group alone is denervated. Thus patients with transplanted hearts have little problem with long-term regulation of blood pressure. Evidently one group of receptors can largely compensate for lack of the other group, at least in controlling *mean* pressure (an illustration of Comroe's principle – 'If a job is worth doing, the body has more than one way of doing it'). If, however, both groups of receptors are denervated, as in the experiment illustrated in Figure 14.7(b), there is sustained hypertension, in addition to the excessive fluctuation in pressure that characterizes arterial baroreceptor denervation alone. This is associated with a sustained rise in renin–angiotensin–aldosterone concentrations.

Reflexes from the heart in man

Indirect evidence indicates that there are sensors of the volume of blood within the human cardiopulmonary region, and that these exert an important reflex control over peripheral vascular tone, though not heart rate. (Arterial baroreceptors seem to dominate the control of heart rate in man.) It is difficult to establish the relative importance of the various types of cardiac receptor in man, for obvious reasons, and general terms such as 'central volume receptors' or 'low-pressure receptors' are therefore often used. The latter term is perhaps best avoided, however, because there is evidence from patients with transplanted, denervated ventricles that left ventricular mechanoreceptors (which are not low-pressure receptors) exert an important reflex control of vascular tone in man.

Reflex control of vascular tone when central blood volume changes Experiments such as that shown in Figure 14.9 suggest that a *rise* in intrathoracic venous pressure and blood volume, accompanied by only slight changes in arterial pressure, evokes a reflex vasodilatation in human skeletal muscle. The reverse experiment, a *fall* in intrathoracic blood volume, can be elicited by a mild blood loss, or by applying moderate suction around the lower body to distend the veins there (simulated hypovolaemia). Even when the lower body negative pressure is so mild as not to change arterial pressure detectably, there is still a reflex vasoconstriction of the muscle, splanchnic and coronary circulations and secretion of renin. Direct neurographic recordings show that the vasoconstriction in muscle is due to a reflex increase in sympathetic nerve activity. In cardiac transplant patients with intact posterior atrial innervation but denervated ventricles, the vascular reflex evoked by mild lower body negative pressure is greatly attenuated. On this basis it is thought that left ventricular mechanoreceptors contribute importantly to the regulation of peripheral vascular tone in man.

Reflex control of human extracellular fluid volume The role of cardiovascular receptors in controlling extracellular fluid volume has been investigated by immersing human subjects in water in a feet-down, head-out position. This shifts about 700 ml of blood into the thorax owing to the pressure of the water on the lower limbs (see Figure 8.18), and thus simulates an expansion of body fluid volume. The total diastolic volume of the heart rises by approximately 180 ml, stroke volume increases by about 30% via the Frank–Starling mechanism and arterial pressure rises approximately 10 mmHg. A

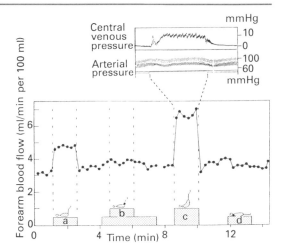

Figure 14.9 Reflex influence of intrathoracic volume on resistance vessels of human forearm muscle. (a) Legs alone raised, raising intrathoracic blood volume: vasodilatation follows. (b) Legs raised but pneumatic cuff around thigh at 180 mmHg prevents blood translocation: no change in forearm flow. (c) Legs and lower trunk raised: inset shows how central venous pressure rises, with little change in arterial pressure; large reflex vasodilatation. (d) Pneumatic cuff around neck inflated to 30 mmHg to reduce carotid sinus distension; very little reflex change in forearm blood flow. Analysis of oxygen content in deep and superficial veins established that the changes in forearm flow did not arise from the skin. (From Roddie, I. C., Shepherd, J. T. and Whelan, R. F. (1957) *Journal of Physiology*, **139**, 369, by permission)

substantial diuresis ensues owing to a reflex renal vasodilatation, a fall in plasma vasopressin concentration and a rise in plasma atrial natriuretic peptide. There is also a slower-acting fall in aldosterone level due to a fall in renin secretion. It is likely that these changes (aside from ANP secretion) are initiated by both myelinated veno-atrial mechanoreceptors and arterial baroreceptors. An analogous chain of events develops in astronauts subjected to *zero gravity*, leading to a diuresis and fall in extracellular fluid volume. The reduction of plasma volume, coupled with a weakened baroreflex, causes severe orthostatic intolerance on returning to earth.

Long-term regulation of arterial blood pressure

As indicated earlier, the baroreflex is concerned with short-term stabilization of blood pressure. In the longer term, maintenance of a normal blood pressure requires maintenance of a normal extracellular fluid volume and sodium mass, since plasma is part of the extracellular fluid compartment. This task is essentially the job of the kidneys and is touched on only briefly here. Renal excretion of salt and water is linked to blood pressure and blood volume both by pressure diuresis (effect of renal peritubular capillary pressure on fluid reabsorption) and by hormonal mechanisms. The chief hormonal links are (a) the renin–angiotensin–aldosterone system, which promotes salt and water retention in response to hypovolaemia and hyponatraemia; (b) vasopressin or antidiuretic hormone, which promotes water retention in response to low blood pressure or hyperosmolarity; (c) atrial natriuretic peptide, promoting salt excretion and diuresis in response to atrial distension; and possibly (d) an endogenous digoxin-like factor that acts as a further natriuretic hormone.

14.3 Excitatory inputs: arterial chemoreceptors and muscle receptors

As well as the ventricular and baroreceptor depressor reflexes, which serve to stabilize the blood pressure, there are excitatory reflexes that help the cardiovascular system to respond positively to stresses such as exercise and hypoxia.

Arterial chemoreceptors and the chemoreflex

Arterial chemoreceptors are nerve terminals that respond to hypoxia, hypercapnia and acidosis of the arterial blood. They are located mainly in the carotid and aortic bodies, which are small, highly vascularized nodules adjacent to the carotid sinus and aorta (see Figure 14.2). Their afferent fibres accompany the baroreceptor afferents in the IXth and Xth cranial nerves. The chief role of the arterial chemoreceptors concerns the regulation of breathing, and their influence on the circulation is slight at normal gas tensions. When excitation is increased by hypoxia and hypercapnia, however, they elicit a sympathetically-mediated constriction of resistance vessels (except in the skin), and constriction of the splanchnic capacitance vessels. If breathing is held constant by artificial ventilation, they also elicit a modest bradycardia, but in spontaneously breathing animals this is overriden as follows. The chemoreflex induces an increase in tidal volume, which in turn excites stretch receptors within the lungs. The pulmonary stretch receptors themselves elicit a *'lung inflation reflex'*, consisting of a modest vasodilatation and a marked tachycardia, and the latter opposes the direct bradycardial effect of the chemoreflex.

The cardiovascular elements of the chemoreflex become very important during asphyxia, producing a rise in blood pressure and thereby enhancing cerebral perfusion. The chemoreflex is also important during severe haemorrhage: severe hypotension impairs the perfusion of the chemoreceptor bodies and the resulting 'stagnant hypoxia' excites the chemoreceptors very strongly. Further stimulation is produced by the metabolic acidosis that develops during clinical hypotension (see Chapter 16), and the chemoreceptor-driven rise in sympathetic vasoconstrictor activity helps to support the blood pressure. This is particularly important in severe hypotension where the baroreflex has reached the limit of its range: the baroreceptor fibres fall silent below about 70 mmHg, whereas the chemoreceptors become progressively more excited the lower the perfusion falls. The support provided by the chemoreceptor input is proved by the sharp plunge in blood pressure when the chemoreceptor nerves are cut in a severely hypotensive animal. The chemoreflex also initiates the rapid breathing that is characteristic of hypotensive shock.

The role of chemoreceptors in the diving response is described in Chapter 15.

Lung stretch receptors

As noted in the preceding section, mechanoreceptors in the lung are stimulated by each inspiration and these receptors have significant reflex effects on the cardiovascular system. The effects are (1) tachycardia, due mainly to reduced vagal outflow, and (2) peripheral vasodilatation due to reduction in sympathetic vasomotor outflow. The increase in heart rate during asphyxia is due to this reflex overpowering the bradycardial effect of the chemoreflex. The lung inflation reflex also contributes to sinus arrhythmia.

The work receptors of skeletal muscle

Exercise elicits a rise in heart rate, myocardial contractility and, in moderate to severe exercise, arterial blood pressure. The rise in pressure is especially marked during isometric exercise and is called the exercise pressor response. The cardiovascular responses to exercise are initiated in part by the higher regions of the brain, but they are also in part a reflex response initiated by receptors in the exercising muscle. In human subjects, local anaesthesia of the major limb nerves to block selectively the sensory input from working muscle, impairs the tachycardia and pressor response to exercise (Figure 14.10). The afferent fibres carrying the excitatory input from muscle are small myelinated fibres (group III) and small unmyelinated fibres (group IV), and not the muscle spindle afferents (group I). Their receptors include both 'metaboloreceptors' activated by chemicals released during exercise, notably K^+ ions and H^+ ions (due to lactic acid formation), and mechanoreceptors stimulated by local pressure and active muscle tension. The

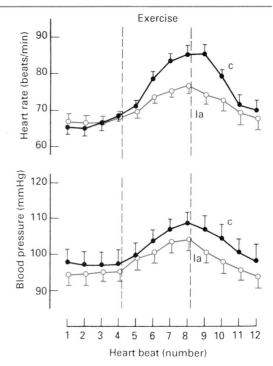

Figure 14.10 Evidence that afferent information from receptors in human working muscle contributes to the rise in heart rate during isometric exercise (4 s maximal voluntary handgrip). Local anaesthesia (la) of the axillary and radial nerves by lignocaine reduces the rate response compared with the control (c). The pressure response however is not significantly changed here. (From Lassen, A., Mitchell, J. H., Reeves, D. R. (1989) *Journal of Physiology*, **409**, 333–341, by permission)

importance of the chemical stimuli is revealed by inflating a pneumatic cuff around the human arm just before forearm exercise is terminated, thereby trapping blood and chemical stimulants within the limb. The exercise pressor response is then partially maintained after the exercise is terminated, and only subsides fully when the cuff is released. The muscle receptor reflex (namely tachycardia, increased myocardial contractility and peripheral vasoconstriction) serves to raise the pressure perfusing the active muscle. The reflex is strongest when the active muscle becomes ischaemic and produces lactic acid, so the reflex is probably best regarded as a system for sensing underperfusion of active muscle.

Influence of external receptors

Cardiovascular responses can also be evoked by receptors not concerned primarily with cardiovascular control. *Somatic pain*, for example, causes tachycardia and hypertension while severe *visceral pain* causes bradycardia, hypotension and even fainting. Ambient *cold* causes a rise in blood pressure, which increases left ventricular work and can trigger angina in susceptible patients. Distension of the *bladder* produces a reflex tachycardia, hypertension and limb vasoconstriction. The *special senses* too influence the cardiovascular system: a sudden loud noise or the sight of a bus bearing down on one produces the alerting or defence response, involving a brisk tachycardia (Section 13.4). *Sexual stimulation* evokes a sharp tachycardia and hypertension (see Figure 8.8). Stimulation of *facial receptors* by cold water elicits a special 'diving response', which is described in Chapter 15.

14.4 Central pathways

In 1854 Claude Bernard showed that transection of the cervical spinal cord causes blood pressure to fall abruptly to around 40 mmHg, due to peripheral vasodilatation. This established that normal sympathetic vasoconstrictor activity depends on a tonic, net excitatory drive from the brain to the spinal sympathetic neurons. This tonic excitatory drive arises within the medulla oblongata, which is the most caudal (tail-end) part of the brainstem (Figure 14.11). The medulla is by no means the only part of the brain involved in cardiovascular regulation; integration of the vast influx of sensory information relevant to the circulation requires the participation of the hypothala-

mus, cerebellum and the cortex. These central pathways are complex and are only partially characterized at present.

Role of the medulla: classic *versus* modern views

Traditionally, the medulla is described as possessing a 'cardiac centre' and a 'vasomotor centre', the latter being a diffuse scattering of cells within the dorsal reticular formation believed to regulate the sympathetic outflow to blood vessels. However, many recent observations have eroded confidence in this classical view. While it is true that cardiovascular changes can be elicited by electrical stimulation of the dorsal reticular region, so too can many non-vascular effects, and the same area has also been described as a 'respiratory centre', 'sleep-walking centre' and 'motor centre'. Its true role may be to regulate the excitability of spinal neurons in general. For this and many other reasons, most workers would now agree with Hilton and Spyer, who in 1980 declared that the classic notion of a medullary vasomotor centre 'though reasonable when first proposed . . . has now become an impediment to research and is in any case untenable'. The modern view emphasizes longitudinal traffic up and down the brain between medulla, hypothalamus and cerebellum (Figure 14.11) as well as transverse traffic within the medulla.

The roles of the medulla in circulatory control may be summarized as follows.

To receive the cardiovascular receptor traffic The dorsomedial medulla contains an elongated nucleus of cells, the *nucleus tractus solitarius* (Figures 14.11 and 14.12), which is the site of first synapse for virtually all the cardiovascular afferents – baroreceptors, cardiopulmonary afferents, arterial chemoreceptors, pulmonary stretch receptors and muscle work receptors. Destruction of the nucleus tractus solitarius causes a sustained hypertension. The muscle afferents also project to a lateral reticular nucleus

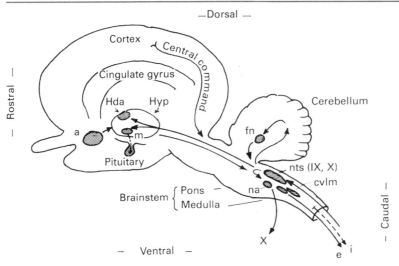

Figure 14.11 Longitudinal arrangement of central cardiovascular pathways in the cat brain. a, amygdala; cvlm, caudal ventrolateral medulla; e, excitatory drive to spinal sympathetic neurons from the rostral ventrolateral medulla; fn, fastigial nucleus; Hda, hypothalamic depressor area; Hyp, hypothalamus; i, descending inhibitory influence on spinal sympathetic neurons; m, magnocellular neurons in supraoptic and paraventricular nuclei of hypothalamus; na, nucleus ambiguus; nts, nucleus tractus solitarius

(Figures 14.12 and 14.14), destruction of which impairs the exercise pressor response.

To relay afferent information to other regions The output of the nucleus tractus solitarius is relayed to various parts of the medulla, hypothalamus and cerebellum (Figure 14.11). Within the medulla, a polysynaptic path relays a signal to the nucleus ambiguus, which contains the vagal cardiac motor neurons. Signals are also relayed to the caudal ventrolateral medulla, which influences sympathetic output (see later). The nucleus tractus solitarius also relays information up to the hypothalamic cells that synthesize vasopressin (the magnocellular neurons of the supraoptic and paraventricular nuclei), and to the hypothalamic depressor area (see later).

To generate the vagal outflow to the heart The cell bodies of the vagal preganglionic fibres controlling the cardiac pacemaker are located chiefly in the *nucleus ambiguus* (Figures 14.12 and 14.13), and to a lesser extent in the dorsal motor nucleus.

These vagal nuclei used to be called, collectively, the 'cardioinhibitory centre'.

To control sympathetic outflow When the anaesthetic pentobarbitone is applied locally to the surface of the *rostral ventrolateral medulla*, a severe fall in blood pressure results. This led to the discovery of a rostral ventrolateral group of neurons that exert a tonic excitatory effect upon the sympathetic preganglionic neurons of the spinal intermediolateral columns. This tonic excitation is carried by bulbospinal fibres that run down the dorsolateral funiculus of the spinal cord (see Figures 12.8 and 14.11). In some species at least, the pre-sympathetic excitatory neurons are spatially organized; for example, the most rostral neurons selectively influence renal sympathetic activity.

The tonic excitatory activity of the rostral ventrolateral medulla is continuously modified by an inhibitory input from the *caudal ventrolateral medulla*, mediated by the inhibitory neurotransmiter γ-aminobutyric acid (GABA). In addition there is a more direct, descending inhibitory influence on the spinal

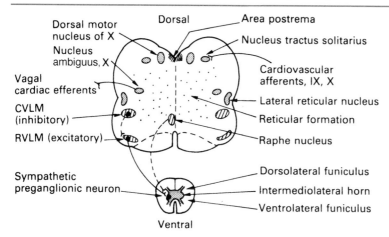

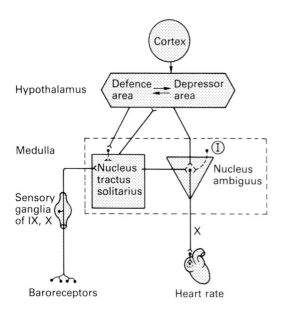

Figure 14.12 Schematic coronal section through the medulla to show relative positions of cardiovascular-related bodies in the dorsoventral plane. RVLM, rostral ventrolateral medulla group; CVLM, caudal ventrolateral medulla group. Dashed lines indicate inhibitory pathways. The structures occur at various rostrocaudal levels and would not in reality all be present in a single anatomical section. Thoracic spinal cord shown on a smaller scale at bottom

Figure 14.13 Central pathways governing vagal efferent activity to the heart. Synaptic complexities are not shown. I, inspiratory neuron input responsible for sinus arrhythmia. The inter-neurons mediating inhibition in the nucleus tractus solitarius are GABAergic; γ-aminobutyric acid is an inhibitory central neurotransmitter. IX, glossopharyngeal nerve; X, vagus. (From Spyer, K. M. (1984), see Further Reading, by permission)

sympathetic neurons, arising from the raphe nuclei of the brainstem.

The *area postrema* is a small patch on the dorsal surface of the medulla where there is no blood-brain barrier. Angiotensin II gains access to area postrema neurons here and increases their discharge rate. Projections to the ventrolateral medulla then lead to an increased vasomotor pre-sympathetic outflow.

Role of the hypothalamus

The hypothalamus contains many regions involved in cardiovascular regulation, including the hypothalamic depressor area, the alerting or defence area, the temperature-regulating area and the magnocellular vaso-pressin-secreting nuclei.

Hypothalamic depressor area This is located in the dorsal part of the anterior hypothalamus and receives an input from the nucleus tractus solitarius (Figure 14.11). When stimulated electrically, the depressor area mimics the baroreflex, i.e. it activates the cardiac vagal fibres and inhibits sympathetic outflow. Although lesions here impair the baroreflex, they do not abolish it, so the region is evidently only one component in the central processing of the baroreflex.

Hypothalamic defence area and 'alerting response' The cardiovascular response in a cat or dog faced with sudden danger is both striking and stereotyped, consisting of tachycardia, acute hypertension, splanchnic and renal vasoconstriction and dilatation in skeletal muscle. The latter is mediated partly by sympathetic cholinergic fibres (see Chapter 12), partly by adrenaline, and partly by reduced sympathetic vasoconstrictor activity. This pattern forms part of a reaction known variously as the defence, alerting, alarm or fear–fight–flight response. Perhaps 'alerting response' is the best description, because the cardiovascular manifestations can be elicited by quite mild arousal in man, such as the performance of mental arithmetic to the beat of a metronome. The response is generated by a discrete 'defence area' of the hypothalamus, the anterior perifornical region, and electrical stimulation here evokes not only the cardiovascular response but also, in a conscious cat, the behavioural manifestations of fear or rage (spitting, snarling and piloerection). The defence area is probably normally activated by the amygdala of the limbic system (Figure 14.11), a system known to be involved in generating emotional behaviour patterns. Stimulation of the defence area indirectly inhibits those neurons in the nucleus tractus solitarius that are excited by baroreceptor traffic (Figure 14.13). The hypothalamic defence area can also, by other pathways, influence the cardiac vagal motor neurons and the rostral ventrolateral medulla neurons that govern sympathetic outflow.

The alerting response does not necessarily occur in exercise; but it does if there is an emotional stress involved. For example, heart rate often increases in anticipation of the start of a race.

'Playing dead' reaction This is exhibited by the opossum and young creatures like the rabbit in the face of danger. It involves a profound bradycardia and hypotension, being in this respect the opposite of the defence response. The response originates in the cingulate gyrus, another part of the limbic system (Figure 14.11). It has been suggested that human fainting in response to intolerable psychological stimuli ('swooning') is really a manifestation of the opossum response – the avoidance of a threatening situation by collapse.

The **temperature-regulating area** in the anterior hypothalamus coordinates the output of the cutaneous vasomotor and sudomotor nerves.

The **supraoptic and paraventricular nuclei** contain the vasopressin-producing magnocellular neurons. The axons of the latter feed vasopressin to the capillary bed of the pituitary gland. Direct electrophysiological recordings show that their activity is controlled by inputs from local osmoreceptors and from the nucleus tractus solitarius.

Role of the cerebellum

The major role of the cerebellum is the coordination of muscular movement, and during exercise this region helps coordinate the cardiovascular response too. The areas involved are the fastigial nucleus and the associated vermal cortex, which receive projections from the medulla. Stimulation of the vermal cortex elicits renal vasoconstriction and muscle vasodilatation, i.e. the pattern seen in exercise, while destruction of the fastigial nucleus reduces the tachycardia and pressor response of dogs to exercise.

Influence of the cerebral cortex: central command

In 1913, Krogh and Lindhard postulated the 'central command' hypothesis to explain the dramatic, rapid cardiovascular response to exercise. The hypothesis proposes that the cerebral cortex, which initiates muscular exercise, also initiates many of the cardiovascular responses by acting on the brainstem. There are undoubtedly areas of cortex (sensorimotor and temporal areas) that initiate cardiovascular changes when stimulated electrically. A subthalamic region capable of evoking the exercise pattern of cardiovascular changes has also been identified.

Biofeedback, the ability of some individuals to exert a degree of voluntary control over their heart rate or blood pressure, could be of cortical origin. The effects of excitement and anxiety on heart rate and blood pressure also presumably involve higher centres, such as the cortex and limbic system.

Overview of central pathways controlling the circulation

Figures 14.13 and 14.14 summarize, in an extremely simplified fashion, the central cardiovascular pathways.

Control of vagal outflow to the heart - There are two main routes linking the *baroreceptor* input with the vagal motor neurons controlling heart rate. One route, of short latency, remains within the medulla and passes from the nucleus tractus solitarius to the vagal motor nuclei, not necessarily directly. The other, of longer latency, passes from the nucleus tractus solitarius up to the hypothalamic depressor centre and from there to the vagal motor neurons.

During *inspiration*, respiratory neurons cause hyperpolarization of cardiac vagal motoneurons. This reduces their discharge rate and leads to tachycardia during inspiration (sinus arrhythmia) and to loss of cardiac responsiveness to the baroreceptors during each inspiration ('gating' of the baroreflex).

Control of sympathetic outflow The central pathways linking the nucleus tractus solitarius to the spinal sympathetic neurons are more complex and less well understood. Higher regions are again involved to some

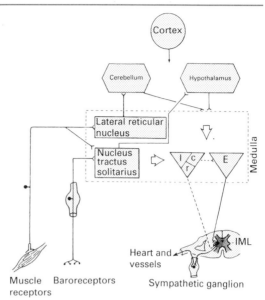

Figure 14.14 Central pathways governing sympathetic nerve activity. The open arrows indicate uncertainty as to exact pathways. Dashed lines denote inhibition. I, inhibitory influences, multifactorial; c, caudal ventrolateral medulla; r, raphe nuclei; E, excitatory neurons: notably those in rostral ventrolateral medulla; IML, intermediolateral horn containing preganglionic sympathetic neurons

degree. Whatever the intermediate pathways, baroreceptor activation leads to inhibition of the neurons in the rostral ventrolateral medulla; indeed, these cells normally fall quiescent during each systole due to the baroreflex. The baroreflex thus inhibits the descending excitatory drive from the rostral ventrolateral medulla to the spinal sympathetic preganglion neurons. This inhibition is mediated partly by the caudal ventrolateral medulla, as illustrated in Figure 14.15. In addition there is a direct descending spinal inhibitory pathway from the brainstem raphe nuclei.

The spinal patient The activity of the spinal sympathetic preganglionic neurons depends partly on the activity of the descending bulbospinal fibres and partly on local inputs from within the spinal cord. As

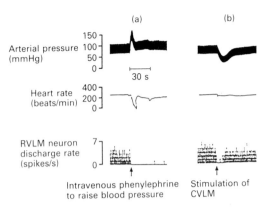

Figure 14.15 Recording of neuronal activity in rostral ventrolateral medulla (RVLM, bottom trace). In (a), blood pressure was raised by an intravenous injection of a vasoconstrictor drug (phenylephrine, α-adrenoceptor agonist). This evokes a baroreflex fall in heart rate (probably vagal) and inhibition of RVLM neuron activity. In (b), the caudal ventrolateral medulla was stimulated by a local injection of glutamate (an excitatory central neurotransmitter), resulting in inhibition of RVLM neurons. This reduced the tonic drive to sympathetic vasomotor neurons in the spinal cord, producing vasodilatation (fall in blood pressure). CVLM, caudal ventrolateral medulla (After Blessing, W. W. (1991), see Further Reading)

Claude Bernard showed, sectioning the cervical spinal cord cuts off the net excitatory influence of the brainstem and causes an abrupt hypotension. Sherrington and others soon pointed out, however, that over several weeks the blood pressure gradually recovers in patients with spinal transections, indicating that the sympathetic preganglionic neurons are capable of generating an output by local mechanisms. Some reflex modulation of this output can occur at a spinal level in these patients; for example, a full bladder or somatic pain cause a reflex rise in blood pressure. Nevertheless, cervical spinal patients lack a baroreflex (except for the vagal control of heart rate) and they therefore suffer from a labile blood pressure and a proneness to postural hypotension.

14.5 Summary

The rate and force of the heart beat, the tone of resistance vessels and the volume of capacitance vessels are controlled by a number of reflexes. The efferent limbs of these reflexes are the autonomic outflows to the heart and vessel, plus hormonal outputs (adrenaline, angiotensin, vasopressin). The central relays lie in the medulla and in higher regions of the brain. The afferent limbs can be considered under two headings – those whose activity evokes a *depressor* (pressure-lowering) reflex, and those whose activity evokes a *pressor* (pressure-raising) reflex.

The *arterial baroreptors* of the carotid sinus and aortic arch are dynamically sensitive stretch receptors. Their afferent fibres, carried in the glossopharyngeal and vagal nerves, respectively, evoke the classic depressor reflex, namely bradycardia, reduced contractility, dilatation of resistance vessels and capacitance vessels, and changes in fluid volumes (via capillary pressure changes, renin–angiotensin–aldosterone activation and ADH suppression). The baroreflex buffers minute-to-minute fluctuations in blood pressure. The above changes in reverse are important safeguards against hypotension. 'Re-setting' of the reflex can make it unsuitable, however, for long-term regulation of blood pressure.

Cardiac receptors fall into several classes. *Veno-atrial stretch receptors* connected to myelinated vagal afferents fire in response to high filling pressures and evoke reflex tachycardia and diuresis. This helps regulate cardiac distension and extracellular fluid volume. *Non-myelinated vagal afferents* from mechanoreceptors in the atria, left ventricle and around coronary arteries elicit a depressor reflex and probably contribute significantly to blood pressure regulation. *Chemosensitive afferents* mediate ischaemic heart pain.

Peripheral arterial chemoreceptors in the carotid and aortic bodies are stimulated by hypoxia, acidosis and asphyxia. They elicit a pressor reflex due to peripheral vasoconstriction. Asphyxia also elicits a tachycardia, but this is a reflex from *lung stretch receptors* stimulated by the concomitant hyperventilation. These reflexes help to sustain blood pressure during severe haemorrhage.

Metaboloreceptors in skeletal muscle are sensitive to K^+ and lactate. Their stimulation evokes tachycardia, increased myocardial contractility and a rise in blood pressure (the exercise pressor response). They help to drive the cardiovascular changes of exercise, especially isometric exercise.

Inputs from all the above receptors relay in the nucleus tractus solitarius of the brainstem (medulla). Projections from the nucleus tractus solitarius pass through the medulla and via higher centres (e.g. hypothalamic depressor area, cerebellum) to modulate (a) the activity of the vagal motor neurons to the heart (nucleus ambiguus or 'cardioinhibitory centre'), and (b) the presympathetic outflow from the rostral ventrolateral medulla. As well as these purely reflex changes, higher centres such as the hypothalamic defence area and hypothalamic temperature-regulating area can elicit complex, coordinated responses (the alerting response and cutaneous vascular responses, respectively).

Further reading

Reviews and chapters

Bisset, G. W. and Chowdrey, H. S. (1988) Control of release of vasopressin by neuroendocrine reflexes. *Quarterly Journal of Experimental Physiology*, **73**, 811–872

Blessing, W. W. (1991) Inhibitory vasomotor neurons in the caudal ventrolateral medulla oblongata. *News in Physiological Sciences*, **6**, 139–141

Calaresu, F. R. and Yardley, C. P. (1988) Medullary basal sympathetic tone. *Annual Review of Physiology*, **50**, 511–524

Coleridge, H. M. and Coleridge, J. C. G. (1980) Cardiovascular afferents involved in regulation of peripheral vessels. *Annual Review of Physiology*, **42**, 413–427

Dampney, R. (1990) The subretrofacial nucleus: its pivotal role in cardiovascular regulation. *News in Physiological Sciences*, **5**, 63–67

De Burgh Daly, M. (1986) Interactions between respiration and circulation. In *Handbook of Physiology II*, Vol. 2, *The Respiratory System* (eds N. S. Cherniack and J. G. Widdicombe), American Physiological Society, Bethesda, pp. 529–594

Dorward, P. K. and Korner, P. I. (1987) Does the brain 'remember' the absolute blood pressure? *News in Physiological Sciences*, **2**, 10–13

Eckberg, D. L. and Sleight, P. (1992) *Human Baroreflexes in Health and Disease*, Oxford University Press, Oxford

Hainsworth, R. (1991) Reflexes from the heart. *Physiological Reviews*, **71**, 617–658

Mancia, G. and Mark, A. L. (1983) Arterial baroreflexes in humans. In *Handbook of Physiology, Cardiovascular System*, Vol. 3 (eds J. T. Shepherd and F. M. Abboud), pp. 755–793. Also Cardiopulmonary baroreflexes in humans, *ibid.*, pp. 794–813. American Physiological Society, Bethesda

Mitchell, J. H. and Schmidt, R. F. (1983) Cardiovascular reflex control by afferent fibres from skeletal muscle receptors. In *Handbook of Physiology, Cardiovascular System*, Vol. 3 (eds J. T. Shepherd and F. M. Abboud), American Physiological Society, Bethesda, pp. 623–658

Rothe, C. F. (1983) Reflex control of veins and vascular capacitance. *Physiological Reviews*, **63**, 1281–1333

Spyer, K. M. (1984) Central control of the cardiovascular system. In *Recent Advances in Physiology*, 10 (ed. P. E. Baker), Churchill Livingstone, London, pp. 163–200

Spyer, K. M. (1994) Central nervous system mechanisms contributing to cardiovascular control. *Journal of Physiology*, **474**, 1–19

Stone, H. L., Dormer, K. J., Foreman, R. D., Thies, R. and Blair, R. W. (1985) Neural regulation of the cardiovascular system during exercise. *Federal Proceedings*, **44**, 2271–2278

Wallin, B. G. and Fagius, J. (1988) Peripheral sympathetic neural activity in conscious humans. *Annual Review in Physiology*, **50**, 565–576

Williams, J. L., Barnes, K. L., Brosnihan, K. B. and Ferrario, C. M. (1992) Area postrema: a unique regulator of cardiovascular function. *News in Physiological Sciences*, **7**, 30–34

Research papers

Al-Timman, J. K. A., Drinkhill, M. J. and Hainsworth, R. (1993) Reflex responses to stimulation of mechanoreceptors in the left ventricle and coronary arteries in anaesthetized dogs. *Journal of Physiology*, **472**, 769–783

Chapleau, M. W., Jianping, L., Hajduczok, G. and Abboud, F. M. (1993) Mechanism of baroreceptor adaptation in dogs; attenuation of adaptation by the K^+ channel blocker 4-aminopyridine. *Journal of Physiology*, **462**, 291–306

Edfeldt, H. and Lundvall, J. (1993) Sympathetic baroreflex control of vascular resistance in comfortably warm man. Analyses of neurogenic constrictor responses in resting forearm and in its separate skeletal muscle and skin tissue compartments. *Acta Physiologica Scandinavica*, **147**, 437–447

Fallentin, N., Jensen, B. R., Byström, S. and Sjogaard, G. (1992) Role of potassium in the reflex regulation of blood pressure during static exercise in man. *Journal of Physiology*, **451**, 643–651

Seagard, J. L., van Brederode, J. F. M., Dean, C., Hopp, F. A., Gallenberg, L. A. and Kampine, J. P. (1990) Firing characteristics of single fiber carotid sinus baroreceptors. *Circulation Research*, **66**, 1499–1509

Chapter 15
Coordinated cardiovascular responses

All the individual elements of the circulation have been covered in the preceding chapters but, as with a jigsaw puzzle, it is not enough to view the individual pieces separately; what matters ultimately is how the pieces fit together to produce an effective whole. The purpose of this chapter is to illustrate how the components of the circulation respond in coordinated patterns to various challenges. One general principle will emerge, namely that *each major adaptation is achieved by the integration of several smaller responses*. To take a specific example, a 13-fold increase in the rate of oxygen absorption by the pulmonary circulation during strenuous exercise is not achieved by a 13-fold change in any one parameter but by the combination of, typically, a 1.5-fold rise in

stroke volume, a threefold rise in heart rate, and a threefold increase in the arteriovenous difference in oxygen concentration across the lung. Other examples of integration will be found below.

An account of the integrated *'alerting response'*, which is elicited by a variety of stresses, was given in Section 14.4.

15.1 Posture

The challenge Movement from a supine to a standing position (orthostasis) is a severe challenge to the human circulation owing to the effect of gravity on the distribution of venous blood. Gravity induces a 10-fold rise in transmural pressure in the most dependent veins, increasing the dependent venous volume by approximately 500 ml. The redistribution of blood causes a 20% fall in intrathoracic blood volume over about 15 s (see Figure 8.18). Cardiac filling pressure falls several cmH$_2$O and the energy of myocardial contraction is reduced by the Frank–Starling mechanism. Stroke volume declines by 30–40% from about 70 ml to 45 ml, so pulse pressure falls substantially (Figure 15.1). Mean pressure falls only transiently owing to reflex corrections (see later), but even so the transient hypotension can be severe enough to impair cerebral perfusion and cause dizziness and visual fading for a few seconds. Most healthy individuals occasionally experience postural giddiness, especially when warm conditions cause cutaneous venodilatation, which further reduces central filling pressure. Postural hypotension is worse after prolonged bedrest or exposure to zero gravity (returning astronauts), but it does not usually progress to postural syncope (fainting) unless the compensatory reflexes are blocked by automatic neuropathy or by pharmacological agents, such as α-adrenergic receptor blockers.

The responses In healthy subjects, reflexes initiated by arterial and cardiac mechanoreceptors quickly restore mean arterial pressure and prevent postural dizziness. Carotid baroreceptor traffic is reduced by both the fall in pulse pressure and by the fall in sinus pressure due to the direct effect of gravity; the sinus is close to the base of the skull and lies 25 cm or so above heart level in orthostasis. Cardiopulmonary receptor traffic is reduced by the fall in cardiac blood volume. The reduced inputs to the nucleus tractus solitarius inform the brain of the gravity of the situation (!), eliciting a reflex reduction in vagal outflow to the heart and an increase in sympathetic outflow to the heart and vasculature. *Heart rate* increases by 15–20 beats/min, due chiefly to the carotid sinus reflex. Combined with a sympathetically-mediated rise in contractility, this limits the fall in cardiac output to approximately 20%.

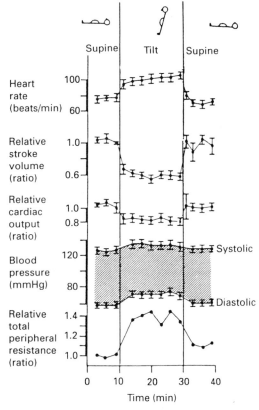

Figure 15.1 Response of young adults to a 20-min head-up tilt. Points represent means, bars are standard errors. (From Smith, J. J., Bush, J. E., Weidmeier, V. T. and Tristani, F. E. (1970) *Journal of Applied Physiology*, **29**, 133, by permission)

Sympathetically-mediated *vasoconstriction* in the skeletal muscle, splanchnic and renal vascular beds raises the peripheral resistance by 30–40% which not only restores mean arterial pressure but even increases it to 10–14 mmHg above the supine value (Figure 15.1). Splanchnic *venoconstriction* partially compensates for the dependent venous pooling, but there is no sustained reflex venoconstriction in muscle or skin during orthostasis.

The above responses normally take less than a minute to complete. The effect of orthostasis on capillary filtration, leading to a 6–12% fall in plasma volume over about 40 min, was described in Section 10.9. Renal *salt and water excretion* is cut down by reflexly-induced increases in plasma vasopressin, renin, angiotensin and aldosterone, acting in combination with the reflex renal vasoconstriction.

The net result of this complex, integrated response is that arterial pressure and therefore cerebral perfusion pressure is safeguarded. It seems perverse that, despite all this physiological 'effort', the cerebral blood flow actually declines by 10–20% during orthostasis. The decline is caused by a rise in cerebral vascular resistance, which may be due partly to the increased ventilation that accompanies orthostasis and lowers the arterial P_{CO_2}, partly to a sympathetically-induced constriction of cerebral vessels and partly to the collapse of the extracranial veins that drain cerebral blood.

15.2 Valsalva manoeuvre

Valsalva was an eighteenth-century Italian physiologist. The eponymous manoeuvre is not, however, an obscure physiological rite but a natural event performed daily by most of us. It is a forced expiration against a closed or narrowed glottis, and this is a normal accompaniment to defaecation, coughing, lifting heavy weights, singing a top A or playing the trumpet. The manoeuvre creates a high intrathoracic pressure which evokes a complex circulatory response with four phases (Figure 15.2). Initially arterial pressure rises because the high intrathoracic pressure presses upon the thoracic aorta (*phase 1*). Mean arterial pressure and pulse pressure then begin to fall because the high intrathoracic pressure impedes venous return, reducing end-diastolic volume and impairing stroke volume by the Frank–Starling mechanism (*phase 2*). As pressure falls, cardiovascular receptors elicit a reflex tachycardia and peripheral vasoconstriction which halts the fall in pressure. When the Valsalva manoeuvre is stopped there is a sudden mechanical drop in blood pressure as periaortic pressure returns to normal (*phase*

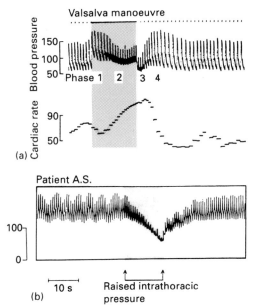

(a)

(b)

Figure 15.2 Effect of Valsalva manoeuvre on blood pressure and heart rate. (a) Normal subject. (b) Patient suffering from idiopathic orthostatic hypotension, caused by an autonomic defect. The patient's pressure failed to stabilize during phase 2, and there was no reflex bradycardia in phase 4. Blood pressure in mmHg; rate in beats/min; top time markers in seconds. ((a) From Bannister, Sir R. (1980) In *Arterial Blood Pressure and Hypertension* (ed. P. Sleight), Oxford University Press, Oxford, pp. 117–121 and (b) From Johnson, R. H. and Spalding, J. M. K. (1974) *Disorders of the Autonomic Nervous System*, Blackwell, London, by permission)

3). The drop in intrathoracic pressure allows venous blood to surge into the thorax, distending the heart and increasing the stroke volume. As a result the pulse pressure and mean pressure rebound rapidly (*phase 4*), causing the baroreceptors to elicit a reflex bradycardia. The Valsalva response, and particularly the sudden heart rate reversal in phase 4, is therefore a useful test of the competence of the baroreflex in man. If the reflex is interrupted by a neurological disorder, the Valsalva test shows a continuing pressure fall in phase 2 and no pressure overshoot or bradycardia in phase 4. Individuals showing such a pattern are prone to postural hypotension.

15.3 Exercise

Overview   From an evolutionary, survival-of-the-fittest point of view, perhaps the most important circulatory adjustment is the response to exercise. Muscular exercise imposes three tasks on the circulation: *pulmonary blood flow* must be increased to enhance gas exchange, *blood flow through working muscle* must be raised, and a reasonably *stable blood pressure* must be maintained. The first requirement, a rise in pulmonary perfusion, is met by an increase in right ventricular output. The second requirement, an increase in muscle perfusion, is met primarily by locally mediated vasodilatation

which reduces the resistance to blood flow through the working muscle. In addition, an increase in left ventricular output is necessary to supply the extra flow. The third requirement, arterial pressure stability in the face of huge changes in systemic vascular resistance and cardiac output, is achieved by controlled vasoconstriction in non-active tissues. The net effect of these changes is the diversion of an increasing fraction of the raised left ventricular output into working muscle, as illustrated in Figure 15.3.

Cardiac output and oxygen uptake during exercise

During exercise the heart shows a remarkable ability to increase its output in direct, almost linear proportion to whole-body oxygen consumption (Figure 15.4). In an

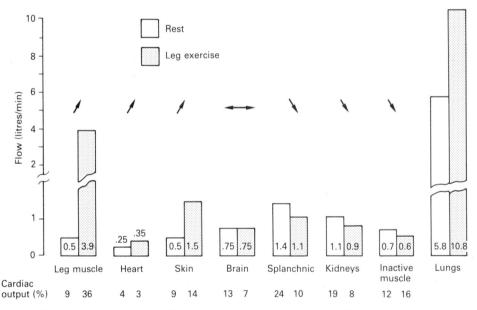

Figure 15.3 Redistribution of cardiac output during light exercise of the legs in the human adult at room temperature. Cardiac output increased from 5.8 litres/min to 10.8 litres/min. Oxygen consumption during the exercise period was 0.4–0.6 litres/min per m². Number at base of each column is blood flow in litres/min. Arrows indicate direction of change. (After Wade, O. L. and Bishop, J. M. (1962) *Cardiac Output and Regional Blood Flow*, Blackwell, Oxford and Blair, D. A., Glover, W. E. and Roddie, I. C. (1961) *Circulation Research*, **9**, 264)

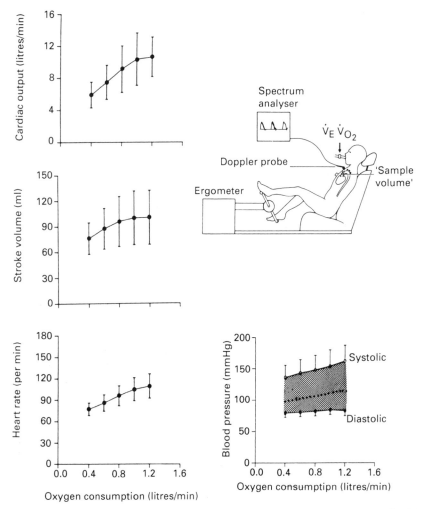

Figure 15.4 Cardiac response to exercise measured by pulsed Doppler method (see Chapter 6) in human adults of mean age 57 years. Bars indicate standard deviation of observations. Note the quantitative, almost linear relation between cardiac output and whole-body oxygen consumption in the steady state. (From Innes, J. A., Simon, T. D., Murphy, K. and Guz, A. (1988) *Quarterly Journal of Experimental Physiology*, **73**, 323–341, by permission)

untrained adult, cardiac output can increase from around 5 litres/min at rest to a maximum of around 20 litres/min, representing roughly a fourfold increase. This increases the rate of absorption of oxygen from alveolar gas in the lungs. The increased oxygen absorption rate is due partly to the rise in *cardiac output* and partly to an increase in the amount of *oxygen added to each litre of*

pulmonary blood. The latter factor can increase just over threefold – not because arterial oxygen content rises (it is normally almost fully saturated) but because the oxygen content of venous blood entering the lungs falls during exercise. Applying the Fick principle (Section 6.1) to the pulmonary blood flow and arteriovenous oxygen difference, we find that the pulmonary oxygen

Table 15.1 Cardiovascular and pulmonary function capacities during maximal exercise in college students and Olympic athletes*

	Exercising students			Olympic athletes
	Control	After bedrest	After training	
Maximal oxygen uptake, litres/min	3.30	2.43	3.91	5.38[†]
Maximal voluntary ventilation, litres/min	191.0	201.0	197.0	219.0
Transfer coefficient for O_2 (ml min^{-1} mmHg^{-1})	96.0	83.0	86.0	95.0
Arterial O_2 capacity, vol %	21.9	20.5	20.8	22.4
Maximal cardiac output, litres/min	20.0	14.8	22.8	30.4[†]
Maximal stroke volume, ml	104.0	74.0	120.0	167.0[†]
Maximal heart rate, beats/min	192.0	197.0	190.0	182.0
Systemic arteriovenous O_2 difference, vol %	16.2	16.5	17.1	18.0

*Mean values, $n = 5$ and 6, respectively. Age, height and weight similar.
[†]Significantly different from college students after training, $P < 0.05$.
(From Blomqvist, C. G. and Saltin, B. (1983) *Annual Review of Physiology*, **45**, 169–189)

uptake rate can increase by around 13-fold, to over 3 litres/min, even in an untrained adult (Table 15.1)*.

Heart rate rises linearly with work rate (Figure 15.4), up to a maximum 180–200 beats/min in adults. The tachycardia is due partly to withdrawal of vagal inhibition of the pacemaker and partly to sympathetic stimulation.

The relative contributions of heart rate and *stroke volume* to the increased cardiac output depend partly on posture, as is shown by the results in Table 15.2. In supine exercise, almost all of the increased output is due to tachycardia; stroke volume increases at most by 10–20%. In the upright position, by contrast, stroke volume starts from a lower value and can increase by 50–100%. Almost all of the increase in stroke volume occurs at low work rates (Figure 15.4).

The enhancement of stroke volume is achieved partly by a rise in *filling pressure* which increases the ventricular end-diastolic volume, and partly by a rise in *ejection fraction* which lowers the end-systolic volume. This can be seen in the echocardiogram of Figure 7.20 and in the results presented in Table 15.3. Filling pressure rises by around 1 mmHg due to the skeletal muscle pump and sympathetically-mediated splanchnic venoconstriction. Ejection fraction and ejection velocity are raised by a sympathetically-mediated improvement in myocardial contractility. Ejection fraction can exceed 80% in heavy exercise. Patients with severe coronary disease cannot achieve this increase in ejection fraction, and partly for this reason their cardiac output during exercise is poor, as shown in Table 15.3.

*The rate of oxygen consumption is widely used as a measure of work rate in the steady state. Resting consumption in an adult is approximately 0.25 litres/min. During light work, such as walking on the level at 3 km/h, oxygen consumption increases to 0.4–0.8 litres/min; moderate work, 0.8–1.6 litres/min; hard work, 1.6–2.4 litres/min; and severe work, such as running at 12 km/h, 2.4–3.0 litres/min. From Pugh, G. (1971) *Journal of Physiology*, **213**, 255.

Changes in blood flow and capillary exchange in active muscle

In a fit human male performing heavy dynamic exercise, the total flow to muscle can increase from 1 litre/min (rest) to around 19 litres/min (comprising >80% of cardiac output), and since many muscle

Table 15.2 Supine exercise *versus* upright exercise in healthy subjects

		Stroke volume (ml)	Heart rate (beats/min)	Cardiac output (litres/min)
Supine	Rest	111	60	6.4
	Exercise	112	91	9.7
Upright	Rest	76	76	5.6
	Exercise	92	95	8.4

Mean cardiac response of 8 healthy males to pedalling at 30% of maximum oxygen consumption. Stroke volume measured by the aortic Doppler flow technique
(From Loeppky, J. A., Green, E. R., Hoekenga, D. E. *et al.* (1981) *Journal of Applied Physiology*, **50**, 1173–1182)

groups are only lightly used even in heavy exercise (e.g. arm muscles during strenuous running, cycling), it is probable that muscle flow in maximally active groups can increase as much as 40 times. This hyperaemia is due chiefly to *metabolic vasodilatation*, aided in upright exercise by the muscle pump's amplification of the *pressure gradient* (Section 13.2). The fall in muscle vascular resistance also has an important permissive effect on cardiac output: without the fall in resistance, left ventricular output would be severely curtailed by a huge rise in arterial pressure which would oppose ejection.

Metabolic dilatation of terminal arterioles also causes *capillary recruitment*, increasing the area available for the exchange of respiratory gases and nutrients (see Figure 9.16). Along with increased blood flow and steepened diffusion gradients, this greatly increases the rate of nutrient transport from blood to tissue. For example, the increased capillary blood flow, capillary recruitment and decreased tissue glucose concentration together raise the glucose transport rate into active fibres by an order of magnitude (see Table 9.2 and Figure 9.17). The case of O_2 transfer was considered in Section 9.10.

Arteriolar dilatation also raises capillary pressure This, coupled with interstitial fluid hyperosmolarity, raises capillary filtration rate. As a result, plasma volume can fall by as much as 600 ml during prolonged heavy exercise (Section 10.9). The resulting haemo-

Table 15.3 Ventricular volume during upright submaximal exercise in normal subjects and patients with multiple coronary artery disease

	Normal		Coronary disease	
	Rest	Exercise	Rest	Exercise
Cardiac output (litres/min)	6.0	17.5	5.7	11.3
Heart rate (beats/min)	81	170	75	119
Stroke volume (ml)	76	102	76	96
End-diastolic volume (ml)	116	128	138	216
End-systolic volume (ml)	40	26	62	120
Ejection fraction	0.66	0.8	0.6	0.46

Means of 30 normal subjects and 20 patients. Upright submaximal bicycle exercise. Left ventricle dimensions determined by radionuclide angiocardiography. (After Rerych, S. K., Scholz, P. M., Newman, G. E. *et al.* (1978) *Annals of Surgery*, **187**, 449–458)

concentration raises the oxygen-carrying capacity of the blood modestly. At the same time, the % saturation of arterial blood falls slightly, due in part to the Bohr shift (effect of increased temperature and pH) and, in endurance athletes, to excessively short pulmonary transit times. The net effect of the haemoconcentration and opposing reduced saturation is that arterial O_2 content is either unchanged (non-athletes) or reduced (athletes) in maximal exercise.

As emphasized above, muscle vasodilatation at the onset of exercise is usually non-autonomic in origin. If, however, onset of exercise involves a stress component (e.g. start of a race, sight of a bus about to hit oneself), then the *alerting response* is evoked, with an initial autonomically-mediated muscle vasodilatation.

Changes in blood flow to other tissues

Blood flow to nearly every tissue in the body is altered during exercise, as shown in Figure 15.3. *Coronary blood flow* increases in proportion to cardiac work owing to metabolic vasodilatation. *Skin* is a battleground of conflicting demands: initially, cutaneous vessels may be constricted to support the blood pressure but if core temperature rises during the exercise the thermoregulatory role of skin becomes dominant and dilatation supervenes. This calls for a further rise in cardiac output, yet at the same time the cutaneous venodilatation is reducing the cardiac filling pressure. Consequently, the stroke volume tends to decline during prolonged heavy exercise and heart rate increases to compensate.

The fall in peripheral resistance occasioned by vasodilatation in skeletal muscle, myocardium and skin is so great during hard exercise that blood pressure would fall by 12–40 mmHg, despite the raised cardiac output, were it not for a *compensatory vasoconstriction* in the splanchnic and renal vascular beds and in non-exercising muscle. During leg exercise, for example, vascular resistance

rises in the forearm. Although textbooks often stress that vasoconstriction in the resting tissues 'diverts' blood to working muscle, a simple tally of the changes in Figure 15.3 shows that the diverted flow is really rather small (0.6 litres) and only accounts for a very small part of the increased flow through the exercising muscle. The true importance of the vasoconstrictor response lies rather in supporting the arterial pressure.

Blood pressure during static and dynamic exercise

Systemic arterial pressure during exercise depends very much on the severity, duration and nature of the exercise. In *dynamic exercise* (i.e. alternating contraction and relaxation), mean pressure rises by 20 mmHg or less. Systolic pressure and pulse pressure increase more than this, owing to the rise in stroke volume and ejection velocity, but diastolic pressure rises little (Figure 15.4) or even falls (Figure 15.5). In *static exercise* such as a sustained handgrip, there is by contrast a large rise in diastolic pressure. Simply supporting a 20 kg suitcase for 2–3 min can raise diastolic pressure by 30 mmHg (the pressor reflex, Section 14.3). This increases left ventricular work considerably, and isometric exercise is therefore best avoided by patients with ischaemic heart disease. The rise in pulmonary blood pressure during exercise was discussed in Section 13.5.

Denervated heart in exercise: role of circulating catecholamines

Normally, the rise in heart rate and ejection fraction are driven chiefly by the cardiac sympathetic nerves: yet patients with denervated, transplanted hearts can still undertake moderate levels of exercise. The cardiac response to exercise after chronic cardiac denervation has been investigated in racing greyhounds. Denervation of the greyhound heart reduces the animal's track speed by

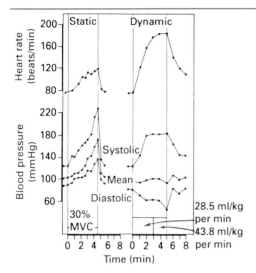

Figure 15.5 Effects of static compared with dynamic exercise. Static exercise caused a bigger rise in mean pressure. Dynamic exercise caused a bigger rise in pulse pressure and heart rate. MVC, maximal voluntary static contraction; arrowed numbers refer to oxygen consumption. (From Lind, R. A. and McNicol, G. W. (1967) *Canadian Medical Association Journal*, **96**, 706, by permission)

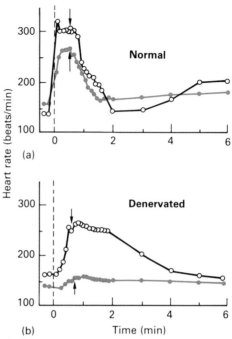

Figure 15.6 Role of circulating catecholamines after cardiac denervation. The heart rate of a greyhound was monitored by telemetry (radio signals) on a race track. Arrows indicate time at which dog passed the 5/16th mile mark. Open symbols: normal heart (a) and denervated hearts (b), without other intervention; denervation impairs but does not abolish the tachycardia. Closed symbols: normal and denervated hearts after β-adrenoreceptor blockade by propanolol; β-blocked, denervated dogs were significantly slowed and became exhausted. Blockade was less effective against normal cardiac nerve activity than against circulating catecholamines. (From Donald, D. E., Ferguson, D. A. and Milburn, S. E. (1968) *Circulation Research*, **22**, 127–133, by permission)

only 5% and there is still a substantial exercise tachycardia, though it is reduced in size and sluggish in onset (Figure 15.6). This tachycardia is produced by a back-up mechanism, namely the rise in plasma adrenaline and noradrenaline that occurs during exercise. If this effect is blocked by a β-adrenoceptor antagonist, the exercise tachycardia is prevented; the denervated greyhound's track speed drops and the dog finishes the lap in a state of extreme exhaustion.

In strenuous human exercise, plasma *noradrenaline* rises from around 1 nM to 10–20 nM, due chiefly to 'spillage' from sympathetic junctional gaps rather than adrenal gland secretion. Plasma *adrenaline* shows little change during light to moderate exercise in man (concentration 0.2 nM) but rises to 2–5 nM during maximal dynamic exercise owing to secretion by the adrenal medulla. These inotropic influences more than offset the concomitant negative inotropic effects of

hyperkalaemia (up to 8 mM K^+) and plasma lactic acidosis (as low as pH 6.9) in severe exercise.

The rise in catecholamine level during exercise benefits *cardiac transplant patients* considerably. A further back-up mechanism of value to such patients is the skeletal muscle pump, which raises the cardiac filling pressure and hence stroke volume by the

Frank–Starling mechanism. These back-ups illustrate a general principle enunciated by the respiratory physiologist, Julius H. Comroe: 'If a job is worth doing, the body has more than one way of doing it.'

What initiates the circulatory adjustments in exercise?

Aside from metabolic vasodilatation, the cardiovascular changes in exercise are caused by altered autonomic nerve activity. It is not entirely clear, however, what causes the brainstem to initiate these changes in autonomic activity. Two main hypotheses have been put forward: the central command hypothesis and the peripheral reflex hypothesis, and there is evidence that both play a part.

The *central command hypothesis* was advocated by Krogh and Lindhard in 1913 and supposes that the cerebral cortex, or a closely related forebrain region, not only initiates the voluntary contraction of muscle but also directly 'commands' the autonomic and respiratory neurons of the brainstem. One observation compatible with central command is that the heart rate begins to increase at the first beat after the onset of exercise (see Figure 14.10), or even before it if there is an emotional component (see 'Alerting response', Section 14.4). Moreover, after *partial* neuromuscular blockade by tubocurarine, voluntary attempts at contracting the partially paralysed muscle (requiring, presumably, a bigger central command signal) produce an enhanced rise in heart rate and blood pressure. Central command does not, however, easily explain a quintessential feature of the cardiac response, the near-linear relation between cardiac output and skeletal muscle oxygen consumption (see Figure 15.4).

A refinement of the 'central drive' hypothesis places the *baroreflex resetting* centre stage in exercise. The idea here is that a central signal raises the set point of the baroreflex. The initial, incoming baroreceptor traffic is therefore interpreted as indicative of too low

a blood pressure, eliciting an immediate reflex tachycardia (withdrawal of vagal activity), increase in cardiac output and sympathetic vasomotor activity.

The *peripheral reflex hypothesis* arose from work carried out by Alam and Smirk in 1938. They found that chemical excitation of receptors in working muscle contributes to the exercise pressor response, i.e. to the increased cardiac output and blood pressure (Section 14.3). Their key observation was that inflation of a pneumatic cuff around a limb, to retain the chemical stimulants within the working muscle, results in a partial maintenance of the pressor response even after exercise is terminated. An attractive feature of this hypothesis is that the chemosensitive endings could provide the necessary, quantitative link between muscle metabolic rate and cardiac output. The progressive interstitial accumulation of chemical factors such as potassium ions and lactate could explain the gradual increase in tachycardia over 1–2 min following the start of exercise, which is clearly seen in Figure 15.5.

It seems likely therefore that both central command and muscle metaboloreceptors drive the cardiac response to exercise, with central command producing the initial tachycardia via suppression of vagal outflow and the muscle chemoreflex contributing to the subsequent slower, sympathetically-mediated rise in cardiac output and peripheral vasoconstriction. There is also a small drive from joint mechanoreceptors.

15.4 Physical training

The circulatory adaptations that accompany fitness training are very important for endurance athletes, though less so for those involved in brief events like sprints and shot-putting, where sheer muscle power is a key factor. In an endurance event such as a medium-distance race, an important factor limiting performance appears to be the maximal rate of oxygen transport from lungs to active muscle. Oxygen transport rate to muscle mitochondria is limited partly by the maximum attainable cardiac output and partly by extracellular resistance to diffusion between red cell and muscle myoglobin.

Training improves oxygen transport in several ways. In skeletal muscle, there is the growth of *new capillaries*. This increases the exchange area and either reduces diffusion distance or, if the muscle fibres hypertrophy, prevents an increase in diffusion distance. Muscle mitochondria become more abundant, especially at subsarcolemmal sites close to capillaries. Muscle myoglobin concentration increases too.

Dynamic training also affects cardiac structure and function. Structurally, the *ventricle wall* grows thicker, *myocardial vascularity* increases and the *ventricular cavities* enlarge. Ventricular end-diastolic volume increases from approximately 120 ml in the untrained resting adult to as much as 220 ml in the resting athlete, and the *stroke volume* is 100–125 ml at rest (cf. normal 70–80 ml). The resting cardiac index (output per unit body surface area) is the same in trained and untrained individuals, but owing to a higher stroke volume the trained subject achieves his resting output at a lower heart rate (40–50 beats/min). The *resting bradycardia* is produced by tonic vagal inhibition of the pacemaker. During exercise, the athlete achieves bigger stroke volumes than the untrained subject, some athletes achieving 170 ml during maximal exercise (see Table 15.1). The athlete's maximum heart rate is about the same as the untrained subject's, but since the athlete starts with a slower heart rate, he can achieve a proportionately greater change. A rise in heart rate from 40 beats/min to 180 beats/min is a 4.5-fold increase, in contrast to a rise from 70 beats/min to 180 beats/min, which is only a 2.6-fold increase. Along with the enhanced stroke volume this enables the athlete to increase his cardiac output up to seven-fold, outputs of up to 35 litres/min having been recorded in certain individuals.

15.5 Feeding and digestion

The arrival of food in the gastrointestinal tract is associated with a marked hyperaemia of the *mucosa* lasting 1–3 h. Fat, which causes slower gastric emptying than carbohydrate, is associated with a milder but longer lasting hyperaemia. The hyperaemia is initiated partly by the actions of local hormones such as gastrin and cholecystokinin, partly by digestion products (glucose and fatty acids, but not undigested food) and partly by vagal parasympathetic activity. *Pancreatic* secretion involves marked hyperaemia too, mediated by parasympathetic neurons that release VIP (Chapter 12). As a result, blood flow to the human splanchnic circulation (i.e. the gastrointestinal tract, spleen and pancreas, fed by the coeliac artery, superior and inferior mesenteric arteries), increases from around 1500 ml/min to 2500 ml/min after a carbohydrate meal. Conversely, splanchnic flow can fall to 300 ml/min during maximum sympathetic-mediated vasoconstriction. The postprandial rise in cardiac work can sometimes trigger angina in patients with severe ischaemic heart disease.

The postprandial rise in splanchnic blood flow evokes an increase in cardiac output (tachycardia) of around 1 litre/min by 30–60 min after the meal. Carbohydrate meals have the greatest effect, and an equal volume of ingested water has no effect. There is also a reflex vasoconstriction in vascular beds such as the forearm and calf. As a result, there is normally no significant change in blood pressure. In some elderly subjects and patients with autonomic dysfunction (e.g. diabetics), however, carbohydrate meals or oral glucose can give rise to postprandial hypotension. This is due to a failure of the reflex tachycardia and limb vaosconstriction. It is thought that in such subjects the glucose load depresses the baroreflex, possibly via insulin release.

15.6 Diving response

Diving animals like the duck, seal and whale show remarkable cardiovascular changes during a dive, and man shows the same responses too to a lesser degree. The diving response comprises three reflexes: apnoea, intense bradycardia and peripheral vasoconstriction. The circulatory changes conserve the limited oxygen store for the benefit of the heart and brain, permitting prolonged survival under water. The Weddell seal can survive up to 70 min immersion and the whale 2 h, though feeding dives are usually shorter than this. By contrast the Amas, the Japanese and Korean women who dive for pearls, remain submerged for only 40–50 s. The vastly superior performance of diving animals is due partly to a larger store of oxygen in blood and muscle myoglobin (Figure 15.7, bottom) and partly to more extreme cardiovascular responses. In addition, diving animals are more tolerant of asphyxia than man; the arterial gas values in a harbour seal after a prolonged dive are 10 mmHg oxygen and 100 mmHg carbon dioxide, which not only vastly exceeds the human breath-hold breaking point but would probably be fatal in man.

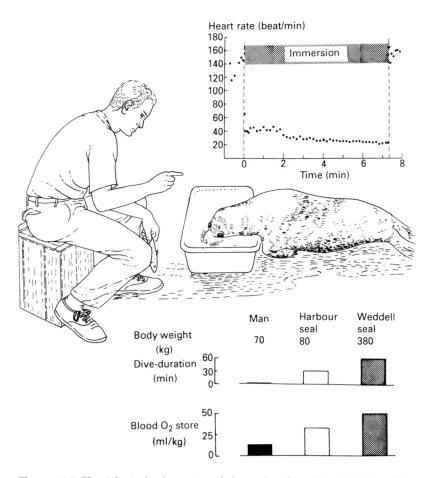

Figure 15.7 Physiological adaptation of the seal to breath-hold diving. Heart rate response of a seal trained to perform voluntary head immersion is shown at top. (Various sources)

The diving response is initiated by cold water touching the facial receptors of trigeminal nerve fibres, especially those around the eyes, nose and nasal mucosa. As the dive progresses, asphyxia develops and arterial chemoreceptor activity reinforces the cardiovascular reflexes.

Bradycardia The seal's heart rate can fall to 20 beats/min during a dive, owing to vagal inhibition of the pacemaker potential. Many human subjects, too, display a pronounced bradycardia during facial immersion in cold water, as shown in Figure 15.8. Facial immersion in cold water has even been used successfully to interrupt human supraventricular tachycardias.

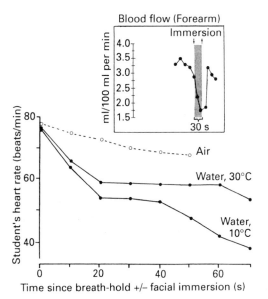

Figure 15.8 Human diving response. Heart rate of a medical student during breath-hold facial immersion. Breath-hold in room air (control) has only a small effect. Cold water evokes a stronger reflex than warm water. The experimenter stopped the experiment in alarm when the subject's heart rate fell below 40 per min. Boxed inset illustrates concomitant peripheral vasoconstriction in human forearm (Unpublished data of J. R. Henderson. Inset from Heistad, D. D., Abboud, F. M. and Eckstein, J. W. (1968) *Journal of Applied Physiology*, **25**, 542–549, by permission)

Peripheral vasoconstriction There is a profound, sympathetically-mediated vasoconstriction in the splanchnic, renal and skeletal muscle circulations, and this outweighs the metabolic vasodilator influence in active muscles. The peripheral vasoconstriction maintains the blood pressure in the face of the extreme bradycardia and at the same time diverts most of the greatly reduced cardiac output to the heart and brain. Large arteries, which are safely upstream of the metabolic vasodilator influence, vasoconstrict strongly. A large quantity of lactic acid accumulates in the swimming muscles and this leads to a sharp vasodilatation when the animal resurfaces. Human subjects also respond to facial immersion with a vasoconstriction in skin and skeletal muscle (Figure 15.8, inset). Forearm blood flow falls by 25–50% and blood pressure rises by approximately 25%. Immersion of the body but not the face, or immersion of the face wearing a breathing tube, fails to elicit this fascinating reflex.

15.7 Changes with ageing

Ageing is associated with changes in both cardiac performance and the peripheral circulation, even in the absence of specific diseases.

In the systemic circulation, the process of arteriosclerosis (hardening of the arteries) leads to a large rise in pulse pressure, which is superimposed on a more modest rise in mean arterial pressure, as illustrated in Figure 15.9

In the heart, the maximum attainable heart rate decreases with advancing age; as a rule-of-thumb, maximum rate is roughly (220 minus age) beats/min. Also, the ability to raise the ventricular ejection fraction during exercise is progressively impaired, despite ample β-adrenoceptor stimulation. Stroke volume can still be raised during exercise, but this is achieved by a rise in end-diastolic volume (Frank–Starling mechanism) rather than a fall in end-systolic volume. The

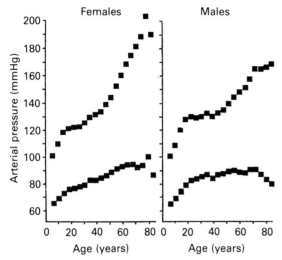

Figure 15.9 Change in systolic and diastolic blood pressure with age in a population from the Rhondda Valley and Vale of Glamorgan. The rule for systolic pressure '100 + age' can be seen to be approximately true. (After Miall and Oldham (1936)), *British Medical Journal*, **I**, 75

impaired sensitivity to β-adrenoceptor stimulation, which underlies the declining maximum rate and ejection fraction, appears to be related to a failure of the β-adrenoceptors to raise intracellular cAMP to the same extent as in younger hearts.

15.8 Sleep

Blood pressure falls substantially during sleep, as shown in Figure 8.8; typical values are 80/50 mmHg. Whole-body metabolic rate and oxygen consumption also fall, the CO_2-ventilation response curve is depressed and P_aCO_2 rises slightly. In non-rapid-eye-movement (non-REM) sleep, as on first falling asleep, the heart rate slows and this largely accounts for the fall in blood pressure. Later, in REM sleep phases, there is also dilatation in splanchnic and renal vascular beds. Cerebral blood flow is increased despite the fall in blood pressure, especially in non-REM sleep and this is attributed partly to the rise in P_aCO_2.

15.9 Summary

Posture   In the standing position, gravity-induced distension of dependent veins causes a redistribution of blood from thorax to lower limbs (~ 500 ml in a man). The fall in cardiac filling pressure leads, via the Frank–Starling mechanism, to a 30–40% fall in stroke volume and arterial pulse pressure. A transient fall in mean pressure at this stage can cause postural hypotension and dizziness, especially if the subject is warm and venodilated. The reduced pulse pressure and carotid sinus mean pressure reduce arterial baroreceptor activity, and there is probably a fall in cardiac mechanoreceptor activity too. The reduced afferent activity quickly evokes a reflex tachycardia of 15–20 beats/min, peripheral vasoconstriction and splanchnic venoconstriction. Together these responses raise the steady-state mean arterial pressure slightly above the supine value. Over longer periods, increased capillary filtration in the dependent limbs can reduce plasma volume by 6–12%. Reflex increases in plasma vasopressin and renin–angiotensin–aldosterone reduce salt and water excretion.

Valsalva manoeuvre   Sustained expiration against a closed glottis raises intrathoracic pressure (phase 1), which impedes venous return and leads to a fall in stroke volume and pulse pressure, with a reflex tachycardia (phase 2). When the manoeuvre is stopped, intrathoracic pressure falls (phase 3) and the inrush of accumulated venous blood raises stroke volume (Frank–Starling mechanism). The resulting rise in pulse pressure produces a dramatic reflex bradycardia (phase 4). This is often used as a clinical test for the autonomic innervation of the heart.

Exercise   This involves (1) increased muscle blood flow for increased nutritional delivery and metabolite removal (flows of up to 19 litres/min in a fit man performing heavy dynamic exercise, cf. 1 litre/min at rest), (2) increased cardiac output, not only to permit increased flow to muscle but also to increase gas exchange rate in the lung, and (3) reflex adjustment of other vascular beds to regulate blood pressure and core temperature:

1. *The increased flow to the exercising muscles* is due to metabolic vasodilatation, aided by the muscle pump in upright exercise and by a small rise in blood pressure. The functional hyperaemia, coupled with capillary recruitment and steepened concentration gradients between blood and tissue, greatly increases the rate of solute exchange between blood and exercising muscle. Plasma volume falls due to increased filtration into exercising muscle.
2. *Cardiac output* rises in almost linear proportion to whole-body oxygen consumption, via increased heart rate and stroke volume. The tachycardia (max. 180–200/min) is driven by vagal tone withdrawal and increased sympathetic activity. The increase in stroke volume is most marked in upright, dynamic exercise; here a doubling can be achieved by a combination of increased ejection fraction (smaller end-systolic volume due to sympathetically-mediated increased contractility) and increased end-diastolic volume (effect of muscle pump and reflex venoconstriction). Maximum output is about 20 litres/min in untrained students (4 × increase), but oxygen uptake can increase much more than this (12 ×) because venous blood entering the lungs has a greatly reduced oxygen saturation (Fick principle). How the cardiac output is linked so precisely to oxygen consumption rate in exercise is unclear; a combination of 'central command' from the forebrain and reflex from peripheral metaboloreceptors in the active muscle has been postulated.
3. *Blood pressure.* Vasodilatation in exercising muscle and myocardium, and later in skin too (for increased heat dissipation), is so marked that it would cause hypotension were it not for compensatory sympathetically-mediated vasoconstriction in inactive tissues, particularly the splanchnic and renal circulations. Mean blood pressure usually rises modestly (up to 20%) in heavy dynamic exercise but rises much more in static (isometric) exercise due to the exercise pressor reflex. Severe isometric exercise is therefore best avoided by patients with ischaemic heart disease. In patients with transplanted and therefore denervated hearts, increased cardiac output in exercise is still possible because circulating levels of noradrenaline rise (sympathetic terminal spillover); adrenaline secretion occurs too in heavy exercise.

Training Improved cardiovascular performance is important for dynamic, endurance events. There is increased capillary density in some trained muscle groups and in myocardium. The ventricular walls thicken, and enlargement of the ventricular cavities produces a bigger end-diastolic volume and hence stroke volume, even at rest. Resting cardiac output is unchanged, owing to a vagally-mediated bradycardia (e.g. 40–50/min). Maximum heart rate is unchanged, so a proportionately greater increase in heart rate than normal is possible, e.g. 4 × (cf. untrained subject's $2\frac{1}{2}$ ×). Maximal cardiac outputs as high as 35 litres/min are possible.

Response to feeding Mucosal hyperaemia is most pronounced after a carbohydrate meal, but is more prolonged after a fatty meal. The hyperaemia is mediated by local hormones (e.g. gastrin, vasoactive intestinal polypeptide) and vagal parasympathetic activity. In man, splanchnic blood flow can increase by 1 litre/min, necessitating a rise in cardiac output. Blood pressure is also supported by vasoconstriction in the limbs. If the latter fails, as in some elderly subjects and those with autonomic neuropathy, postprandial hypotension can develop.

Diving response Stimulation of facial and nasal mucosal receptors by cold water evokes a reflex bradycardia, peripheral vasoconstriction and apnoea. Chemoreceptor discharge reinforces the cardiovascular changes as asphyxia develops. The cardiovascular changes conserve the blood's oxygen store for the benefit of the brain and heart. In man, dives of up to 40–50 seconds are possible; in whales, up to 2 h.

Ageing Pulse pressure rises markedly with age due to arteriosclerosis, and mean pressure also rises. The ability to raise the ejection fraction during exercise is impaired in the elderly due to decreased coupling between β-adrenoceptors and second messenger production. Stroke volume can nevertheless be raised by increasing the end-diastolic volume. Maximum exercise-induced heart rate also decreases with ageing.

Further reading

Reviews and chapters

Blix, A. S. and Folkow, B. (1983) Cardiovascular adjustments to diving in mammals and birds. *Handbook of Physiology, Cardiovascular System*, Vol. 3, Part 2, *Peripheral Circulation* (eds J. T. Shepherd and F. M. Abboud), American Physiological Society, Bethesda, pp. 917–946

Blomqvist, C. G. and Saltin, B. (1983) Cardiovascular adaptations to physical training. *Annual Review of Physiology*, **45**, 169–189

Blomqvist, C. G. and Stone, H. L. (1983) Cardiovascular adjustments to gravitational stress. *Handbook of Physiology, Cardiovascular System*, Vol. 3, Part 2, *Peripheral Circulation* (eds J. T. Shepherd and F. M. Abboud), American Physiological Society, Bethesda, pp. 1025–1063

Bove, A. A. (1989) Hormonal responses to acute and chronic exercise. *News in Physiological Sciences*, **4**, 143–146

Christensen, N. J and Galbo, H. (1983) Sympathetic nervous activity during exercise. *Annual Review of Physiology*, **45**, 139–153

de Burgh Daly, M. (1984) Breath-hold diving: mechanisms of cardiovascular adjustments in the mammal. In *Recent Advances in Physiology 10* (ed. P. F. Baker), Churchill Livingstone, London, pp. 210–245

Eckberg, D. L. and Sleight, P. (1992) *Human Baroreflexes in Health and Disease*, Clarendon Press, Oxford

Herd, J. A. (1991) Cardiovascular response to stress. *Physiological Reviews*, **71**, 305–326

Lakatta, E. G. (1993) Cardiovascular regulatory mechanisms in advanced age. *Physiological Reviews*, **73**, 413–460

Lind, A. E. (1983) Cardiovascular adjustments to isometric contractions: static effort. *Handbook of Physiology, Cardiovascular System*, Vol. 3, Part 2, *Peripheral Circulation* (eds J. T. Shepherd and F. M. Abboud), American Physiological Society, Bethesda, pp. 947–966

Mathias, C., da Costa, D. and Bannister, R. (1988) Postcibal hypotension in autonomic disorder. In *Autonomic Failure* (ed. Sir R. Bannister), Oxford University Press, Oxford, pp. 367–368

Rowell, L. B. (1993) *Human Cardiovascular Control*, Oxford University Press, New York

Stone, H. L., Dormer, K. J., Foreman, R. D., Thies, R. and Blair, R. W. (1985) Neural regulation of the cardiovascular system during exercise. *Federation Proceedings*, **44**, 2271–2278

Vatner, S. F. (1984) Neural control of the heart and coronary circulation during exercise. In *Nervous Control of Cardiovascular Function* (ed. W. C. Randall), Oxford University Press, New York, pp. 414–424

Wieling, W. (1988) Standing, orthostatic stress and autonomic function. In *Autonomic Failure* (ed. Sir R. Bannister), Oxford University Press, Oxford, pp. 308–320

Research papers

Gandevia, S. C. and Hobbs, S. F. (1990) Cardiovascular responses to static exercise in man : central and reflex contributions. *Journal of Physiology*, **430**, 105–117

Honig, C. R., Gayeski, T. E. J. and Groebe, K. (1991) Myoglobin and oxygen gradients. In *The Lung – Scientific Foundations* (eds R. G. Crystal and J. B. West), Raven Press, New York, pp. 1489–1496

Chapter 16

Cardiovascular responses in pathological situations

16.1	Systemic hypoxaemia	16.4	Essential hypertension
16.2	Shock and haemorrhage	16.5	Chronic cardiac failure
16.3	Fainting (syncope)	16.6	Summary

In the previous chapter, specific coordinated patterns of response were recognized to different physiological challenges. In this final chapter it seems appropriate to consider how the circulation reacts to pathological situations, drawing some examples from the field of human disease. The first example, systemic hypoxaemia, occurs both in disease (e.g. chronic lung disease) and in healthy individuals at high altitudes.

16.1 Systemic hypoxaemia

Systemic hypoxaemia is a subnormal partial pressure of oxygen in arterial blood. It can arise from many causes – high altitude, impaired uptake of oxygen by diseased lungs (pulmonary oedema, chronic emphysema) and right-to-left shunts through congenital heart defects. In severe, chronic lung disease, arterial P_{O_2} can be reduced to 27–60 mmHg, in contrast to the normal 100 mmHg. Low arterial P_{O_2}s also occur in asphyxia (Section 14.3), the diving response (Section 15.6) and local ischaemia (e.g. myocardial infarct, arm during sphygmomanometry), but are then accompanied by a *rise* in P_{CO_2}. By contrast, P_{CO_2} *falls* in the systemic hypoxaemia described below, namely systemic hypoxaemia of high altitudes. This is readily simulated in the laboratory by lowering the oxygen content of inspired gas, or by using a hypobaric chamber.

The effect of local hypoxaemia on blood vessels is described in Section 12.2 (mechanisms) and Chapter 13 (heart, muscle, lungs).

Altitude and partial pressure

Atmospheric pressure at sea level is close to 760 mmHg, inspired P_{O_2} is 160 mmHg (21%

of the inspired gas), arterial P_{O_2} is 100 mmHg in young adults, and arterial haemoglobin is 98% saturated with oxygen. With increasing altitude, atmospheric pressure falls, reducing the inspired P_{O_2} and therefore the arterial P_{O_2}. Because of the plateau on the oxyhaemoglobin dissociation curve (see Figure 13.2), oxygen saturation does not begin to fall significantly until arterial P_{O_2} falls below approximately 60 mmHg. This corresponds to an altitude of around 3000 m. Above this height, ventilatory and cardiovascular changes can be detected even at rest, and exercise becomes increasingly difficult.

Heights of 3000 m or more are commonly attained these days, not only by Alpinists but also by cable-car-borne tourists. Major peaks in the European Alps are 3000–4000 m high, and arterial P_{O_2}s on such summits are roughly half normal, 55–45 mmHg. Permanent human habitations exist in the Andes as high as 5000 m, and the summit of Mount Everest is 8848 m above sea level.

The cardiovascular responses of a non-acclimatized human to low oxygen pressures are considered first, followed by the adaptations that occur during residence at high altitude.

Responses to acute hypoxaemia at rest

These vary markedly between species, and the following account concentrates on man. Man responds to acute hypoxaemia with hyperventilation, tachycardia and peripheral vasodilatation, as illustrated in Figure 16.1.

Hyperventilation Acute hypopoxaemia increases arterial chemoreceptor activity and this stimulates ventilation. Increased ventilation raises alveolar P_{O_2} closer to the inspired level but also lowers alveolar P_{CO_2}. The fall in arterial P_{CO_2} has two important effects: (a) it shifts the oxyhaemoglobin dissociation curve to the left (*Bohr shift*, Figure 13.2), thereby raising the arterial oxygen content at a given arterial P_{O_2}; (b) it reduces central chemoreceptor activity and attenuates the increased

peripheral chemoreceptor activity (i.e. reduces the discharge frequency caused by a given P_{O_2}), thereby reducing the ventilatory response. This is one of the marked differences between *asphyxia* (where arterial P_{CO_2} rises) and hypoxaemia (where P_{CO_2} falls).

Tachycardia and increased cardiac output Hypoxaemia not only reduces arterial oxygen content but also reduces the arteriovenous oxygen difference; less oxygen is extracted by the tissue from each millilitre of blood, because the blood-to-tissue P_{O_2} gradient is reduced. This is compensated for by an increase in cardiac output and peripheral blood flow, enabling resting oxygen consumption to remain close to the normal level of 250 ml/min. At an inspired O_2 content of only 7.5% (severe, Himalayan-equivalent hypoxaemia), typical responses at rest are a rise in cardiac output to 8 litres/min, fall in arterial oxygen concentration to 120 ml/litre (normal 195 ml/litre) and in venous oxygen concentration to 89 ml/litre (normal 150 ml/litre). Thus, the increased cardiac output compensates for the reduced arteriovenous oxygen difference to give a normal *resting oxygen consumption* of 250 ml/min (Fick principle, Section 6.1). There is a resting *tachycardia* of up to 100 beats/min, the cause of which is unclear. The arterial chemoreflex itself produces bradycardia (Section 14.3), as does sinoatrial node hypoxia. The possibility that the tachycardia is driven by the lung inflation reflex (as in asphyxia, Section 14.3) is not supported by controlled breathing experiments. Possible explanations include inhibition of cardiac (SA node) vagal motoneurons by central inspiratory neurons (Section 14.4), whose activity is increased; and stimulation of sympathetic outflow by brainstem hypoxia (as in the Cushing reflex, Section 13.4; but resting plasma noradrenaline is not raised, Figure 6.1).

Reduced peripheral resistance and increased blood flow The systemic resistance vessels are a battleground of conflicting influences, but vasodilatation predominates in man. *Local* hypoxaemia causes arteriolar

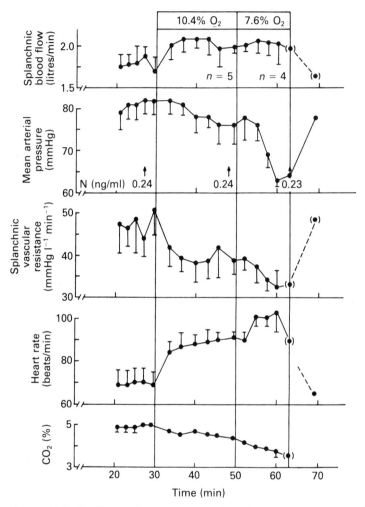

Figure 16.1 Cardiovascular response to lowering oxygen content of inspired gas from 21% to 10.4% (equivalent to 5500 m; arterial P_{O_2} 35 mmHg; moderate hypoxaemia) and 7.6% (major Himalayan summit; arterial P_{O_2} 27 mmHg; severe hypoxaemia). Note fall in alveolar CO_2 content, caused by hyperventilation. N, noradrenaline. (After Rowell, L. B. (1986), see Further Reading)

vasodilatation in many tissues, directly or indirectly, as described in Section 12.2. The effect is most potent in the *coronary* circulation. In the *cerebral* circulation, vasodilatation is largely or completely offset by the strong vasoconstrictor effect of the reduced P_{CO_2}. In human *limbs*, blood flow and conductance are increased by severe hypoxaemia (e.g. 7.5% inspired oxygen, arterial P_{O_2} 28–30 mmHg, 8000 m) but not by moderate hypoxaemia (10% oxygen, arterial P_{O_2} 35 mmHg, 5500 m).

Systemic hypoxaemia increases sympathetic vasomotor activity via the chemoreflex in many laboratory animals, causing vaso-constriction of some resistance vessels, though not the majority. In man, by contrast, there is little evidence of increased sympa-thetic activity at *rest*; for example, plasma noradrenaline concentration is not raised even at arterial P_{O_2} of 27 mmHg. In both man and animals, the non-reflex vasodilator effect of hypoxia predominates and there is vasodilatation in resting muscle, skin and the splanchnic circulation (see Figure 16.1).

Blood pressure Systemic arterial pressure falls only a little in man subjected to moderate hypoxaemia (10% oxygen) because peripheral vasodilatation is largely balanced by the rise in cardiac output. In the *lungs*, by contrast, there is marked pulmonary hyper-tension, owing to hypoxic vasoconstriction (Chapter 13). This can double the mean pulmonary artery pressure, to approximately 30 mmHg. While this increases the work load for the right ventricle, it also has the beneficial effect of increasing blood flow to the upper portion of the lungs and so improving the ventilation:perfusion ratio in that region. If prolonged, however, as in chronic lung disease such as emphysema, the pulmonary hypertension can cause *right heart failure.* This is exacerbated by the direct depressant effect of hypoxaemia upon myocardial contractility.

Exercise during acute hypoxaemia

The changes described above are the cardio-vascular responses to hypoxaemia at rest. When exercise is undertaken in a hypoxae-mic state, the cardiac output is higher than normal at any given exercise intensity as measured by oxygen consumption rate. The same is true for blood flow to the exercising muscle. The heart's *maximal* output is not increased, however, so the maximal attain-able oxygen transport rate and hence max-imal exercise intensity are reduced by hypoxaemia.

Acute mountain sickness

Unacclimatized subjects who ascend too rapidly to >3000 m (10 000 ft) often experi-ence acute mountain sickness after 8–24 h. Acute mountain sickness consists of head-ache, dizziness, sweating, nausea and vomit-ing, sleeplessness and irritability. The condition appears to be of cerebral origin and is attributed to the reduced cerebral P_{O_2} coupled with acute respiratory alkalosis (low P_{CO_2}). Treatment includes descent to a lower altitude, supplementary oxygen and CO_2, acetazolamide (to stimulate renal excretion of bicarbonate and so counterbalance the re-spiratory alkalosis) and in severe cases the synthetic steroid dexamethasone (to reduce cerebral oedema).

Acute pulmonary oedema is another pro-blem of high altitude. It can develop in subjects with predisposing factors (e.g. ischaemic heart disease) who are transported rapidly to high altitude, or in climbers exposed for too long to extreme altitude.

Acclimatization to chronic hypoxaemia

Slow, progressive exposure to altitude over several days allows time for acclimatization and usually avoids acute mountain sickness. The process of acclimatization involves a gradual increase in *ventilation* at any given altitude and hence an increase in alveolar and arterial P_{O_2}. The additional drive to breathing is due to correction of the respiratory alka-losis; a textbook of respiration physiology should be consulted for details.

In addition, the *oxygen-carrying capacity* of the blood gradually increases with acclimati-zation, due to a rise in haematocrit. The haematocrit can reach 0.6 (which also in-creases the risk of thrombotic events). In-creased red cell production is stimulated by renal secretion of the hormone erythropoie-tin. Production of 2,3-diphosphoglycerate in the red cell tends to shift the oxygen dissociation curve to the right, thereby counteracting the leftward shift caused by respiratory alkalosis.

16.2 Shock and haemorrhage

Meaning of 'shock', and its causes

The term 'shock' is used by the medical profession and general public alike, but with quite different meanings. In general conversation the term refers to a withdrawn psychological state, often with physical manifestations such as a muscular tremor, but without an underlying organic cause. To the physician and surgeon, however, 'shock' is a serious, potentially fatal, pathophysiological disorder characterized by an acute failure of the cardiovascular system to perfuse the tissues of the body adequately. The state is recognized by a characteristic pattern of physical signs. The skin is pale, cold and sweaty with constricted veins. The pulse is rapid and weak, due to a tachycardia and low stroke volume. Mean arterial pressure may be reduced or normal, but pulse pressure is always reduced. Breathing is rapid and shallow, urine output is impaired and the general condition is one of muscular weakness and reduced mental awareness or confusion.

Clinical shock falls into four categories. *Hypovolaemic shock* is caused by a fall in blood or plasma volume, which may be due to external fluid loss (haemorrhage, diarrhoea and vomiting, dehydration) or to internal fluid loss (extensive burns, crushing injuries, pancreatitis). *Septic shock* is caused by bacterial infections, the organisms releasing powerful cardiovascular toxins such as endotoxin. *Cardiogenic shock* is caused by an acute organic impairment of cardiac function such as myocardial infarction, myocarditis or an arrhythmia. *Anaphylactic shock* is an immunologically-triggered event caused by an intense allergic reaction to antigens to which the patient had prior exposure, e.g. foodstuffs, antibiotics, insect bites. Although the details of the physiological response vary to some degree with the cause, there is a shared pattern, and this will be illustrated by considering the response to haemorrhage.

Haemorrhagic shock

A 10% blood loss (the volume withdrawn during a blood donation) elicits little change in mean blood pressure and does not produce the shock syndrome. A rapid 20–30% blood loss can lower mean pressure to some degree (depending on the level of compensation) and produces the shock syndrome, but does not usually threaten life. A 30–40% blood loss lowers pressure to 50–70 mmHg and causes severe, sometimes irreversible shock, with anuria and impaired cerebral and coronary perfusion. The arterial hypotension is mediated by the *Frank–Starling mechanism*: acute hypovolaemia lowers central blood volume and hence ventricular end-diastolic volume, which reduces the energy of contraction. Stroke volume therefore declines, and if severe enough this reduces the arterial pressure. Arterial hypotension is thus an indirect rather than direct consequence of a bleed; it is quite unlike the loss of pressure in a punctured tyre in this respect.

Hypovolaemia initiates a series of reflex responses that help preserve mean blood pressure and therefore the perfusion of the brain and myocardium. Cardiopulmonary volume-receptor activity and arterial baroreceptor activity decline or cease (Figure 16.2), while arterial chemoreceptor activity increases, owing to metabolic acidosis (see Figure 16.3, bottom) and impaired chemoreceptor perfusion (stagnant hypoxia). The chemoreceptor input stimulates the rapid ventilation that characterizes shock. The altered inputs to the nucleus tractus solitarius evoke a reflex increase in *sympathetic outflow* and reflex secretion of renin, leading to *angiotensin II* formation. After a severe haemorrhage (30% or more), there is also significant secretion of *adrenaline* and *vasopressin*. Reflexes thus play a vital role in the immediate defence against hypovolaemia.

In moderate hypovolaemia, or the early stages of severe progressive hypovolaemia, reflex tachycardia and peripheral vasoconstriction succeed in maintaining mean blood

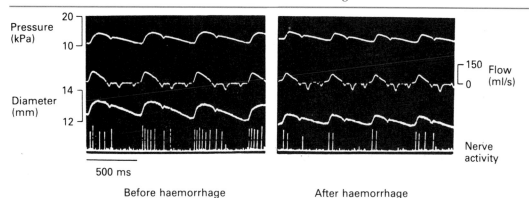

Figure 16.2 Aortic baroreceptor discharge (single fibre), aortic diameter and aortic pressure before (left) and after (right) a slow haemorrhage of 20% blood volume in dog. Note that *mean* pressure is unchanged (compensated phase). The reduced baroreceptor activity is attributed to the reduction in aortic diameter and increased wall stiffness (presumably the result of active constriction), and to the fall in pulse pressure. (After Hartikainen, J. *et al.* (1990) *Acta Physiologica Scandinavica*, **140**, 181–190)

pressure near normal (*compensated phase*; dashed line at the top of Figure 16.3). If blood volume falls by over 30%, however, a distinct second phase can occur, in which blood pressure falls rapidly (*decompensated phase*), as described later. In the milder cases that do not progress to decompensation, the body's defences can be divided into three stages: responses that are effective within seconds, those that act more slowly (5–60 min) and those that act over longer periods (days–weeks).

Compensated (non-hypotensive) phase

Immediately effective responses

The increased *sympathetic outflow* constricts the resistance vessels in the cutaneous, skeletal muscle, splanchnic and renal vascular beds, raising the total peripheral resistance and supporting arterial pressure. The reduced perfusion of the tissues leads, however, to muscular weakness, lactic acidosis, oligura (low urine flow) and pallor. Increased sympathetic cholinergic discharge to skin causes sweating and produces the 'clammy' skin characteristic of shock. A secondary factor, thought to impair tissue perfusion in severe shock, is the adhesion of white cells to the walls of microvessels.

The sympathetic outflow helps to support cardiac output by causing tachycardia, increased myocardial contractility, and active venoconstriction in the splanchnic and skin circulations. The peripheral venoconstriction partially restores thoracic blood volume and cardiac filling pressure. The attending physican becomes acutely aware of cutaneous venoconstriction when he attempts to cannulate a vein for intravenous fluid replacement.

The above neurally-mediated responses can be reinforced by increased levels of circulating *vasoconstrictor hormones*, namely angiotensin II, adrenaline and vasopressin. The contribution of vasopressin is probably important only in cases of severe (i.e. hypotensive) haemorrhage, whereas angiotensin II and catecholamines play a part in normotensive (compensated) haemorrhage too. Angiotensin II contributes to the peripheral vasoconstriction by both local and central actions (Section 12.6) and accounts for about 30% of the initial recovery in blood pressure in venesected dogs. The renin–angiotensin system is activated strongly by the combination of high renal sympathetic nerve activity, reduced renal artery pressure and reduced sodium load at the macula densa. Vasopressin is secreted by the hypothalamic magnocellular neurons as a reflex

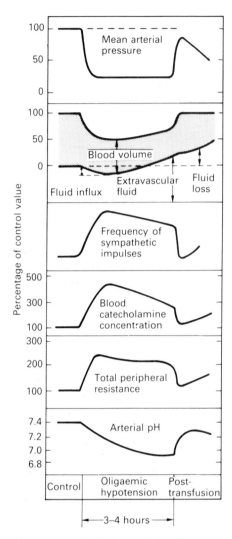

Figure 16.3 Shock induced by 50% blood withdrawal in the dog. The remaining blood volume is indicated by the shaded region in the second panel; the dip below the zero line indicates fluid transfer from the interstitial space into the bloodstream. In this very severe case of hypovolaemia, the fluid transfer begins to reverse again after approximately 2 h as vasoconstriction fails, and blood volume declines further, leading to irreversible shock. Dashed line in top panel indicates preservation of mean pressure by peripheral vasoconstriction that would follow a less severe 'compensated' haemorrhage. (Adapted from Chien, S. (1967) *Physiological Reviews*, **47**, 214–288, by permission)

response to the fall in cardiac receptor and baroreceptor inputs and enhances the peripheral vasoconstriction.

Because of the compensatory changes in peripheral resistance, venous capacitance and cardiac performance, the arterial pressure may not fall much after a moderate haemorrhage, making arterial pressure an unsafe guide to the severity of shock.

Intermediate term response: the 'internal transfusion'

The fall in blood pressure and the sympathetically-mediated increase in pre- to postcapillary resistance ratio (R_A/R_V) together reduce capillary pressure substantially in shock. As a result, the osmotic pressure of the plasma proteins predominates across the capillary wall for a while, and a transient absorption of interstitial fluid ensues (see Figure 10.11). Up to 500 ml of interstitial fluid can be absorbed into the vascular compartment in a human adult, partially restoring the plasma volume but reducing the haematocrit and plasma protein concentration. This 'internal transfusion' of fluid explains why most haemorrhage patients have a low haematocrit by the time they reach hospital. The amount of fluid absorbed is limited by changes in the other three Starling pressures: a reduction in plasma COP due to haemodilution, a rise in interstitial COP and a fall in interstitial pressure. Nevertheless as much as half a litre is absorbed from the interstitial compartment during the first hour after a severe haemorrhage. Much of it comes from skeletal muscle, since this is 40% of the body weight.

A second factor aiding the internal transfusion of fluid is post-haemorrhagic glycogenolysis in the liver, induced by sympathetico-adrenal stimulation and glucagon. The output of glucose by the liver rises sharply and raises the osmolarity of plasma and interstital fluid by as much as 20 mOsm. The rise in interstital osmolaity draws fluid osmotically from the huge intracellular compartment into the interstital compartment and this replenishment of the interstital compartment allows capillary absorption to continue for 30–60 min, much longer than would otherwise be possible. It is estimated that, overall, about half the internal transfusion comes, ultimately, from the intracellular compartment.

While the internal transfusion is of value in preserving blood pressure and, by lowering blood viscosity, improving tissue blood flow, it also reduces the oxygen-carrying capacity of blood.

Long-term responses

Although the above responses preserve cerebral and myocardial perfusion in moderate 'compensated shock', the patient is left with a reduced perfusion of most major organs and a reduced body content of water, electrolytes, plasma protein and red cells. These deficiencies are corrected gradually over days and weeks. The water and salt deficits are corrected first, by reduced renal excretion and increased fluid intake. *Glomerular filtration rate* is cut down by a sympathetically-mediated constriction of the afferent arterioles, while *salt and water reabsorption* is stimulated by a rise in plasma aldosterone and vasopressin (antidiuretic hormone). The high plasma concentration of angiotensin II not only stimulates aldosterone secretion but also stimulates the subfornicular organ of the brain, producing the intense *thirst* that patients experience after a haemorrhage. The resulting increase in water intake, in combination with the oliguria, quickly replenishes the body water content. Salt retention by the renal tubules, combined with a normal dietary intake of salt (2–10 g/day), replenishes the extracellular salt mass within a few days.

The synthesis of *albumin* by the liver gradually restores plasma protein mass over the course of a week. *Red cell* production by the bone marrow is stimulated by an erythropoietic factor secreted by the kidney, restoring the haematocrit to normal over a period of some weeks, provided that iron intake is adequate.

Outcome: decompensated phase and other complications

The above sequence of events occurs in reversible, compensated shock, such as might be produced by a 25% blood loss. If, however, the loss exceeds 30% and has lasted over 3–4 h before fluid replacement begins (as in Figure 16.3), shock enters a second phase that is often irreversible, even if the whole loss is subsequently made good by transfusion. In such cases, blood pressure may be maintained for a while by the high sympathetic outflow (compensated phase), but pressure then begins to fall (decompensated phase), leading to myocardial hypoperfusion and possibly death.

The collapse of blood pressure in the decompensated phase is caused by a relative slowing of the heart rate and, more importantly, a profound peripheral vasodilatation, except in skin. The changes resemble those in fainting (next section), which can in fact occur at this stage. The switch to vasodilatation is chiefly due to a reduction in sympathetic vasoconstrictor drive; this outweighs the effects of plasma angiotensin II, adrenaline and vasopressin, which increase markedly in this phase. There is uncertainty as to what inhibits the sympathetic vasoconstrictor outflow; vagal afferents in the heart can initiate the inhibition in some species (e.g. cats) but not others (e.g. dogs). Central pathways in the brain involving δ-opiate receptors and 5-hydroxytryptamine have also been implicated. For example, administration of the opioid antagonist naloxone into the fourth ventricle helps to restore sympathetic outflow and so prevent decompensation.

Several other serious complications can arise during severe, prolonged hypotension. Probably the commonest of these is acute tubular necrosis, a form of acute renal failure caused by hypoxic damage to the renal tubules. This is heralded by failure of the urine output to improve after a day or so. For this reason the urine output of a patient in shock is closely monitored. Another serious complication in patients with pre-existing ischaemic heart disease is myocardial infarction or acute cardiac failure, triggered by the fall in perfusion pressure. In the most severe cases multi-organ failure can develop, leading to death.

16.3 Fainting (syncope)

A faint is a sudden, transient loss of consciousness that occurs when cerebral blood flow falls to less than half normal owing to an abrupt fall in arterial pressure. The critical cerebral artery pressure is approximately 40 mmHg, which corresponds in an upright subject to approximately 70 mmHg mean pressure at heart level. The initiating factor may be a pathophysiological stress such as severe hypovolaemia or orthostasis, as in Figure 16.4; or it may be a psychological stress such as fear, pain or horror, as in Figure 16.5. The sight of blood, especially one's own, often induces emotional fainting in young adults. In such psychogenic fainting, the circulation initially evinces a normal alarm response, namely tachycardia, muscle vasodilatation, cutaneous vasoconstriction and sweating. During this pre-faint period the subject looks pale and sweaty, hyperventilates and, very characteristically, yawns. Then a sudden increase in vagal outflow causes a profound bradycardia (there was no heart beat for 8 s in Figure 16.4) and at the same time the peripheral resistance vessels dilate, due probably to a fall in sympathetic vasoconstrictor drive. As a result, blood pressure falls precipitously, and reduced cerebral perfusion is followed within seconds by loss of consciousness. This sequence is sometimes called a 'vasovagal attack'. The cause of the sudden changes in vagal and vasomotor activity is not certain; in the case of psychogenic fainting, the response could be related to the 'playing dead' response of small animals, which emanates from the cingulate gyrus (Section 14.4). In the case of post-haemorrhagic syncope, the response may be initiated by activation of left

ECG

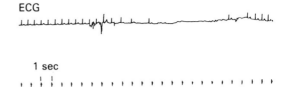

1 sec

Figure 16.4 ECG taken during a faint (vasovagal attack) in a healthy medical student. The student had received the vasodilator nitroglycerine and was then tilted from supine to upright. There was a period of 8 s asystole during the faint. The student quickly recovered on being restored to a supine position

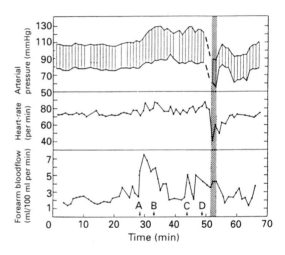

Figure 16.5 Circulatory changes in a male student during an emotional faint. The student showed forearm vasodilatation (alarm response) while watching the preparation for venepuncture (A) and venepuncture of a colleague (B), but did not faint as on an earlier occasion (and as the experimenter intended). Insertion of a needle into his arm (C) again produced vasodilatation, but no faint. The subject was therefore asked to drink some of the blood taken from his colleague (D). He became pale, yawned, said 'I'm going' and fainted (stippled area). No heart beat was detected by ECG for 11 s and heart rate then averaged 37 per min. Forearm blood flow remained above resting level despite the slump in blood pressure, showing that vasodilatation had occurred. Consciousness was regained after 2 min. (From Greenfield, A. D. M. (1951) *The Lancet*, p. 1303, by permission)

ventricular mechanoreceptors in the near-empty heart at end-systole.

The supine position resulting from a faint raises the intrathoracic blood volume and filling pressure. This, along with the baro-reflex, quickly restores the cardiac output and arterial pressure (except of course in hypovolaemia). Consciousness is recovered in about 2 min. It is a mistake, albeit a well-intentioned one, to prop up the patient during a faint, since this deprives him of the benefit of the Frank–Starling mechanism. Ordinary faints occur almost solely in the upright position, i.e. they require a low CVP, so it is sound advice for a person feeling faint to sit or lie down.

16.4 Essential hypertension

Definition and classification

The medical condition 'hypertension' can be defined as a chronic, usually progressive, raised arterial pressure. To some extent this definition begs the question, for the dividing line between normal and raised pressure is a rather difficult issue, the distribution of pressure in the population being unimodal. Most physicians would diagnose hypertension if repeated measurement of resting pressure exceeded 140/90 mmHg in a patient under 50 years old, or 160/95 mmHg in an older patient. The disease is in itself almost symptomless, and it may come to light only as a result of a routine medical examination; or it may present later with one of its many sequelae, namely heart failure, coronary artery disease, a cerebro-vascular accident (stroke), retinopathy or chronic renal failure. Distinct identifiable causes are relatively uncommon but they include hyperaldosteronism (Conn's syndrome), renal artery stenosis (which activates the renin–angiotensin–aldosterone system) and phaeochromocytoma (a catecholamine-secreting tumour); such cases are termed 'secondary hypertension'. In 90% or more cases, however, no such cause is found and the disease is classed as primary or essential hypertension.

The course of essential hypertension, untreated, can be 'benign', meaning only slowly progressive, or more rarely 'malignant', meaning rapidly progressive with renal damage (proteinuria), cardiac failure (oedema) and cerebral damage (papilloedema, retinopathy).

A distinctive form of hypertension occurs in pregnancy called pre-eclamptic toxaemia (because it is due to toxins arising from the placenta and can lead to fits – eclampsia – if untreated). The condition can be serious but resolves rapidly after delivery.

Pathophysiology of essential hypertension

Since blood pressure depends on the balance between cardiac output and peripheral resistance, hypertension must be regarded as an imbalance in cardiovascular regulation. In the early stages of the disorder, when hypertension is both marginal and labile, the cardiac output is raised while the peripheral resistance is only slightly above normal. When the disease is well established, however, the cardiac output is normal or slightly reduced and the hypertension is therefore due to an increase in peripheral resistance (Table 16.1). The increase in vascular resistance affects virtually every organ, including the kidney, and is caused partly by a narrowing of the small arteries and partly by rarefaction. *Rarefaction* is a reduction in the number of vessels present in unit volume of tissue, and the occurrence of rarefaction has recently been confirmed in both the retina and the intestine of hypertensive patients. *Narrowing* of the small arteries is due to increased vascular tone in the early stages, and is fully reversible by vasodilator drugs at this stage. As time passes, however, the smooth muscle of the tunica media responds to the chronically raised pressure load by hypertrophying, and this leads to organic narrowing of the lumen. The elevated resistance can then no longer be fully abolished during maximal vasodilatation

Table 16.1 Vascular resistance of the hand in hypertension. (Percentage change from normal in parenthesis)

	Normal	Hypertensive
Mean arterial pressure (mmHg)	82 (100%)	116 (141%)
Peripheral resistance $(PRU_{100})^*$	3.8 (100%)	5.9 (156%)
Peripheral resistance at maximal vasodilatation $(PRU_{100})^*$	1.6 (100%)	2.5 (163%)
Sensitivity of resistance to noradrenaline (slope of response curve)	100%	178%

(Hypertensive vessels can dilate and contract but even at maximal dilatation their resistance is higher than normal maximally dilated vessels.)
*PRU_{100} is a peripheral resistance unit, mmHg/(ml/min)100 g.
(After Sivertsson, R. and Olander, B. 1968, *Life Science*, **7**, 1291–1297)

(Table 16.1). Medial hypertrophy takes only a few weeks to develop in rats subjected to experimental hypertension by clipping one of the renal arteries (which stimulates the renin–angiotensin–aldosterone system).

The baroreflex is still operative in hypertensive patients but operates around a higher set point (resetting). Also, in severe cases stiffening of the artery wall reduces the sensitivity of the baroreflex. It is generally accepted that the changes in the baroreflex are an effect rather than a cause of the hypertension.

What initiates the hypertension?

Despite enormous research efforts, the answer to this question remains uncertain. There is a strong familial tendency to hypertension and also an epidemiological association with a high salt intake. These observations, coupled with direct experimental work, have led to a number of causative theories.

Neurogenic (stress) hypothesis This proposes that an excessive sympathetic outflow in response to stress initiates bouts of reversible hypertension, which gradually induce a structural reaction (medial hyper-

trophy) that perpetuates the condition. Experimental lesions of the nucleus tractus solitarius raises the sympathetic outflow and leads to chronic hypertension in experimental animals. Moreover, repeated exposure of laboratory animals to psychogenic stress can cause chronic hypertension.

Kidneys and salt imbalance hypothesis Here the proposition is that a small but sustained discrepancy between renal salt excretion and dietary intake leads to an increase in extracellular salt mass and, owing to the osmotic effect of the salt, an increase in extracellular water. This leads to a rise in plasma volume, filling pressure, stroke volume and blood pressure, which in turn evokes medial hypertrophy and the non-reversible rise in peripheral resistance. The association of hypertension with a high-salt diet fits this hypothesis. Also, a genetic strain of rat exists in which a salt diet, harmless to ordinary rats, causes hypertension.

Normally one would expect that a high salt intake, and the associated fluid retention, would inhibit the renin–angiotensin–aldosterone system and so reduce salt and water reabsorption by the renal tubules. However, the renin–angiotensin–aldosterone system is actually found to be stimulated rather than depressed in many (but not all) human hypertensives. Extracellular fluid volume is found to be increased or normal in hypertension, but plasma volume is reduced in the established disease.

Depressed transport by cell membrane Na^+–K^+ ATPase The activity of the Na^+–K^+ ATPase pump of the cell membrane is reduced in red and white cells taken from the blood of hypertensives. The extent to which this is due to a circulating digoxin-like factor or to intrinsic membrane abnormalities is unclear. It has been suggested that if reduced Na^+–K^+ pump activity also occurred in vascular smooth muscle cells, the knock-on effect on the Na^+–Ca^{2+} exchanger might elevate free cytosolic Ca^{2+}, leading to increased vascular tone and hypertension. This hypothesis remains unproven, however.

Multifactorial hypothesis The long-term control of blood pressure involves neural, endocrine and renal mechanisms and many workers suspect that hypertension develops only if more than one regulatory process is abnormal, usually in a genetically susceptible individual. Whatever the initial cause, the process is thought to become self-perpetuating once medial hypertrophy develops, since a rise in pressure evokes further hypertrophy.

Treatment of hypertension This is based on *diuretic drugs* to lower extracellular fluid volume, *captopril* to block the angiotensin-converting enzyme and therefore reduce angiotensin and aldosterone levels, *peripheral vasodilators* such as calcium-channel blockers (nifedipine) and α_1-adrenoreceptor blockers (prazosin) to lower peripheral resistance, and *β-adrenoreceptor blockers* like propranolol to reduce cardiac output. The aim is to reduce systolic pressure to 135–145 mmHg and diastolic to 85 mmHg. This greatly reduces the mortality and morbidity. Untreated the outlook is grave, with about 50% of patients eventually developing heart failure, 25% renal failure and 25% cerebral complications (retinopathy, encephalopathy, strokes).

16.5 Chronic cardiac failure

Definition and causes

Chronic or congestive cardiac failure (CCF) may be defined as an intrinsic inability of the heart to maintain an adequate perfusion of the tissues at a normal filling pressure. This contrasts with the disorder 'shock', where the low output state is secondary to a low filling pressure. Starling, working with the isolated heart preparation, noted long ago that when a heart begins to fail, it requires a higher filling pressure and higher end-diastolic volume to maintain its stroke volume; at a normal filling pressure the stroke volume became subnormal. Thus the immediate cause of cardiac failure is a fall in the energy of contraction at any given end-diastolic volume; in other words, a reduction in contractility.

In many patients, a recognizable pathological condition initiates the chronic failure; for example, diffuse coronary artery disease, reduction in functional muscle mass after a myocardial infarct, or chronic work overload caused by hypertension. In other cases there is no obvious precipitating pathology and the cause is related to myocyte biochemistry. Studies of myocardium from failing hearts indicate that although contractility is impaired, energy production is normal, judging by the normal levels of ATP and creatine phosphate. Energy utilization, however, is impaired: both myofibrillar ATPase activity and myofibril content per gram of myocardium are low. The most serious abnormality may involve intracellular calcium, the key factor in excitation–contraction coupling (Section 3.5); calcium transport into the sarcoplasmic reticulum is impaired, so the internal calcium store may be low. Possible impairment of the affinity of troponin for calcium is also being investigated.

Impairment of cardiac performance

Owing to the reduction in contractility, the ventricular function curve of the failing ventricle(s) is depressed and its slope is reduced (Figure 16.6). The pump function curve (stroke volume against arterial pressure, Figure 7.13) is depressed too. The rate of tension development is slow, and the ejection fraction falls from the normal 66% to as little as 10–20%. In severe failure this reduces the stroke volume, but in mild failure the stroke volume may be almost normal owing to a compensatory increase in end-diastolic volume (see later). Consequently, the cardiac output at rest may be either within the normal range (compensated failure) or subnormal (decompensated failure; mean 3.8 litres/min in one series). The impaired cardiac performance becomes much more obvious during an exercise test, because the failing heart cannot increase its output to a normal extent, as shown by the data in Table 15.3. The patient's exercise tolerance is poor and he/she complains of excessive fatigue. The poor response to exercise is interesting, because it is not only due to impairment of the stroke volume response but also to impairment of the heart rate response. The inability of *stroke volume* to rise to a normal extent is caused by the decreased sensitivity to filling pressure (i.e. the reduced slope of the ventricular function curve), by the decreased ability to cope with a rise in arterial pressure, and by a decrease in the responsiveness of contractility to catecholamines (see later). The impaired *heart rate* response (see Table 15.3) is caused partly by a depletion of noradrenaline from the cardiac sympathetic nerve terminals due to a fall in tyrosine hydroxylase activity, and partly by 'down-regulation' of the myocyte β_1-adrenoreceptors. Down-regulation of the β_1-adrenoreceptor is due to a fall in receptor density and/or uncoupling of the receptor from cAMP production caused by changes in the G proteins of the cell membrane.

Pathophysiological responses to heart failure

The responses of the circulation and other systems to heart failure include compensa-

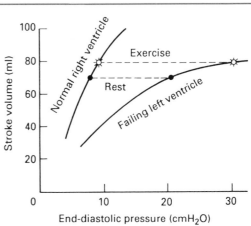

Figure 16.6 Diagram illustrating the operation of the Frank–Starling mechanism in a patient with a failing left ventricle but relatively healthy right ventricle. The left ventricle function curve is depressed and its slope is reduced. Under resting conditions (closed circles) the left ventricle requires an elevated filling pressure to match the right ventricle's stroke volume. In exercise (open symbols) the disparity in filling pressure becomes extreme owing to the near-plateau on the function curve of the failing left ventricle

tory influences on the heart, redistribution of cardiac output, renal retention of salt and water, and oedema.

Compensatory influences on the heart

The output of the failing heart is supported by two compensatory mechanisms, namely an increase in filling pressure and an increased level of circulating catecholamine.

Raised ventricular filling pressure: good and bad aspects Filling pressure rises to well over 12 cmH$_2$O, distending the failing ventricle and, in mild failure, improving its contractile energy by the Frank–Starling mechanism. The rise in filling pressure is due to a combination of increased plasma volume and peripheral venoconstriction (see later). The resulting cardiac dilatation can be gross, and is readily detected in chest radiograms (Figure 16.7). Although the increase in end-diastolic volume shifts the ventricle along the ventricular function curve, this is

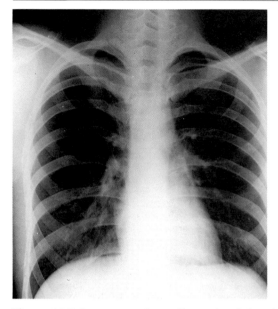 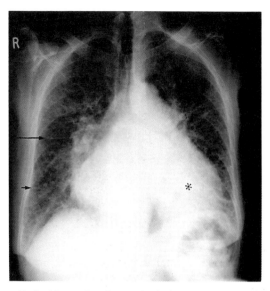

Figure 16.7 Anteroposterior radiograph of the chest. Left: Normal subject. Right: Patient with left ventricular failure. Asterisk marks grossly dilated left ventricle. Upper, long arrow: line of oedema fluid in fissure between upper and middle lobes. Lower, short arrow: septal line caused by interstitial oedema (Kerley B line). Radiating opacities due to pulmonary interstitial oedema are also present in the left lung field (Kerley A lines). (Courtesy of Dr A. Wilson, St. George's Hospital, London)

of little benefit beyond a certain point because the curve reaches a virtual plateau (see Figure 16.6). Moreover, excessive cardiac dilatation can be harmful because contraction becomes mechanically inefficient: the active tension required to generate systolic pressure increases with ventricular diameter (see 'Laplace effect', Figure 7.12), raising the energy cost of systole in a ventricle that can ill afford extra energy costs. In addition, gross dilatation can widen the atrioventricular orifice to such an extent that the atrioventricular valve becomes functionally incompetent, further reducing the ventricular ejection fraction. A further ill-effect of a high filling pressure is the generation of oedema (see later). There are thus several reasons for trying to reduce the filling pressure in severe cardiac failure, even though this does shift the ventricle back along the Starling curve.

Stimulation by circulating catecholamines
The cardiac nerves themselves become depleted of catecholamine, as mentioned

earlier, but there is a marked rise in plasma adrenaline and noradrenaline levels in severe failure which helps to support the inotropic state. The support is somewhat mitigated, however, by a down-regulation or un-coupling of myocardial β_1-adrenoreceptors as the disease progresses.

Changes in peripheral vascular beds

The limited cardiac output is preferentially distributed to the coronary, cerebral and skeletal muscle circulations at the expense of other peripheral tissues, as shown in Figure 16.8. The perfusion of the renal, splanchnic and cutaneous vascular beds is severely reduced, owing to sympathetic vasoconstrictor nerve activity coupled with a rise in plasma angiotensin II. This peripheral vasoconstriction maintains the arterial pressure, which would otherwise be threatened by a low cardiac output. The increases in sympathetic outflow and circulating angiotensin II also induce cutaneous and

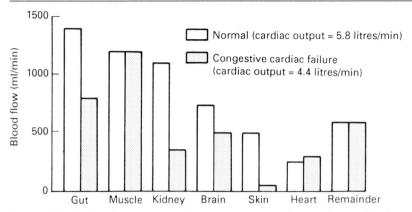

Figure 16.8 Redistribution of cardiac output in a resting patient with chronic cardiac failure and an output of 4.4 litres/min (filled columns). Note the poor perfusion of kidney, gut and skin. (From Wade, O. L. and Bishop, J. M. (1962) *Cardiac Output and Regional Bloodflow*, Blackwell, Oxford, by permission)

splanchnic venoconstriction, which contributes to the rise in cardiac filling pressure. The increased sympathetic outflow is thought to be the result of cardiopulmonary and arterial baroreceptor reflexes.

Although these changes may be beneficial in mild failure, they cause problems in severe failure, partly because of the harmful effects of excessive cardiac dilatation and partly because stroke volume is reduced when a failing ventricle has to eject against a normal arterial pressure.

Renal retention of salt and water

The kidneys retain salt and water in isotonic proportion in cardiac failure, expanding the extracellular fluid compartment by up to 30% and contributing to cardiac dilatation and oedema formation. The mechanisms underlying the salt and water retention are only partially understood but they include altered renal haemodynamics and stimulation of the renin–angiotensin–aldosterone system due to increased sympathetic discharge to the kidney. Plasma aldosterone is further elevated by a reduced degradation rate in the congested, underperfused liver.

Peripheral and pulmonary oedema in cardiac failure

Oedema of the lungs and/or periphery is a prominent clinical feature in cardiac failure. The oedema is caused primarily by a rise in capillary pressure following the rise in venous pressure; pressure in the venous limbs of human finger capillaries reaches 20–40 mmHg in right ventricular failure. Another contributory factor is the fall in plasma colloid osmotic pressure by approximately 7 mmHg due to plasma volume expansion. These changes tip the balance of Starling forces across the venous capillary wall in favour of an excessive filtration rate, leading to oedema. The oedema may be worse in the periphery or in the lungs, depending on whether the right side or left side filling pressure is more severely affected.

Pulmonary oedema If the left ventricle is weakened more than the right (as is common in ischaemic heart disease), the pressure in the pulmonary veins is raised. This is due to the operation of the Frank–Starling mechanism which ensures that left output equals right output, even in failure. If the left side transiently pumps out less blood than the right, more blood enters the left side, raising left ventricular filling pressure until by the Frank–Starling mechanism the left ventricle output achieves parity with the right (see Figure 16.6). Because pulmonary venous pressure is raised, oedema develops in the lungs and such patients display pulmonary vein congestion (see Figure 16.7), reduced lung compliance, pulmonary interstitial oedema and dyspnoea (difficulty in breathing). This form of dyspnoea is especially marked during the night (paroxysmal nocturnal dyspnoea) because the supine position increases pulmonary congestion and pulmonary capillary filtration pressure. Such patients find it more comfortable to sleep propped up by pillows. In moderate pulmonary oedema the excess fluid collects mainly in the pulmonary interstitium around the bronchi and larger vessels, but in severe pulmonary oedema the fluid floods into the alveolar spaces too, impairing oxygen transport with potentially fatal results.

Peripheral oedema If the right ventricle fails (for example secondary to pulmonary hypertension caused by lung disease), the combined effects of the Frank–Starling mechanism and renal salt-and-water retention is to raise the systemic venous pressure. This gives rise to peripheral oedema in the dependent tissues, namely the ankles in ambulant patients and over the sacrum in bed-ridden patients. Such patients show a combination of distended jugular veins and pitting ankle or sacral oedema. Not infrequently both ventricles fail and oedema occurs both in the periphery and the lungs.

Principles of treatment

The treatment of cardiac failure merits a mention here because it is an exercise in applied physiology. The aims of treatment from a physiological point of view are (1) to reduce cardiac work, (2) to reduce the excessive plasma volume and cardiac dilatation, and (3) to improve myocardial contractility if possible.

Cardiac work can be reduced by rest, by reducing arterial pressure and by reducing filling pressure. To this end, peripheral vasodilator drugs can be used, such as the α_1-adrenoreceptor blocker prazosin. By reducing the arterial pressure opposing ejection such drugs improve the cardiac ejection fraction. Peripheral venodilators like nitroglycerine and nitroprusside lower filling pressure and relieve pulmonary congestion. Captopril and enalapril (angiotensin-converting enzyme inhibitors) are now very widely used, to lower tone in resistance and capacitance vessels.

Cardiac dilatation, plasma volume and oedema can be reduced by diuretic drugs like frusemide and the thiazides. ACE inhibitors like captopril exert their therapeutic action partly in this way too; by lowering angiotensin II levels, they also reduce aldosterone levels. The advantage of reducing gross cardiac dilatation is that the heart can then operate at a better mechanical advantage (Laplace's law), which makes up for the concomitant movement down the ventricular function curve. (It is interesting to note that both vasodilator and diuretic drugs are partially reversing the natural compensatory responses to cardiac failure; one can view the natural compensations as 'overdone' in cardiac failure.)

The third line of attack is to enhance *myocardial contractility* by the inotropic drug digoxin. The discovery of this agent by William Withering in 1785 makes an interesting story. Dr. Withering was journeying through Shropshire when he was asked to see a woman suffering from severe 'dropsy' (cardiac failure). He could do little for her and on his return journey was astonished to find her not only alive but much improved. On enquiring, he discovered that she had been taking a local folklore remedy, an infusion of the leaves of the foxglove, *Digitalis purpurea*. The efficacy of a digitalis infusion is illustrated in Figure 3.13, and its mechanism of action (enhancing the intracellular store of calcium) is explained there. However, digoxin is also rather cardiotoxic and difficult to control therapeutically, and its use has fallen out of favour recently. An exception is made in cases of failure associated with atrial fibrillation (a common association), where digoxin also helps to slow and regularize the heart beat. In other cases, however, good responses are often obtained simply by a combination of rest, ACE inhibitor and diuretic therapy.

16.6 Summary

Systemic hypoxaemia occurs at high altitude, in chronic emphysema, severe pulmonary oedema and right-to-left shunts through congenital heart defects. Taking high altitude as an example, the cardiovascular responses are a compound of local effects of hypoxaemia on vessels (systemic vasodilatation, pulmonary vasoconstriction) and reflex effects of increased peripheral chemoreceptor activity. The result is a resting *hyperventilation*, driven by increased peripheral chemoreceptor activity; *tachycardia and increased cardiac output at rest*, the cause of which is not entirely clear; and *peripheral vasodilatation*, due to the local action of hypoxaemia on vessels. The increase in cardiac output and tissue blood flow compensates for the reduced arterial oxygen content. In the brain, however, vasodilatation is largely offset by the vasoconstrictor effect of hypocapnia (arising from hyperventilation) and this can lead to acute mountain sickness. Maximum cardiac output in exercise is not increased, so maximal work rate is impaired. *Pulmonary hypertension* results from the vasoconstrictor response of pulmonary vessels to hypoxia, improving perfusion of the lung apices but increasing the work load on the right ventricle and sometimes leading to cardiac failure. *Acclimatization* to high altitude involves correction of the respiratory alkalosis, further increase in ventilation, a rise in haematocrit and shifts in the oxygen dissociation curve.

Shock and haemorrhage Acute circulatory failure ('shock') can arise from hypovalaemia, septicaemia, acute cardiac failure or anaphylaxis. Taking haemorrhage as an example, the acute hypovolaemia reduces CVP and hence stroke volume and pulse pressure (Frank–Starling mechanism). Reduced afferent input from the cardiac and arterial baroreceptors, and increased peripheral chemoreceptor activity, evoke a reflex rise in sympathetic activity and in circulating levels of angiotensin II and, in severe cases, adrenaline and vasopressin. The immediate effects are tachycardia, increased cardiac contractility, peripheral vasoconstriction and venoconstriction, which can restore mean blood pressure after moderate haemorrhages. The skin is pale and sweaty, there is muscular weakness and impaired consciousness, and hyperventilation due to lactic acidosis.

The subnormal capillary pressure allows plasma oncotic pressure to dominate and absorb interstitial fluid into the circulation over the course of half-an-hour or so. This internal transfusion is aided by a shift of intracellular fluid into the interstitial compartment caused by a rise in extracellular fluid osmolarity; the latter is due to adrenaline-induced hepatic glycogenolysis.

Oliguria and salt retention are the result of increased renal sympathetic nerve activity, vasopressin (ADH) and aldosterone secretion. The renal conservation of salt and water, coupled with increased fluid intake (thirst is stimulated by angiotensin II) and adequate salt intake, restores the lost salt and water over a few days. Plasma proteins and red cells are resynthesized more slowly.

The above events occur in well-compensated hypovolaemia. In severe or late-treated haemorrhage, an irreversible, decompensated phase is entered in which peripheral vasoconstriction suddenly gives way to a relative vasodilatation, causing a sharp collapse of blood pressure. This can be fatal. Other possible sequelae include acute renal failure (signalled by anuria) and acute cardiac failure in patients with pre-existing ischaemic heart disease.

Fainting Here, a sudden brief loss of consciousness arises from an abrupt, vagally-mediated bradycardia coupled with sudden peripheral vasodilatation (vasovagal attack).

Essential hypertension Resting blood pressures in excess of 140–160/90–95 mmHg (depending on age) are harmful, leading to cardiac, cerebral, retinal and renal disease. The high pressure in established disease is due to increased total peripheral resistance, caused by narrowing of small arteries (initially by reversible vasoconstriction, later by medial hypertrophy too) and some rarefaction. The aetiology is probably multifactorial, with the following factors implicated: genetic predisposition, stressful lifestyle, high salt intake, inappropriate activity of renin–angiotensin–aldosterone system, impaired renal regulation of salt excretion, and possibly depression of cell membrane Na^+–K^+ ATPase. Treatment is by angiotensin-converting enzyme inhibitors, peripheral vasodilators, diuretics, and β-adrenoreceptor blockers (to reduce cardiac output).

Chronic cardiac failure Failure of the heart to maintain a normal stroke volume at a normal filling pressure can arise from ischaemic heart disease, chronic overload by pulmonary or systemic hypertension, valvular defects, and intracellular biochemical defects as yet poorly defined. Signs and symptoms include exercise intolerance, pulmonary oedema (left ventricular failure), dependent oedema (right ventricular failure) or a combination of these.

Cardiac pathophysiology. Cardiac contractility and the Starling curve (ventricular function curve) are depressed and ejection fraction is reduced; but, despite this, stroke volume and cardiac output at rest can be near normal in compensated failure, due to a rise in filling pressure and cardiac distension (Starling's law of the heart). If distension is gross, however, its effect is deleterious (Laplace's law). During exercise, both stroke volume and heart rate fail to increase adequately. The latter is due to noradrena-line depletion in cardiac sympathetic fibres, and to β-adrenoceptor down-regulation and uncoupling.

Peripheral circulatory changes. In the peripheral circulation there is sympathetic vasoconstriction of the cutaneous, splanchnic and renal circulations, which helps support blood pressure in a face of a reduced cardiac output. Venoconstriction contributes to the rise in CVP. Raised angiotensin II levels contribute to vasoconstriction both directly and indirectly. Aldosterone levels are raised and there is renal retention of salt and water, leading to a rise in cardiac filling pressures and to oedema.

Treatment is based on reduction of plasma volume and excessive cardiac dilatation (diuretic drugs, ACE inhibitors); reduction of cardiac work by rest and by peripheral vasodilator drugs; and in some cases enhancement of myocardial contractility by inotropic drugs such as digoxin.

Further reading

Reviews and chapters

Bohr, D. F. (1989) Cell membrane in hypertension. *News in Physiological Science*, **4**, 85–88

Cowley, A. W., Barber, W. J., Lombard, J. H., Osborn, J. L. and Liard, J. F. (1986) Relationship between body fluid volume and arterial pressure. *Federal Proceedings*, **45**, 2864–2870

Eckberg, D. L. and Sleight, P. (1992) *Human Baroreflexes in Health and Disease*, Clarendon Press, Oxford

Francis, G. S. and Cohn, J. N. (1990) Heart failure: mechanisms of cardiac and vascular dysfunction and the rationale for pharmacologic intervention. *FASEB Journal*, **4**, 3068–3075

Haddy, F. J. (1989) Humoral factors in hypertension. *News in Physiological Sciences*, **4**, 202–205

Homy, C. J., Vatner, S. F. and Vatner, D. E. (1991) β-adrenergic receptor regulation in the heart in pathophysiological states: abnormal adrenergic responsiveness in cardiac disease. *Annual Review of Physiology*, **53**, 137–159

Ludbrook, J. and Evans, R. (1989) Posthemorrhagic syncope. *News in Physiological Science*, **4**, 120–133

Mulvany, M. J. and Aalkjaer, C. (1990) Structure and function of small arteries. *Physiological Reviews*, **70**, 921–961 (Hypertension)

Prewitt, R. L., Stacy, D. L. and Ono, Z. (1987) The

microcirculation in hypertension: which are the resistance vessels? *NIPS*, **2**, 139–141

Rowell, L. B. (1986) *Human Circulation Regulation During Physical Stress*, Oxford University Press, New York (Hypoxaemia)

Schadt, J. C. and Ludbrook, J. (1991) Hemodynamic and neurohumoral responses to acute hypovolaemia in conscious mammals (Review). *American Journal of Physiology*, **260**, H305–318

Research papers

Hartikainen, J., Ahonen, E., Nevalaines, T., Sikanen, A. and Hakumaki, M. (1990) Haemodynamic information encoded in the aortic baroreceptor discharge during haemorrhage. *Acta Physiologica Scandinavica*, **140**, 181–189

Länne, T. and Lundvall, J. (1992) Mechanisms in man for rapid refill of the circulatory system in hypovolaemia. *Acta Physiologica Scandinavica*, **146**, 299–306

Marshall, J. M., Thomas, T. and Turner, L. (1993) A link between adenosine, ATP-sensitive K^+ channels, potassium and muscle vasodilatation in the rat in systemic hypoxia. *Journal of Physiology*, **472**, 1–9

The end but not the end

'Begin at the beginning', said the King, very gravely, to the White Rabbit, 'and go on till you come to the end: then stop'. Heart failure seems to offer a natural ending to this text, but the scientific investigation of the circulation is far from at an end – too many mysteries remain unsolved. The discerning reader will have recognized the superabundance of unresolved problems from the frequent use of 'perhaps', 'may be', 'probably', 'is thought to' and so on. Our subject began essentially with the work of William Harvey over three centuries ago, yet a comment by Harvey still makes an apt conclusion to today's textbook: 'I see a field of such vast extent . . . that my whole life perchance would not suffice for its completion.' (A Mallock (1929) *William Harvey*, Hoeber, New York.)

Appendix I
Learning objectives

Although this book presents only a basic account of the cardiovascular system, it does contain more than the bare minimum of material needed to pass a preclinical medical examination. In order to help the hard–pressed medical student preparing for an examination to focus on the most vital, fundamental points, the following chapter-by-chapter learning objectives are suggested. The level of the learning objectives is set with medical students sitting a preclinical examination in mind.

Chapter 1   Overview of CVS

The student should have a clear understanding of the following:

- The distance limitation for diffusional transport, and the roles of both diffusional and convective transport.
- The organization of the CVS into low-pressure pulmonary and high-pressure systemic circulations lying in series, each served by a pump.
- The distribution of cardiac output to different tissues in a resting man.
- The basic physical factors governing blood flow (basic law of flow). What simple evidence shows that resistance lies chiefly in the arterioles and smallest arteries?
- The functional categories of blood vessel.
- The basic triple-layered composition of vessel walls and the functional importance of the vascular smooth muscle.
- The meaning of 'portal circulation' and its functional implications.

Chapter 2   Cardiac cycle

The student should understand:

- The gross structure of the heart, especially functionally important aspects (valves, fibro-tendinous ring, wall thicknesses, papillary muscles, site of pacemaker).
- The sequence of valve positions in the four phases of the cardiac cycle and the corresponding changes in volume and pressure in each chamber.
- The ventricular pressure–volume loop.
- The meaning of 'ejection fraction' and typical values.
- The origin of clinical signs, namely apex beat, central venous pressure waveform and heart sounds.
- The relative timing of different phases of cycle, and how this changes during tachycardia.

Chapter 3   Excitation and contraction of a myocyte

- The fine structure of a cardiac myocyte (sarcomere structure, contractile machinery, sarcoplasmic reticulum, etc.) and functions of the main components.
- The student should be able to explain how the contractile machinery produces shortening/tension and how it is activated by Ca_i^{2+}.
- The main features of the resting potential and action potential of a myocyte, their ionic basis and functional significance.

- The role of Ca_i^{2+} and the myocyte's calcium cycle.
- The effect of diastolic length on contractile force, and its underlying mechanisms.
- The action of catecholamines and digoxin on contractile force.

Chapter 4   Initiation of the heart beat and its neural control

The student should be able to:

- Sketch the anatomy of the excitation–conduction system of the heart.
- Explain 'pacemaker dominance'.
- Draw a sino-atrial node action potential and pacemaker potential, and explain their ionic basis.
- Explain how depolarization propagates through the myocardial mass.
- Describe the chronotropic actions of the sympathetic and parasympathetic nerves upon the electrical system of the heart, and the mechanisms that underlie these actions.

Chapter 5   Electrocardiogram and arrhythmias

- Draw, label and scale a typical ECG.
- Explain the origin of the P, QRS and T waves, and the PR and ST intervals.
- Give the meaning of 'cardiac dipole'.
- Explain why different leads (I–III) show different QRS patterns for the same systole.
- Explain how the dipole changes with time and how this gives rise to the QRS pattern.
- Understand the meaning of 'sinus arrhythmia', 'ectopic beat', 'heart block', 'pathological tachycardia', 'atrial fibrillation', 'ventricular fibrillation', 'circus mechanism', and 'afterpotential'.

Chapter 6   Measurement of cardiac output

- Define the Fick principle (cf. law of diffusion) and explain how it can be used to calculate pulmonary blood flow. What samples need to

be taken? What are the limitations of the method?
- Explain the basis of the dye dilution or thermal dilution method. Draw a typical concentration *versus* time curve and explain how the recirculation problem is circumvented.
- Give an outline of modern 'high-tech' methods, namely pulsed Doppler ultrasound measurement of aortic blood velocity, and radionuclide angiography for determining stroke volume and ejection fraction.
- Give an account of the relation between pulse pressure and stroke volume.

Chapter 7   Regulation of stroke volume and cardiac output

- State the Starling law of the heart and explain how it influences stroke volume in an isolated heart.
- Define 'stroke work' and draw a ventricular function curve (Starling curve; stroke work *versus* an index of diastolic stretch)
- What intracellular mechanisms underlie the Frank–Starling effect (length–tension curve)?
- What factors determine central venous pressure?
- State the roles of the Frank–Starling mechanism in man.
- What does Laplace's law tell us about the deleterious effects of excessive cardiac distension?
- Give a working definition of 'contractility' and draw a graph showing how a rise in contractility affects the Starling curve.
- Describe the several effects of cardiac sympathetic nerve stimulation upon cardiac performance, and explain the mechanisms.
- Outline the important positive inotropic factors, and the negative ones.
- Explain why a coordinated control of both the heart and peripheral circulation is necessary to achieve optimal cardiac output.

Chapter 8   Haemodynamics

- The following fundamental relations should be understood: relation between mean arterial pressure and pulse pressure; relation between mean arterial pressure, cardiac output and total peripheral resistance; Poiseuille's law for flow in tubes; Laplace's law relating tube radius to wall tension.

- What are laminar, turbulent and bolus flow patterns and in what vessels do they occur?
- Describe the principal methods for measuring blood flow in man.
- Draw, label and scale the arterial pressure pulse (waveform). Explain its principal features. How is the aortic pulse propagated to the radial artery?
- Outline the factors that influence human arterial blood pressure.
- Explain how arteriolar radius is used to regulate flow and arterial blood pressure.
- What factors influence the viscosity of blood, and what is the physiological or clinical significance of each?
- What factors affect the volume and distribution of blood in peripheral veins?

Chapter 9   Solute transport between blood and tissue

The student should be able to:

- Differentiate between the process responsible for transfer of metabolized solutes like glucose and oxygen (diffusion) and that responsible for net water transfer (hydraulic flow).
- Describe the structure of the three main types of capillary, and the ultrastructural features involved in permeation (intercellular clefts, fenestrations, vesicles, glycocalyx).
- Define 'solute permeability', and explain how permeability is affected by the presence of a porous membrane (pore area, restricted diffusion, etc.).
- Classify solutes into three main classes according to ease and route of transcapillary permeation.
- Describe the special properties of exchange across the blood-brain barrier.
- Explain how the rate of exchange of metabolized solutes can be increased in exercising muscle. What is the meaning of 'flow-limited' and 'diffusion-limited' exchange?
- Briefly outline the active, metabolic functions of vascular endothelium.

Chapter 10   Fluid exchange between plasma, interstitium and lymph

- What is the Starling principle of capillary fluid exchange? Write down an expression that summarizes the principle.
- What is an osmotic reflection coefficient and what is its importance?
- What are typical values for capillary pressure and what factors determine the pressure?
- What are typical values for human plasma colloid osmotic pressure and interstitial colloid osmotic pressure? Explain how the latter varies with filtration rate and why this is important.
- Why does normal interstitial fluid not flow readily under gravity? Draw the pressure–volume relation and explain its significance.
- Describe the circumstances that cause capillaries to reabsorb interstitial fluid.
- Explain why lymph flow is important, how lymph is propelled along, and how it is returned to the circulation.
- What is oedema? Give a systematic outline of the causes of oedema. Explain what is meant by 'safety factors against oedema'.
- Outline the basic microvascular changes involved in inflammation.

Chapter 11   Vascular smooth muscle

- Describe the main ultrastructural features of a VSM cell, including the arrangement of the contractile machinery.
- Explain how the initiation of contraction (via Ca-calmodulin and MLCKase) differs from that in cardiac muscle. What is the 'latch state'?
- State the roles of the principal ion channels governing VSM tone (e.g. K^+ channels, VOCs, ROCs and Cl^- channels).
- Explain how sympathetic stimulation produces contraction in action-potential generating VSM cells (electromechanical coupling).
- Explain how sympathetic stimulation or agonists such as angiotensin produce contraction in non-spike-forming VSM cells (pharmacomechanical coupling).
- Describe the three main mechanisms by which VSM relaxation can be induced.

Chapter 12 Control of blood vessels

The student should be able to give an account of:

- The effect of distension on active vascular tone (myogenic response).
- The importance of metabolic vasodilatation (functional hyperaemia) and outline of factors involved.
- Thumbnail sketches of key autacoids.
- EDRF, its production and physiological roles.
- Control phenomena of local origin. Autoregulation, shape of autoregulated pressure–flow relation and how this is affected by functional hyperaemia. Reactive hyperaemia and mechanisms involved.
- The sympathetic vasoconstrictor system: its anatomy, pharmacology of neuromuscular transmission, and physiological roles.
- Vasodilator nerves of limited distribution (sympathetic cholinergic fibres, parasympathetic vasomotor nerves, nociceptive sensory nerves), their roles and modes of action.
- Principal vasoactive circulating hormones, namely adrenaline, angiotensin II and vasopressin; their actions and factors controlling their release.

Chapter 13 Special circulations

The learning objectives for the coronary, skeletal muscle, cutaneous, cerebral and pulmonary circulations are indicated by the entries in the Summary tables (Tables 13.1–13.5).

Chapter 14 Receptors and reflexes

The student should be able to describe the anatomy, chief characteristics of the receptor and the reflex effects, for the following cardiovascular neural receptors:

- Arterial baroreceptors (in some detail).
- Veno-atrial stretch receptors (peripheral terminals of myelinated vagal afferent fibres).
- Mechanoreceptors in the atria, left ventricle and around coronary vessels (terminals of non-myelinated vagal afferents).
- Chemosensitive afferents in the myocardium.
- Peripheral chemoreceptors in the carotid and aortic bodies.
- Metaboloreceptors in skeletal muscle.

The student should have an outline knowledge of the primary central relay station (n. tractus solitarius), 'vertical' relaying, the role of the hypothalamus, and the medullary regions controlling the vagal and sympathetic outflows to the cardiovascular system (n. ambiguus, rostral ventrolateral medulla).

Chapter 15 Coordinated cardiovascular responses

- Posture:
  Explain how orthostasis reduces cardiac output.
  Describe the reflexes involved in maintaining blood pressure in orthostasis
- Valsalva manoeuvre:
  What effects does it have on the heart and blood pressure (the four phases)? How is it clinically useful?
- Exercise:
  Describe the vascular changes in the exercising muscles and their mechanisms.
  Explain how the rate of solute exchange between blood and active muscle increases.
  Describe the changes in cardiac activity and how they are produced.
  How is pulmonary oxygen uptake increased?
  What vascular changes occur in other tissues during muscle exercise?
  Contrast the blood pressure changes in static and dynamic exercise.
  Explain the 'central command' and 'peripheral reflex' theories for cardiac control in exercise.
  Explain how cardiac output can still rise in patients with transplanted hearts.
- Training:
  Describe the changes in capillarity, stroke volume and heart rate that result from training.
- Feeding:
  What happens to splanchnic blood flow, limb blood flow and cardiac output after a meal?
- Diving response:
  What are the three key features and what receptors initiate the reflex?
- Ageing:
  How does mean blood pressure change with age, and why does the pulse pressure rise so markedly?

What happens to the performance of even healthy hearts with increasing age?

Chapter 16   Cardiovascular pathophysiology

- Systemic hypoxaemia:
  What circumstances can give rise to this?
  Describe the immediate responses of ventilation, the heart, the systemic circulation and the pulmonary circulation.
- Shock and haemorrhage:
  List the main causes of acute circulatory failure ('shock').
  Explain how hypovolaemia leads to clinical shock.
  Describe the reflexes that help preserve blood pressure during hypovolaemia.
  What longer-term responses occur after the compensated phase?

What are the possible outcomes of clinical shock?

- Fainting:
  Explain the cardiovascular changes responsible for fainting.
- Hypertension:
  How is this defined and in what ways is it harmful?
  Describe the vascular changes in hypertension.
  Outline the aetiological theories for hypertension.
- Chronic cardiac failure:
  Describe the changes in cardiac performance in heart failure.
  Describe the physiological changes in the peripheral circulation in heart failure.
  Explain how and where oedema arises in failure.
  Outline the principles underlying the treatment of heart failure.

Appendix II
Technicalities

The units employed below are in the main 'standard international units', based on metres, kilograms and seconds (the SI system). Some of the literature uses the older system of units based on centimetres, grams and seconds (c.g.s. system).

Arterial input impedance. Resistance is the ratio of a mean pressure drop to mean flow: but arterial pressure and flow oscillate, and do so out of phase owing to the distensibility of the arterial tree (see Figure 8.9). Consequently, the ratio of pressure to flow alters from moment to moment. To take account of this, the concept of 'impedance' has been adapted from the theory of alternating electrical currents. Arterial input impedance is a measure of the opposition of the circulation to an oscillating input (i.e. stroke volume). The input impedance depends not only on peripheral vascular resistance but also on arterial viscoelastic compliance and the frequency of oscillation (i.e. heart rate).

Avogadro's number (N, N_A). This is the number of molecules in 1 mole (1 gram-molecule) of a substance: 6.0×10^{23}/mole.

Brownian motion. Tiny random movements of supramolecular particles suspended in a fluid. First observed in a pollen suspension by the Scottish botanist Robert Brown in 1828.

Density (ρ, rho). Density is mass per unit volume. Important values in physiology are water 1.00 g/ml; blood 1.06 g/ml; mercury 13.55 g/ml; these values are at 20°C.

Electrical conductance of a membrane permeable to ions. The relation between the electrical conductance of a membrane (G) and its permeability to an ion (P) is given by:

$$G = \frac{P(V_m C_o F)}{(RT/F)^2 \cdot (1 - e^{-V_m F/RT})}$$

where V_m is the membrane potential, R the gas constant, F the Faraday constant, T the absolute temperature and C_o is ion concentration.

Equilibrium. A system is said to be in equilibrium when its components have the same free energy level, for example, two solutions containing solute at the same concentration or, more accurately, at the same chemical potential. Equilibrium should not be confused with steady state (see later).

Faraday's constant (F). This is the charge carried by one mole of monovalent ion; 96 484 coulombs/mole.

Flux. Flux is the rate of movement of a material (e.g. a diffusing solute) across unit area of surface. In physiology the word is sometimes used loosely, omitting the 'per unit area of surface' aspect.

Force, work, energy and power. A force of one newton (N) is one that accelerates 1 kg mass at 1 m/s²; $1N = 1 \text{ kg m/s}^2$. The c.g.s. unit of force, the dyne (1 g cm/s²), equals 10^{-5} N. *Work* is defined as force times distance moved by the point of application of the force. *Energy* is defined as the capacity to do work and has the same units as work. One joule of work or energy (J) equals a force of 1 newton displaced over 1 metre (1 Nm).

It equals 10^7 ergs (the c.g.s unit, 1 dyne cm). *Power* is defined as rate of work or rate of change of energy; its unit; the watt (W), equals 1 J/s.

Gas constant (R). This quantifies the relation between energy level and absolute temperature for one mole of substance; 8.316 joules K^{-1} $mole^{-1}$.

Gravity (g). The force of gravity varies at different points on the earth's surface, depending on latitude and altitude. It is 9.81 m/s^2 at latitude 50°N (e.g. Land's End, Cornwall).

Laplace in a tube. Love's equation (equation 8.8) gives the total force in the wall of a tube, but in physiology and medicine we are usually more interested in the tension in the fibrous elements of the wall (both passive and active) due to blood pressure, rather than absolute wall force, which depends partly on atmospheric pressure too. An example should make the distinction clearer, comparing an artery first with no pressure drop across its walls (both sides atmospheric) and then with the internal pressure raised. Taking first a small artery of outer radius $r_o = 1$ mm (10^{-3} m) and wall thickness $w = 0.2$ mm when internal and outside pressures are both atmospheric ($P_1 = P_o = 1$ atmos $= 760$ mmHg $= 101$ kPa $= 10^5$ N/m^2), then from Love's equation the wall force per unit length is $(10^5 \times 0.8 \times 10^{-3}) - (10^5 \times 1.0 \times 10^{-3})$ or -0.2×10^2 N/m. Note that the 'tension' is negative, i.e. the wall is under a compressive force, because the atmosphere is acting on a bigger external surface than internal surface. The stress S in the wall is T/w, so the stress is -10^5 N/m^2, i.e. an atmosphere, just as one would expect intuitively. Now consider the artery when internal pressure is raised by 76 mmHg or one-tenth of an atmosphere, i.e. to an absolute P_i of 1.1 atmos or 1.1×10^5 N/m^2. This distends the vessel to, say, $r_o = 1.2$ mm (the exact value depends on wall stiffness), and assuming constant wall volume r_i becomes 1.04 mm; the stretched wall is thinner. Love's equation now gives $(1.1 \times 10^5 \times 1.04 \times 10^{-3}) - (10^5 \times 1.2 \times 10^{-3})$ or -0.056×10^2 N/m. Two things are notable. The *absolute* wall force is still dominated by atmospheric pressure in this thick-walled vessel and is still compressive (note the minus sign), albeit less so than before. But if we consider how the force in the wall has been *changed* by raising the blood pressure, we see that 0.144 N/m of *tension* has been added to the wall [i.e. $(-0.056) - (-0.2)$].

Much of this extra tension is carried by the fibres and cells of the wall, as expressed by equation (8.9).

Osmole. An osmole is defined by analogy with the ideal gas law; it is the mass of a substance which when distributed in 22.4 litres of solvent at 0°C exerts an osmotic pressure of 1 atmosphere. This definition stems from van't Hoff law's, osmotic pressure $\pi = RTC$, where C is molal concentration (moles/kg solvent), T is absolute temperature and R is the gas constant. A one *osmolar* solution contains 1 osmole of solute per litre of solution. A one *osmolal* solution contains 1 osmole per kilogram of solvent. Mammalian body fluids contain approximately 0.3 osmoles/ kg water and have a potential osmotic pressure of 5800 mmHg at body temperature ($22.4 \times 0.3 \times 310/273 = 7.6$ atmospheres). Human plasma protein (60–80 g/l) by contrast exerts an osmotic pressure of only approximately 25 mmHg.

Pressure. Pressure is the force exerted by a gas or liquid upon unit area of surface. Pressure acts equally in all directions, unlike stress. The SI unit of pressure, the pascal (Pa), equals 1 newton per square metre (N/m^2). One atmosphere of pressure is 100 100 Pa or 100.1 kPa (kilopascals). This pressure will support a column of mercury 760 mm high, so an atmosphere is commonly quoted as 760 mmHg pressure. Body fluid pressures are conventionally expressed relative to atmospheric pressure; a venous pressure of '0 mmHg' really means an absolute pressure of 760 mmHg, and an interstitial pressure of '−5mmHg' means an absolute pressure of 755 mmHg. The pressure exerted by a 1 mm tall column of mercury (1 mmHg) is 133 Pa or 1.36 cmH$_2$O at 20°C, being fluid height × density × gravity. The pressure exerted by a 1 cm tall column of water (1 cmH$_2$O) is 98.1 Pa (981 dynes/ cm^2) at 20°C.

Quantity of ions exchanged during an action potential. A cylindrical myocyte of length 10^{-2} cm and radius 10^{-3} cm has a volume of 3.14×10^{-8} cm^3 and a surface area of 6.28×10^{-5} cm^2. Each cm^2 of cell membrane requires 1 microcoulomb of charge to alter its potential by 1 volt; this is its capacitance. An action potential of 0.1 V (from −80 mV to +20 mV) requires a net transfer of 6.28×10^{-6} microcoulombs per cell. One mole of monovalent ion carries 96 500 coulombs (the Faraday constant), so the quantity of ions transferred works out to be 6.51×10^{-17} moles or, applying Avogadro's number, 3.9×10^7 ions. From the cell volume and intracellular concentrations in Table 3.1, the cell actually contains 1.9×10^{11} sodium ions and 2.6×10^{12} potassium ions. The fractional change in ion concentration after a single action potential is thus miniscule.

Second messengers. The 'first messenger' is a hormone such as noradrenaline, which binds to a cell surface receptor. The receptor is an integral membrane protein and undergoes a conformational change upon binding to the ligand (first messenger). This conformational change can have two main effects. (1) It may open up a nearby ionic channel, to which it is linked via a GTP-binding protein (guanosine triphosphate-binding proteins or G proteins). This can lead to a major influx of ions (e.g. receptor-operated calcium channels in vascular smooth muscle). (2) It may activate a class of GTP-binding protein which in turn activate membrane-bound enzymes (adenylate cyclase, guanylate cyclase or phospholipase C). The latter catalyse production of intracellular 'second messenger' at the cytoplasmic boundary. The main second messengers are cyclic adenosine monophosphate (cAMP), cyclic guanosine monophosphate (cGMP) and inositol trisphosphate (IP3). The second messenger activates enzymes called protein kinases which acts on ion channels in the surface membrane or on intracellular organelles to achieve the response associated with the ligand. (Robinshaw, D. and Foster, K. A. (1989) Role of G proteins in the regulation of the cardiovascular system. *Annual Review of Physiology*, **51**, 229–244.)

Sodium–calcium exchanger. This exchanges $3 \, Na^+$ ions for $1 \, Ca^{2+}$ ion and can operate in either direction. Under resting conditions, the direction of exchange is Ca^{2+} removal from the cell in exchange for Na^+ entry. Since there is then a net entry of positive charge into the cell, the exchanger creates an inward current too. Because the exchanger is electrogenic, its rate and direction are affected not only by the ion concentration gradients but also by the transmembrane potential. The effects of the sodium gradient, calcium gradient and membrane potential together govern the rate and direction of operation of the exchanger. These can be brought together by noting that, for a given ion species X, the force driving ion flux is proportional to $(V_m - E_x)$, where V_m is intracellular potential and E_x is the Nernst equilibrium potential, which depends on the ratio of extracellular to intracellular ion concentration (Chapter 3). Since the exchanger transports $3 \, Na^+$ in the opposite direction to 1 Ca^{2+}, the net outflow current through the exchanger is proportional to $3(V_m - E_{Na}) - 2$ $(V_m - E_{Ca})$. For example, at rest $V_m = -80 \, mV$, $E_{Na} = 69 \, mV$ and $E_{Ca} = 130 \, mV$, so the result is $(-447) - (-420)$, denoting a net force driving Na^+ into the cell. This expression can be used to understand how the rate and direction of operation of the exchanger alters as membrane potential changes during the action potential and as intracellular Ca^{2+} concentration varies during the action potential. For example, a rise in intracellular calcium during the action potential reduces E_{Ca}, which allows the sodium electrochemical gradient to dominate and drive the expulsion of Ca^{2+} at an increased rate. The increasing negativity of V_m during repolarization helps to speed the rate of expulsion. If intracellular Na^+ rises, as when digoxin impairs the Na–K pump, then E_{Na} declines, the net force driving Na^+ entry declines and Ca^{2+} expulsion declines.

Steady state. If two components at different energy levels are brought into contact, material or energy will flow from the higher level to the lower. If this transfer is occurring at a steady rate and without any change in the energy level at either end, the system is said to be in a steady state. This should not be confused with an equilibrium state (see earlier). If there is a very slow, almost negligible change in the energy levels, the system is said to be in a quasi steady state (L. *quasi* = as if).

Stokes–Einstein radius (a, r_{se}). The hydrodynamic resistance which a solute particle experiences as it diffuses through a solvent depends partly on the size of the solute particle. The hydrodynamic resistance encountered by a sphere of known radius was worked out by Stokes and Einstein, and this enables the average dimension of a solute (whatever its true shape) to be represented by a sphere of equal hydrodynamic resistance (the Stokes–Einstein radius). The equation relating the free diffusion coefficient of the solute, D (a measure of its hydrodynamic drag), to the Stokes–Einstein radius is:

$$a = RT/DN_a6\pi\eta$$

where η (eta) is the solvent viscosity and T is absolute temperature.

Strain and stress. When a solid body is subjected to a force, the force per unit cross-sectional area of material is called the stress (N/m^2). The change in size, divided by the original size, is called the strain (dimensionless). The ratio, stress/strain, is Young's modulus of elasticity.

Viscoelasticity. When a solid, perfectly elastic body is subjected to a deforming stress (e.g. a spring with a suspended weight) the strain is linearly proportional to stress and is independent of time; and on removing the stress the body reverts exactly to its original conformation, without any dissipation of energy. Virtually all biological materials, e.g. artery wall, behave differently. After the application of a stress, there is an initial rapid deformation, but this is followed by a slower, ever-decreasing deformation as time passes ('creep'). On removal of the stress, the recovery of shape follows a non-symmetrical pathway (hysteresis) owing to a dissipation of energy. This form of mechanical behaviour can be mimicked by an arrangement of elastic elements (springs) and viscous flowing elements (dashpots), and is called viscoelasticity.

Index